Orthodontic Laboratory Techniques

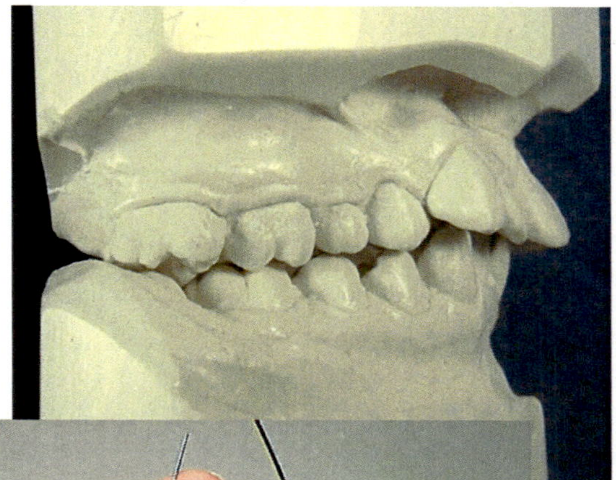

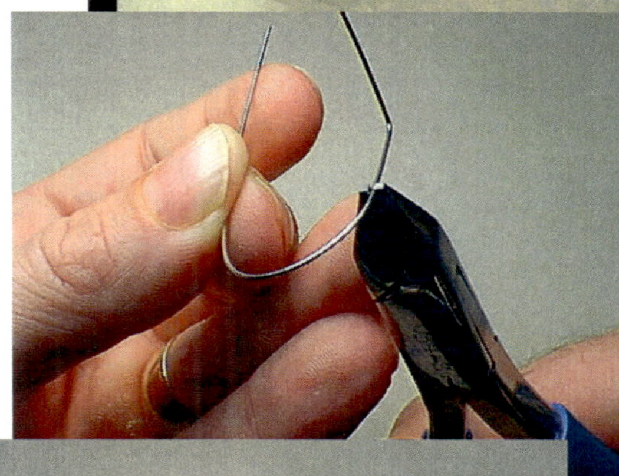

Al McOrmond, RDT, DD
George Brown College
Dental Technology Department
Faculty of Health Sciences
Toronto, Ontario

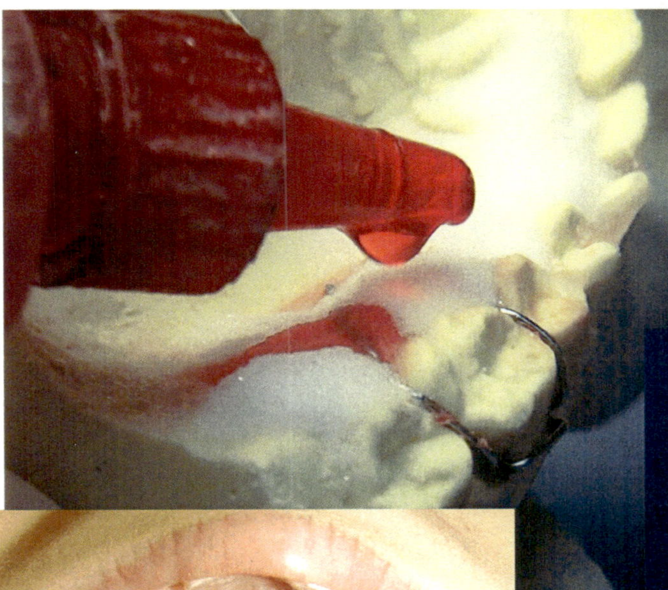

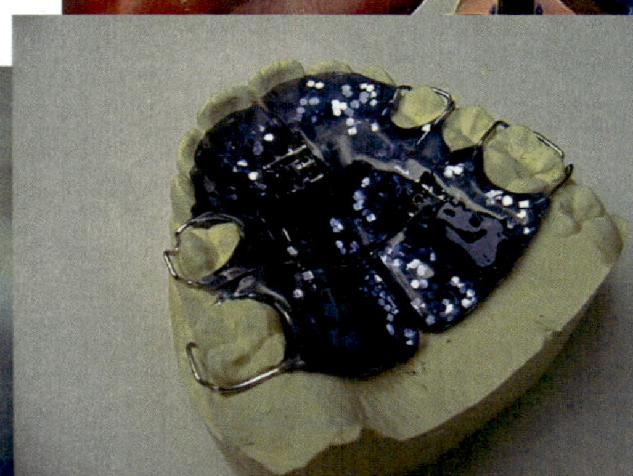

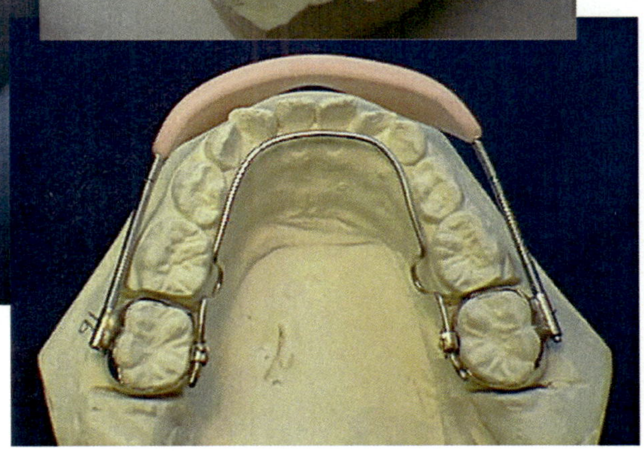

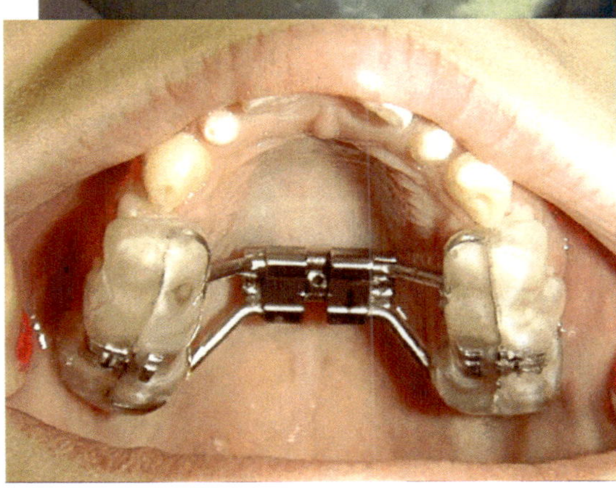

WD PUBLISHING
Whitby, Ontario 2003

Orthodontic laboratory techniques

Printed and bound in Canada.

First edition published in 1996
ISBN 0-9681430-0-8
Second edition published in 2003
by
WD Publishing
A division of
McO Dental Technology Services Inc.
517 Powell Rd
Whitby, Ontario
Canada
L1N 2H5
(905) 725-4652
North America 1-800-668-4652
Fax (905) 725-9348
www.mcodental.com

ISBN 0-9681430-0-9

First Edition

To my wife, Linda.
Proofreader, editor, cheerleader, partner and friend.
Without whom this book could not have happened.

Second Edition

To my son, Stephen

Just before Christmas 2002, I took my almost 18 year old son to see The Lord of the Rings - The Two Towers. We loved it. My wife then got him a beautiful, illustrated hardcover compilation of the three books for Christmas. As I wrapped his present, I thought about trolls and orcs and elves and journeys, then wrote this incription for him. I hope that it has meaning for him and all of us.

"In our lives we all have demons to fight, mountains to climb, and good and worthy companions.
May you vanquish your demons, scale your mountains and remember your friends.
There will be triumph and despair.
Be humble in your victories and strenghtened by your defeats, for neither will last.
At the end of the road you will stand alone with the man that you have become.
May he be another good and worthy companion."

To Stephen, Al McOrmond 2003

About the author

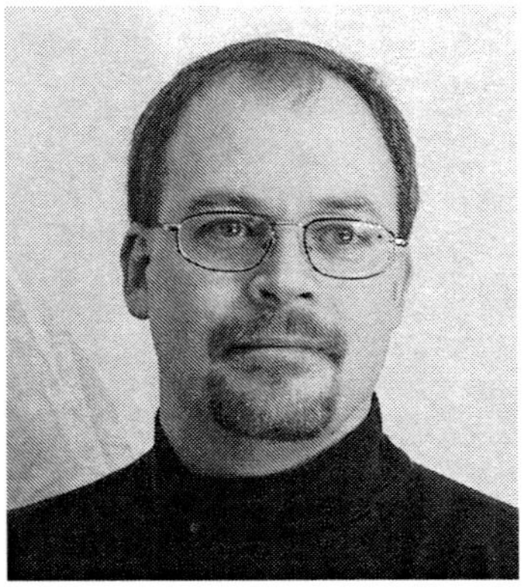

Al McOrmond RDT, DD, CDLI

My first edition had a 6 line, very impersonal biography. Linda, my wife, teased me that I don't like to talk about myself. Which is true.

Then a a few years ago, while I was in an appeals meeting, a young technician who didn't know me quoted my book in her case. Someone must have pointed out to her who she had been presenting against (I'm sorry to say that she lost), because afterwards she came to me and said, "Your book is very good, but I thought you'd be really old."

So here is a photo and a little more personal story

I was born in Sudbury, Ontario in 1958 so I'm not that old yet. My Dad was in the Air Force so by 1964, when we settled in Edmonton for ten years, I had lived in Quebec, Nova Scotia, Ontario and France. We returned to Ontario in 1973 to live in Toronto.

I became involved in Dental Technology in 1979. In 1981 I was accepted into the Dental Technology Program at George Brown College. When I tried to resign from the laboratory for whom I worked, they convinced me to continue with them and they would help to train me and assist with my education. At that time it was possible to gain a Registered Dental Technologist Licence through an apprenticeship in a laboratory. I accepted and attended all the educational opportunities that I could find while working with several well-known Ontario laboratories. I have worked to production levels in all areas of the lab; dentures, crown & bridge, ceramics, partials and orthdontics.

Since 1985 I have specialized in Orthodontics. I passed the RDT examination in Ontario in 1988 and in 1990 opened McO Dental Technology Services, a speciality orthodontic laboratory in Whitby, Ontario.

In 1990, I began teaching courses at George Brown College in Toronto, becoming a full-time Professor in the Dental Technology Department in 1991. I teach: full and partial denture fabrication, orthodontics, dental materials and have taught crown & bridge and anatomy. Recent additions to the faculty have allowed me to concentrate on the dentures, orthodontics and dental materials courses.

Seeing a lack of teaching texts for laboratory orthodontics, I formed WD Publishing and wrote and published "Orthodontic Laboratory Techniques" in 1996. My textbook is used by all Dental Technology programs in Canada and has been adopted by numerous colleges and universities in North America and around the world. It was translated into French, "Les techniques de laboratoire en orthodontie", in 2000.

From 1995-98 I took courses with Oklahoma State University on using technology in the classroom and become a Certified Distance Learning Instructor. In 1996, after teaching Dental Technology for six years, I wanted to earn the diploma which I had forgone in 1981. So I joined my students and completed all the courses for which I had not already completed an equivalance. I graduated with the Diploma of Dental Technology in 1998.

I love to learn and wanted to upgrade my denture skills to improve my teaching, so in 1999 I enrolled as a full-time student in the Denturism program at George Brown College. I completed the program and the licencing examination to become a Denturist in 2002. I continued to teach Dental Technology as a full-time Professor throughout all of this.

I am active in a number of professional associations and capacities. I have served as the President and Vice-President of the Association of Registered Dental Technologists of Ontario, the President of the Canadian Association of Dental Technology, and a founding member and Co-Chair of the Orthodontic Technology Study Group. I have contributed a number of articles to professional journals, and have worked with the College of Dental Technologists of Ontario as an invigilator and examiner for the RDT examination.

I do have a life outside of the lab. I love to run but don't do it enough, especially in the winter. Taking my computers apart is great fun, Linda gets frustrated when I'm using 3 computers at a time and have another couple disected on the pool table. I have also done my best in the challenging areas of husband to Linda, and father to Christyne and Stephen, but you will have to ask them how well I have succeeded there.

Table of Contents

Chapter 6 - Components of removable appliances

Chapter 7 - Removable appliance designs

Chapter 8 - Fixed appliances designs

Chapter 9 - Nightguards

Chapter 10 - Colour and Patterns in Acrylics

Chapter 11 - Appliance Glossary

References

Index

Acknowledgments

A project like this has the contributions of many people in its pages. I cannot possibly thank all of them for they include almost everyone with whom I have worked, or attended courses over the past 18 years. Each and every one has generously given of their time and knowledge, and I have yet to meet anyone from whom I cannot learn. This is one of the great strengths of our profession, and one that must continue, the sharing of knowledge and experience with our colleagues.

There are some people who have stood out in their generosity of spirit and professionalism, and them I would like to especially thank.

Richard Hack R.D.T. is the most knowledgeable and skilled all-round technologist that it has been my honour to work with. He is the true Master Technician, and a model for all that I have learned.

Bernie Mullen R.D.T. is a tireless champion of our profession, working with students and industry to improve the teaching of technologists to come. Bernie has been generously encouraging to me throughout this project and it is a true honor to share the teaching of our program at George Brown College with this dedicated man.

Swiss NF-Forestadent of Toronto, was extremely generous in letting me use their photographs and knowledge. And Orthopli of Philadelphia, PA for their information about and samples of their orthodontic pliers.

Aaron Carr helped me with the preparation of many of the appliances pictured in this book and more than once was pressed into service as a reluctant model.

Derek Keoughan of Finnegan Software for making sure that our computers, cameras, printers and all the other electronic gizmos attendant to this endeavor worked the way they were supposed to, when they were supposed to.

Jennifer Bolt, and my wife; Linda, who worked to edit this book and keep it understandable.

All my students, who are continually teaching me about the joy of learning and the wonders of our profession.

The Wicks family for giving me a writing refuge, their cabin in the forest, which they generously gave me the undisturbed use of.

And finally my family, especially my children; Stephen and Christine, who endured the ordeal of these months with hardly a protest and gave me so much encouragement.

My thanks to you all.
Al McOrmond R.D.T.

Second edition, 2003

The people that I would like to thank are those of you who have read and used this book and the one before it. It is amazing and heartwarming the number of wonderful responses that I have received from you. It has made all of the labour that goes into a project like this worthwhile.

Thank you, Al McOrmond, RDT, DD

Introduction

1

"Practice and thought might gradually forge many an art"
Virgil (Publius Virgilius Maro)
70-19 B.C.

"First things first, but not necessarily in that order."
Doctor Who

This book will guide you in learning the design and fabrication of a number of commonly used orthodontic appliances.

There are a number of areas in which you must have a basic working knowledge in order for this book to be most useful to you. Therefore, I'm going to start off with reviews of basic concepts and techniques in these areas. They include: anatomy, dental materials, wire and acrylic manipulation, and the tools and equipment found in the orthodontic laboratory.

If you don't feel that you need this review, skip ahead to the details of appliance fabrication. If you need it later, the review section will still be there.

The content of the book progresses from the simple to the more complex. However, with this subject, that does not necessarily refer to the difficulty of the fabrication processes.

As far as I'm concerned — once you have mastered the basic techniques required — no appliance is really much harder than any other. It is only during the learning stage that you will find them so difficult and frustrating.

Therefore, the more advanced appliances described in this book are not necessarily harder to make, only less common, or they require a more in-depth knowledge of the clinical objectives of the appliance to achieve an appliance that functions correctly.

The specific techniques that are described were chosen because they are the way I like to do things. For some tasks, I will present different methods of accomplishing the same objective. Remember, there is only one correct way to do anything, and that is the way that works best for you.

Any method that you want to use that conforms to the basic laws of chemistry and physics, and accomplishes the objectives, sounds right to me. However, a knowledge of the basics is useful because once you know the fundamentals, you will know when the rules may be bent or broken without harm to the objectives of a specific appliance.

Why Ortho?

You may be asking yourself, why should I be interested in ortho?

The amount of restorative dentistry that is required has generally decreased in recent years. Dentistry has done an exceptional job of educating the public. Consequently, with better oral hygiene, more patient awareness, and fluoridated water, in some areas the rate of tooth decay has fallen dramatically.

DMF is the statistic used to determine the dental history of a patient. It stands for Decayed, Missing or Filled teeth A study was conducted comparing the DMF ratings of groups of children in Toronto and Montreal between the years 1963 and 1984.

Between 1963 and 1984 the DMF of children in Toronto between the ages of 9 and 13 had dropped by over 60%. In the same time period, the percentage of 11 year olds with no cavities in their permanent teeth increased from 7% to 50%. What do these statistics tell us?

They tell us that with the improvements constantly being brought to preventative dentistry such as fluoridated water, fluoridated toothpaste, fissure sealant and better dental hygiene and education, the amount of restorative dentistry needed will sharply drop as today's caries-free children approach adulthood. The future focus of the average dental operatory will, therefore, shift from restorative dentistry to preventative and cosmetic dentistry. Orthodontics is a component of both cosmetic and preventative dentistry.

The importance of a "nice smile" has also come into vogue world wide.

Watch a movie or T.V. program and compare the actors' smiles to those of the stars of the 40's, 50's or even 60's. In older movies you will see smiles which are far from perfect. Today, the only bad teeth you will see are on the villains and are supplied by the props department. This emphasis on the "perfect smile" is encouraging adults who did not have orthodontics as children to seek treatment in ever increasing numbers.

Orthodontics has suddenly become "cool"; braces seem to have become a fashion accessory as much as a medical procedure to some children.

The popular concept of orthodontics is "straightening of teeth". However, orthodontics really undertakes a much more comprehensive approach, taking into consideration cranial norms, growth or treatment tendencies, and most importantly, the patient's facial appearance.

I firmly believe that to be an effective part of the orthodontic team the dental technician must have an understanding of the basic principles and clinical procedures employed in orthodontic treatment, as well as a thorough knowledge of the laboratory procedures involved in their fabrication. Therefore, we will touch upon the theory behind the design of the appliances, as well as some clinical considerations. I'm not going to pretend that this book will cover orthodontic theory in depth; it won't. But it will give basic information on the whys and wherefores that will make our interaction with the dentist easier, more exact and more interesting.

"Experience is the name everyone gives to their mistakes."
Oscar Wilde
1854-1900

"Good judgement comes from experience. Experience comes from bad judgement."
Jim Horning

The basics

2

"Men occasionally stumble over the truth, but most of them pick themselves up and hurry off as if nothing ever happened."
Winston Churchill
1874-1965

"Verbosity leads to unclear, inarticulate things"
Dan Quayle

2a: Planes of reference

In any body of knowledge, the first requirement of effective communication is a common language or nomenclature for the expression of exact concepts.

When we wish to visit a place we have never been before, we use a map to help direct us. We can understand the necessary direction of travel from its north, south, east, west co-ordinate system.

To find our way around the anatomical structure of the body a mapping system has been developed which allows us to define exact relationships between bodily structures.

The common language of up, down, right, left, front, back does not suffice. The relationship of your body parts can change depending upon the changing positions of your body. Your head and feet have different vertical relationships when you are standing than when you are lying down.

We use defined imaginary planes called *planes of reference* to provide us with the mapping system that we need to describe anatomical relationships.

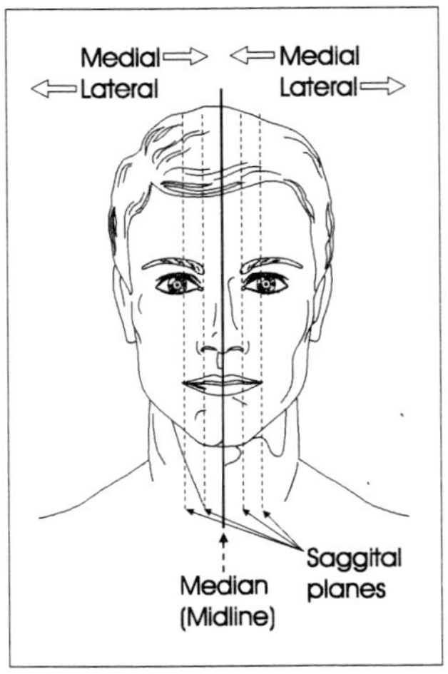

Fig. 2.1 Saggital planes

The *median (or midsaggital) plane* divides the body vertically into equal, mirror image left and right halves. In dentistry this plane is also referred to as the *midline* with relation to the head and the mouth. Any plane parallel to the median plane that does not produce equal halves is called a saggital plane.

The positions of structures with reference to the median are defined as *medial (or internal)* and *lateral (or external)*. These describe the distance of objects from the median, the object closer to the median being medial (internal) and the further object being lateral (external). For example, the ear is lateral (external) to the eye, while the eye is medial (internal) to the ear.

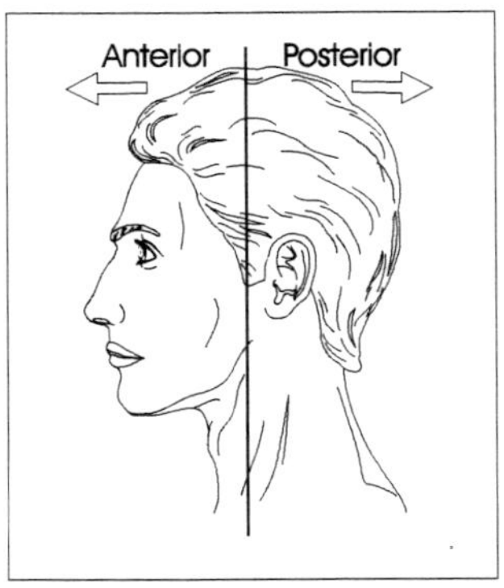

Fig. 2.2 Frontal plane

The *frontal (or coronal) plane* divides the body into front and back portions. The coronal plane is perpendicular to the medial plane. The terms that describe relationships in the coronal plane are *anterior* and *posterior*. Anterior refers to the front of the body, while posterior refers to the back. The eye is anterior to the ear, while the ear is posterior to the eye.

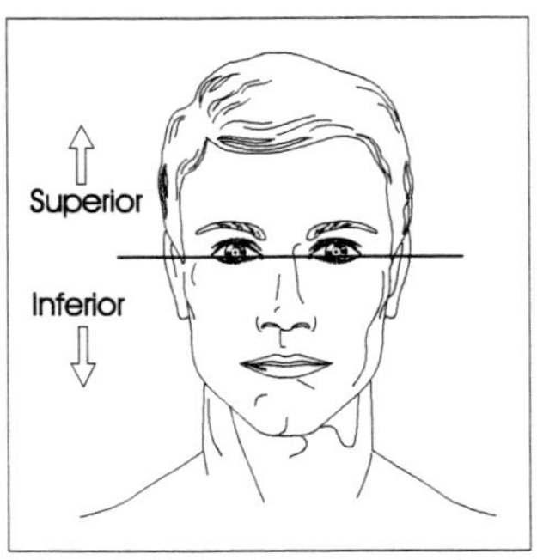

Fig. 2.3 Horizontal plane

The *horizontal (or transverse) plane* is perpendicular to both the medial and the coronal planes. It divides the body into top and bottom. The positions of structures are defined as *superior* or *inferior*. Structures which are closer to the top of the head are the superior. Therefore, the eyes are superior to the mouth, and the mouth is inferior to the eyes.

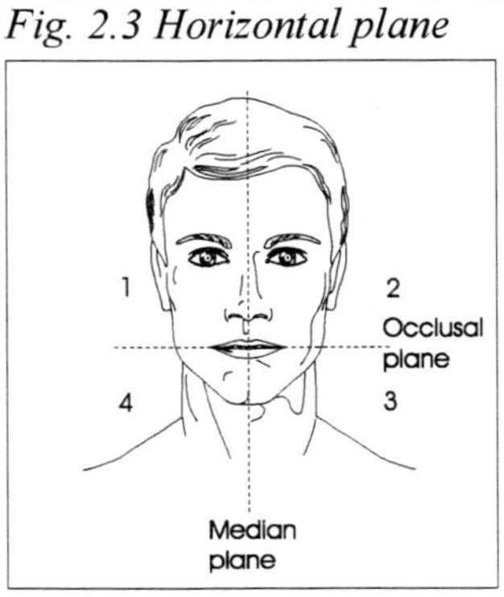

Fig. 2.4 Quadrants

Oral nomenclature

We also need terms to allow us to define exact positioning in the mouth.

The *occlusal plane* is the plane where the occlusal surfaces of the upper (*maxillary*) and lower (*mandibular*) teeth meet (*occlude*). The occlusal is generally assumed to be perpendicular to the midline, even when it is not.

The mouth is divided into four quadrants by the intersection of the midline and occlusal plane: upper-left, upper-right, lower-right, and lower-left. In the primary dentition each quadrant contains 5 teeth, in the permanent 8.

We can now look at the terms that are used to describe position in the oral cavity.

The front of mouth is the *anterior*. The back of the mouth is the *posterior*.

The midline, which helps to define the quadrants, is used as a reference for the terms defining some of the surfaces of the teeth. However, we use only the midline as it passes between the two centrals for these definitions. Most tooth surfaces are defined as opposing pairs.

The surface of the tooth that is closer to the midline is the *mesial*, the surface farther from the midline the *distal*. The surface of a tooth that contacts the tooth beside it in the arch is the *proximal*, whether it is mesial or distal.

The surface of the tooth that faces the tongue is the *lingual;* the surface facing the lips (in the anterior) is the *labial* and the surface facing the cheek (in the posterior) the *buccal*. Any labial or buccal surface can also be referred to as a *facial* surface.

The surface of the tooth which meets the tooth in the opposing arch and is used for chewing is the *occlusal surface*. The portion of the tooth that is closer to the apex of the root is *cervical* or *apical*.

In orthodontics, we are concerned with the movement of the teeth, so we describe movement using the surface of the tooth towards which it is moving. When an anterior tooth is pushed out toward the lip, we call this *labializing* the tooth. To *lingualize* is to move toward the tongue, to *mesialize* is to move toward the midline, and to *distalize* is to move away from the midline.

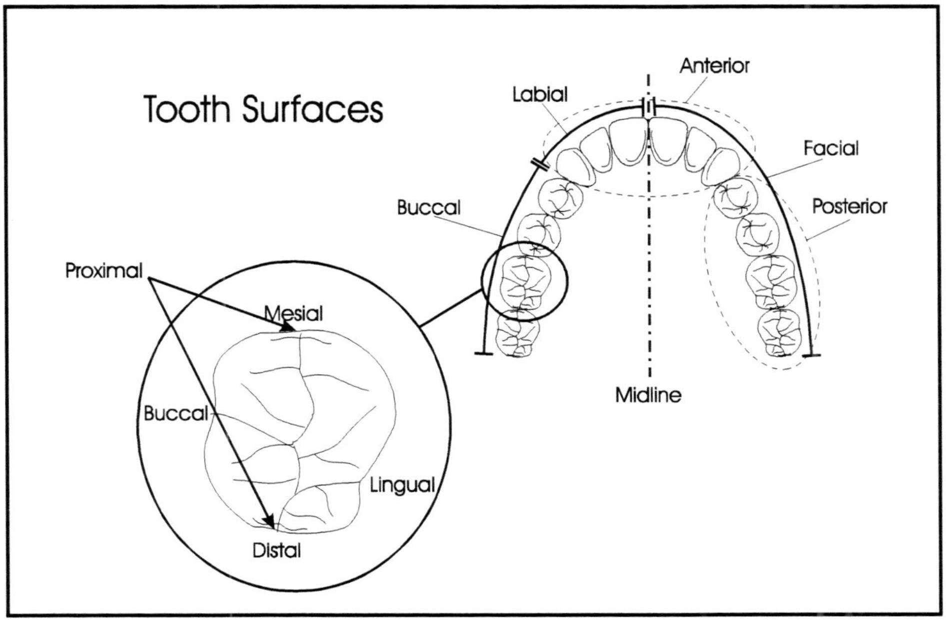

Fig 2.5 Identifying tooth surfaces

"Aristotle maintained that women have fewer teeth than men; although he was twice married, it never occured to him to verify this statement by examining his wives' mouths."
Bertrand Russell

"It's what you learn after you know it all that counts."
John Wooden

2b: The oral environment - an overview

The oral environment consists of: the teeth, two bony arches that support the teeth, an articulated joint to allow movement, the surrounding muscles and tissues that provide the motive power and supporting structures, blood vessels, nerves and glands, as well as, the fluids that occur in the oral cavity.

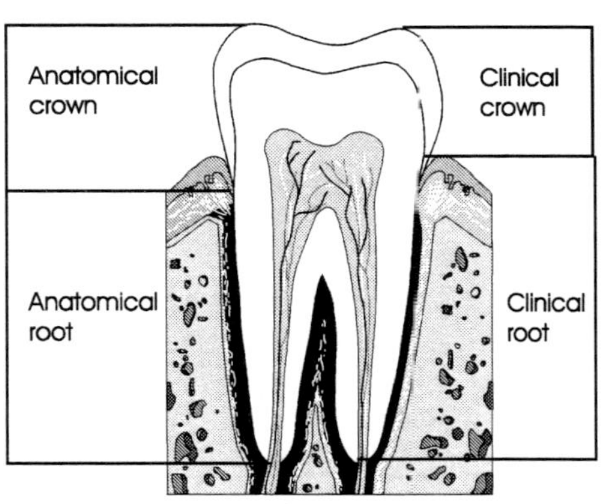

Fig. 2.6 Crown and root

The teeth and anatomy

The teeth, when viewed from the exterior, have a *crown* and a *root*. In the mouth, these are called the *clinical crown* and *clinical root*. The clinical crown is the portion of the tooth that is exposed above the tissue (*gingival margin*) — the part that we see — while the clinical root is everything under the tissue. The size of the clinical crown and root changes throughout the course of a person's life.

When a tooth is removed from the mouth it is divided into the *anatomical crown* and *anatomical root*. These are divided by the junction between their covering materials, the crown being covered by the *enamel* and the root being covered by the cementum. This junction is called the *cemento-enamal junction (or CEJ)*.

The surfaces of the teeth that meet those on the other jaw are called the *occlusal surfaces*. These are the surfaces that work when you chew. Chewing is referred to as *mastication or function*. When the jaws are together in the position of maximum contact between the teeth it is called *centric occlusion* or simply *centric*.

The two bony arches supporting the teeth are called the *alveolar ridges*. The teeth are each set with their roots in individual sockets in the ridges. They are supported in the sockets by a network of short elastic ligaments called the *periodontal ligaments*. The periodontal ligaments are attached to the root of the tooth and the wall of the socket in bundles resembling braided rope. This arrangement gives the teeth excellent "shock absorption" in resisting the forces placed upon them during mastication to prevent damage.

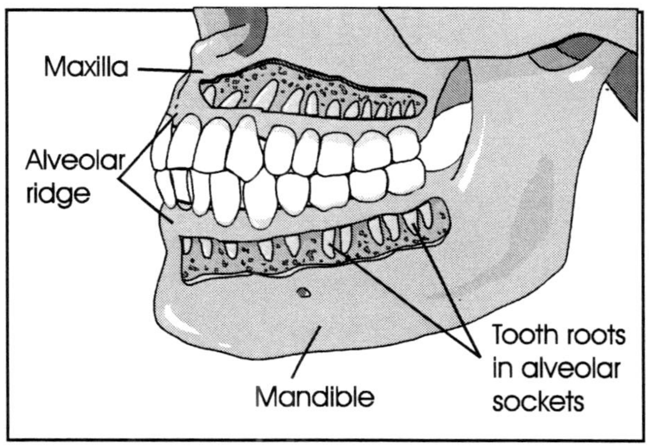

Fig. 2.7 Bones of the mouth

The fixed upper arch is called the *maxilla*. It is solidly attached to the base of the skull or cranial base. The mobile lower arch is called the *mandible*. The mandible moves or articulates on *the temporomandibular joint (or TMJ)*, which is located just in front of the ear.

The TMJ is similar to a ball and socket joint. The ball-like structure is attached to the mandible and is called the *condyle*. The socket is called the *glenoid fossa* and is found under the temporal bone of the skull. Between the ball and socket is a disk of dense collagen tissue called the *meniscus or articular disk*. The rounded prominence at the anterior of the glenoid fossa is the *articular eminence*. From

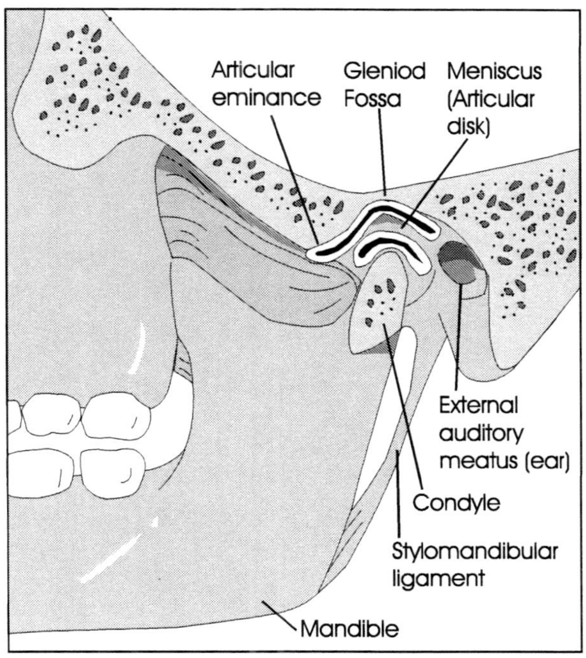

Fig. 2.8 Temporomandibular Joint

the *styloid process* to the posterior of the mandible extends the *stylomandibular ligament*, which limits the forward movement of the mandible. This ensures that the condyle does not pass anterior to the articular eminence.

The TMJ is really two joints joined together. It is capable of two types of movement. The condyle can rotate in place in the glenoid fossa. This allows a rotation of the jaws for the first few millimeters of opening. The condyle can also translate, or move forward, down the front (anterior) slope of the glenoid fossa. This results in full opening of the mouth, as well as a protruding of the mandible on opening.

Dentition

All of the teeth in the mouth, their general arrangement and positioning are called the dentition. There are two sets of dentition, the primary and secondary, that occupy the mouth at different times. Each of these sets is divided into two arches, one on the upper jaw (maxillary arch) and the other on the lower jaw (mandibular arch). The arches are divided into mirror image quadrants, left and right, by the median line.

Primary (Deciduous) dentition

The first teeth to erupt into the mouth are the primary dentition. They are also know as the deciduous teeth, or baby teeth. Deciduous in teeth, as in trees, refers to the fact that these teeth fall out after a period of growth. There are 20 teeth in the deciduous arch, 5 in each quadrant. These teeth are the *central, lateral, cuspid, first deciduous molar and second deciduous molar*. The deciduous teeth begin their formation or germination in the womb and may start erupting at any time from birth to 12 months of age. The deciduous teeth are similar in appearance to their permanent successors, although they are smaller. The deciduous anterior teeth are shorter from CEJ to incisal in proportion to their permanent equivalents. The deciduous posterior teeth tend to be more narrow buccolingually than the permanent teeth, with a small occlusal table and an exaggerated buccal slope caused by a large cervical ridge.

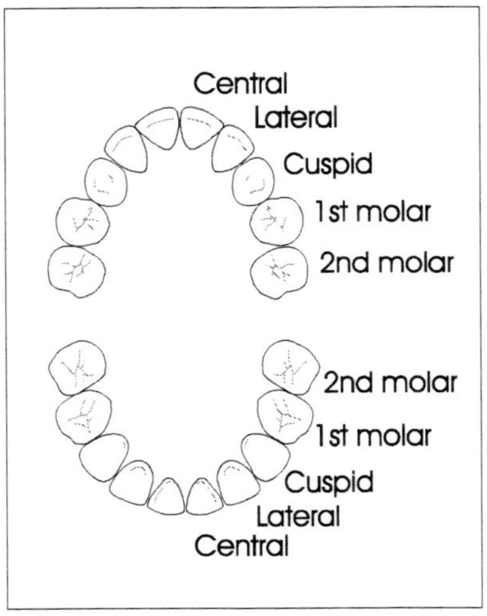

Fig. 2.9 Deciduous dentition

Mixed Dentition

At approximately six years of age, the first of the permanent teeth begin to erupt into the mouth. These are usually the upper first permanent molars or *six year molars*. The six year molars erupt immediately distal to the second deciduous molars. Once the permanent teeth have begun to erupt into the mouth, the child enters a stage known as the mixed dentition stage, when both deciduous and permanent teeth are present in the mouth. This stage will last until all of the deciduous teeth are lost and the permanent teeth have erupted, at approximately 11 years of age.

Permanent Dentition

The remainder of the permanent teeth form under the deciduous teeth. The teeth form starting with the crown and the growth continues to build the tooth apically (towards the apex of the root). As the more apical portions of the root are deposited, the crown of the tooth moves occlusally. This occlusal migration of the permanent teeth as they form causes the deciduous roots to resorb. As the permanent teeth near the surface, the deciduous roots almost completely disappear causing the deciduous teeth to fall out. This allows the permanent teeth to erupt into the space shortly afterwards.

The centrals are usually the next teeth to erupt, followed by the laterals, cuspids on the lower, bicuspids on the upper and second molars. The eruption sequence can vary widely in different children. The third molars (wisdom) erupt several years after the other teeth.

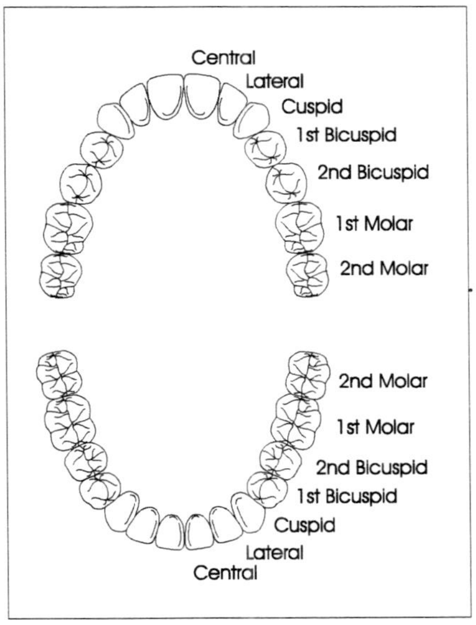

Fig.2.10 Permanent dentition

Overjet, overbite and crossbites

Overjet and overbite represent horizontal and vertical relationships between the upper (maxillary) and lower (mandibular) teeth.

Overjet is a horizontal measurement. In normal occlusion, the upper teeth fall outside of the lower teeth when we bite. To put that another way, the facial surfaces of the maxillary dentition rest buccally or labially to the facial surfaces of the mandibular dentition when the teeth are in centric occlusion.

Overjet is most commonly measured at the central incisors. Overjet is the distance in millimeters from the labial surface of the lower central to the lingual surface of the upper cen-

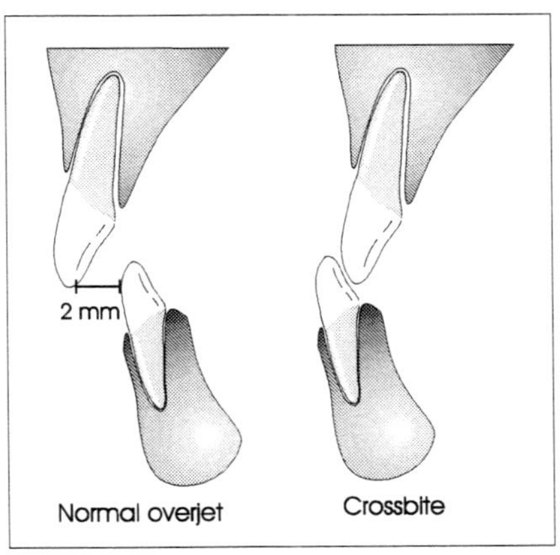

Fig. 2.11 Overjet and crossbite

tral. In practice, we normally only measure this at the level of the incisal edge of the upper central. However, each person has two overjets; the second is at the level of the incisal edge of the lower central. These two measurements taken together give a record of the inclination of the upper central.

Overjet is not generally measured in the posterior. Only when there is an obvious discrepancy do we worry about measuring it. In normal occlusion this horizontal overlap, the fact that the upper cusps are outside of the lowers, keeps us from biting our cheeks.

Overbite is a vertical measurement. It is the amount that the upper anteriors cover the lower anteriors in centric. Overbite is measured in percentage. Normal overbite is 10-20% or 1 or 2 mm of the lower centrals are covered by the upper centrals. If half of the lowers are covered that is a 50% overbite, all of them covered would be 100% and called a *"deep bite"*. When the uppers do not cover the lowers or when there is a gap between the upper and lower anteriors, that is called an open bite. When you have an anterior deep bite, it is common for the lower posterior teeth to be very short. This can be called a collapsed vertical.

Crossbite is when a maxillary tooth is positioned lingual to a mandibular tooth. A single tooth or a group of teeth can be in crossbite. A few teeth can be in cross bite due to *ectopic eruption*, meaning the teeth came up in the wrong place. An entire quadrant or all of the maxillary teeth in crossbite points to a small or deficient maxilla or an oversize mandible.

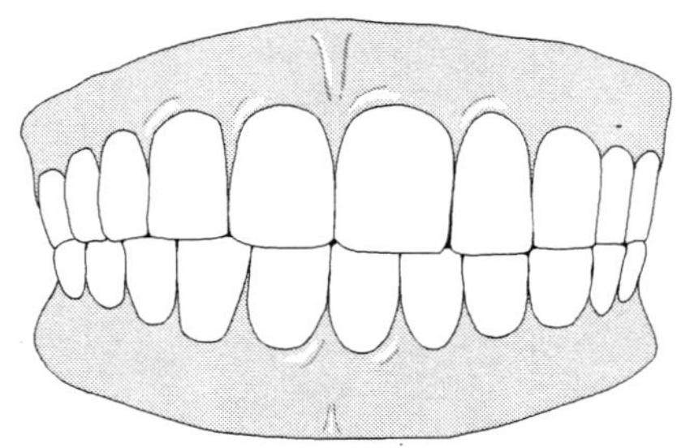
20% overbite

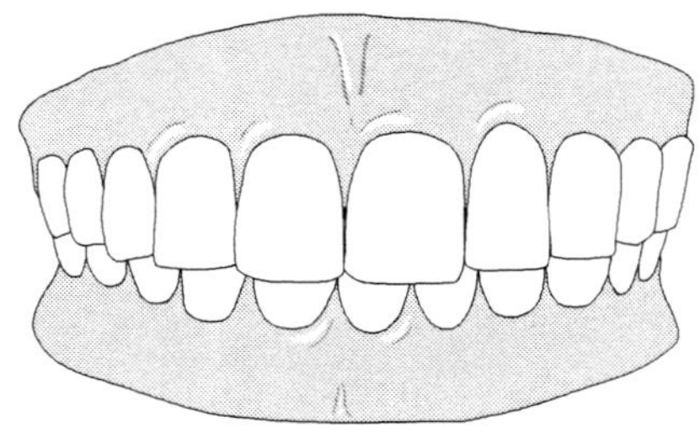
80% overbite

Fig. 2.12 Overbite

Angle Classification of Malocclusions

The Angle classification of malocclusions is a basis on which a patient's dental and skeletal relationships may be judged in relation to a perceived normal condition. There are three major classes in the system. They represent the spatial relationship that exists between the bone structure of the patient's maxilla and mandible (skeletal classification), as well as the anterior-posterior relationship of the patient's first molars and cuspids (dental classification). In the mouth or on models, we can visually distinguish the dental classifications.

At their most basic level a *Class I (Orthognathic)* is a normal lower face, a *Class II (Retrognathic)* is a retruded lower face, and a *Class III (Prognathic)* is a protruded lower face.

More explicitly, the mesial buccal cusp of the maxillary first molar and its relationship with the mandibular first molar is used as the gauge for the positioning of the mandible.

A Class I occlusion is taken to be a normal "bite". In this position, the mesial buccal cusp articulates in the buccal groove of the first mandibular molar. In a Class II, the mesial buccal cusp articulates in the embrasure between the mandibular first molar and the second bicuspid. In a Class III, the mesial buccal cusp articulates in the distal groove of the mandibular first molar. When the teeth occlude exactly in these positions, the occlusions are all referred to as full cusp Class II or III. Greater or less anterior-posterior discrepancies would be 1½ or ½ cusp Class II or III occlusions.

Class II has two subdivisions. Class II division 1 (div. 1) indicates that the anterior teeth are protrusive or flared. This is commonly called "buck teeth". Class II division 2 (div. 2) indicates that the central incisors are retroclined (pointing back), and the laterals are usually protrusive.

The approximate division of the different classifications is:

Class I - 60-65%

Class II - 25-30%

Class III - 3-5%.

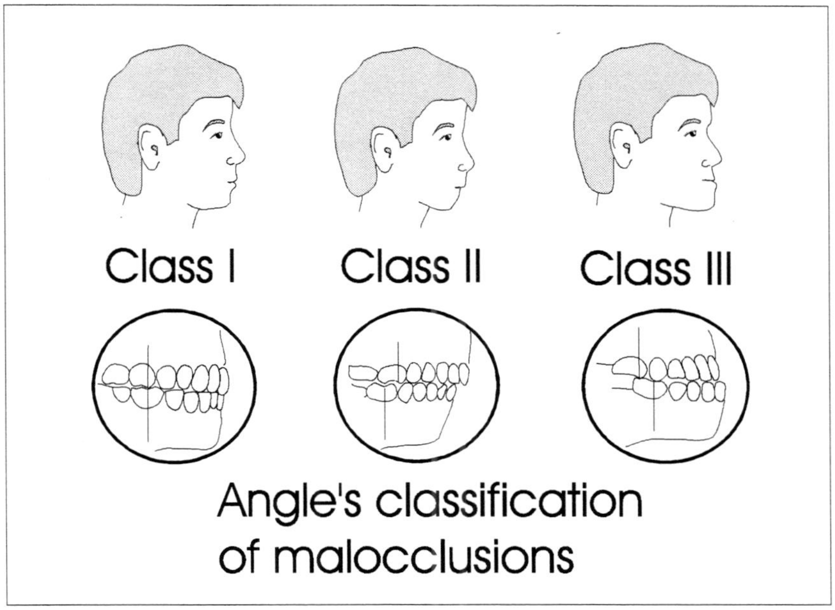

Fig. 2.13. Angle's classification of malocclusion - Class I is normal profile, Class II has retruded chin, Class III prominant chin. Note line indicating alignment of maxillary mesio-buccal cusp with mandibular buccal groove.

Approximately 60% of orthodontic cases exhibit a Class II malocclusion.

This is the classic system developed by Dr. Angle. Mesial movement of the first molars can cause the observer to be unsure of the true relationships of the teeth. We can supplement this classification system by observing the positioning of the canines in conjunction with the molar positioning. This helps to overcome any discrepancies that may be introduced by the movement of the molars.

In a Class I, the maxillary canines articulate in the mandibular cuspid/1st bicuspid embrasure. In a Class II occlusion, the canines articulate to the mesial of the mandibular canines, and in Class III to the distal of the cuspid/1st bicuspid embrasure.

It is interesting to note that artificial teeth for dentures are designed to articulate and balance in a Class I occlusion. Knowledge of the positions of the teeth in these classes of malocclusion can be of great help when setting teeth for an edentulous patient with a skeletal Class II or III.

Biomechanics of tooth movement

Orthodontic movement is accomplished by exerting a force on the crown of the tooth that is to be moved. The actual biological mechanism that allows this to occur without damaging the teeth is still a matter of debate and research. However, after almost a century of successfully moving teeth, we have some ideas and guidelines.

The classical view of how teeth move through the alveolar process involves pressure and tension exerted on the socket wall by the periodontal ligaments. Bones change or remodel when a constant or repeated stress is placed on them in a consistent direction. When a force is placed (a simple pushing force) on a tooth this produces a pressure on the root of the tooth on the opposite side from the point of exertion, and a tension on the root on the same side

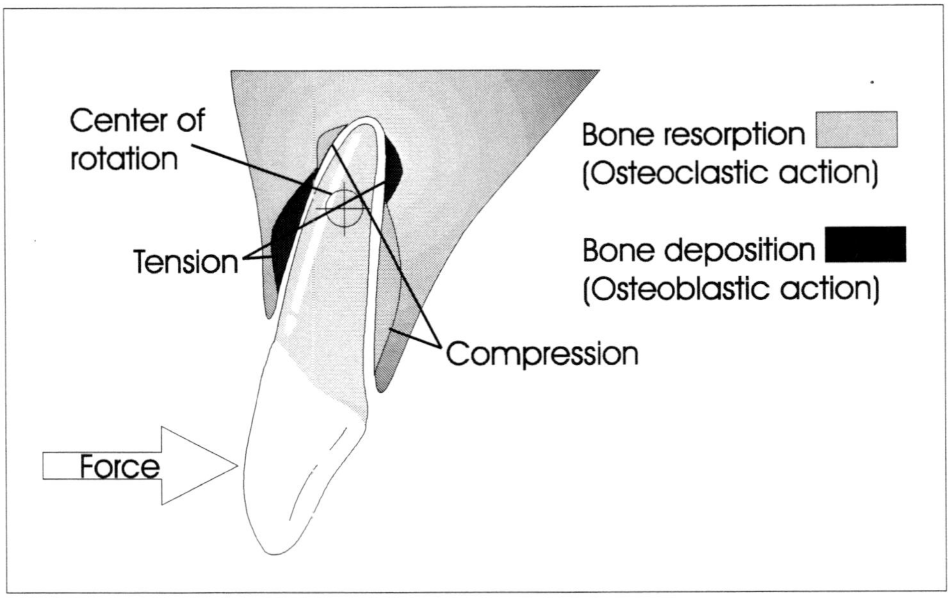

Fig. 2.14. Action of a simple force on tooth.
A simple force acting on the buccal surface of the central will cause an area of compression on the opposite side from the force, and tension on the same side as the force. In the apical region the forces will be reversed due to the rotation of the tooth about a point of rotation. The point of rotation is approximately 2/3's the depth of the socket. Bone deposition will occur in the areas under tension, and resorption will occur in the compressed areas.

as the exertion. The pressure on the alveolar socket causes resorption (osteoclastic activity) to occur on the socket wall, while the tension causes deposition of new osteoid tissue on the opposite side (osteoblastic activity). This mechanism allows the movement of the tooth through bone.

Degrees of efficiency

The amount of force that is placed on the tooth is important. In 1932 Dr. Schwarz produced his "Degrees of Efficiency", four levels of force application and the effect of these forces on the tissue and tooth movement.

First Degree of Efficiency - this represents a force too weak to induce tooth movement. It may also be a force which is of too short a duration. First degree force will move a tooth if it is applied constantly for a long enough time, but is not generally efficient.

Second Degree of Efficiency - this is the most favourable force for the efficient movement of a tooth without damage. The resorption and deposition of bone can occur at the same rate. The forces involved, by Schwarz's definition, are less than the capillary blood pressure in the periodontium. This means that blood flow to the tissues is never stopped.

Second degree movement can also occur when a large magnitude force is exerted over a very short distance. An expansion screw exerts great pressure, but the distance of activation is only 0.2-0.25 mm. Because this force acts bilaterally, each side of the arch is displaced 0.1-0.125 mm, half of the 0.2 mm thickness that Schwarz attributed to the periodontal membrane. This simply means that the tissues were not crushed between the root and socket wall before the periodontium could adjust.

The optimum force that he defined is 15-20 grams per square centimeter (g/cm^2).

Third Degree of Efficiency - these are medium level forces, 20-50 g/cm^2, enough force that the blood circulation to the periodontium is interrupted, but the tissue is not crushed. If the force is removed before permanent damage is done to the tissues, they will recover. Applying such a force repeatedly, while giving the tissue time to recover, will cause tooth movement. Too long application of the force will lead to necrosis (death) of the periodontal tissue. This can cause damage to the alveolar socket and root resorption.

Fourth Degree of Efficiency - these forces are so strong that the periodontal membrane is simply crushed between the root and the alveolar socket. If the force is continued for any length of time, the damage becomes irreparable.

Types of movement

There are several different types of movement which can be achieved. These are:

- tipping
- rotational
- bodily
- torquing
- vertical.

Tipping movement

Tipping is the easiest of the movements to accomplish and the type used by removable appliances. Any force applied to a single point on a tooth will cause the tooth to tip, with its center of rotation being near the apical third of the root.

Rotation movement

Rotation requires either two points of force application or one point of force application and one stop. Rotational movement is the most prone to relapse because the periodontal ligaments attached to the free gingiva take a longer time to adjust to the new position. In a rotation, these ligaments are stretched and they continue to place a force on the tooth once it is in its new position.

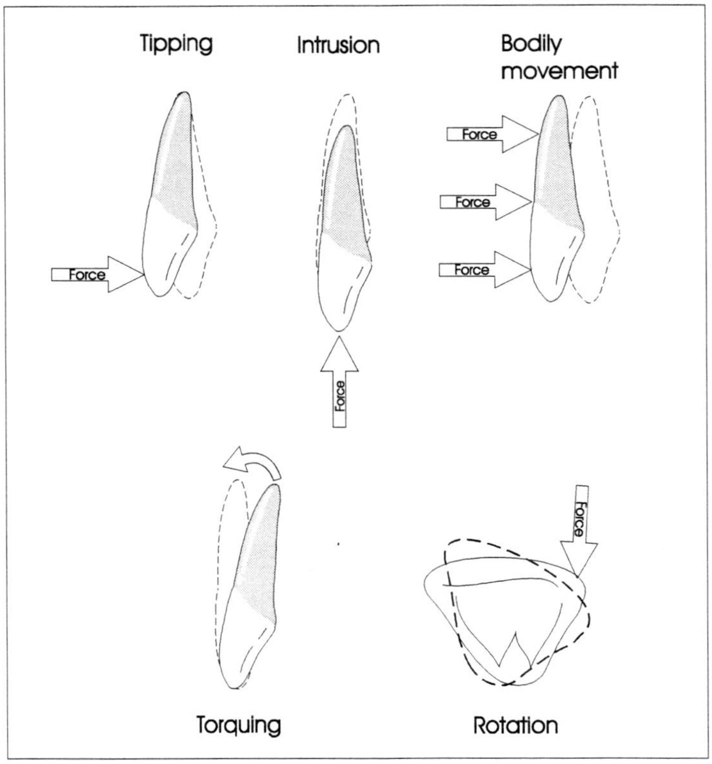

Fig. 2.15. Types of tooth movements

Bodily movement

Bodily movement is when the teeth are translated through the alveolar bone. That means that all parts of the teeth move equally with no tipping or rotation. This is only practically achievable with brackets.

Torquing movement

Torquing is the moving of only one part of the tooth, commonly the root, while maintaining another portion of the tooth in its position.

Vertical movement

Vertical movement refers to the intrusion or extrusion of a tooth. Extrusion is an easily accomplished movement because the tooth has a tendency to erupt naturally. Intrusion can be one of the most difficult movements to achieve.

Name that tooth!

Tooth identification systems

Maxillary left second permanent molar is a very accurate way to identify the tooth which you want to discuss. But it's a bit long. If this were the only way we had to name teeth, we would all be spending our time doing nothing but writing and reading prescriptions.

Fortunately for us there have been a number of naming conventions developed that give us a dental shorthand for accurately naming the teeth. In Canada the F.D.I. and Palmer systems are popular, while in some other countries and with the military the universal system is frequently used.

Palmer

The Palmer system is based on dividing the mouth into quadrants. The quadrants are represented by a cross; the upright is the midline, the crossbar the occlusal plane. Each of the four quadrants contain eight teeth, central to the third molar.

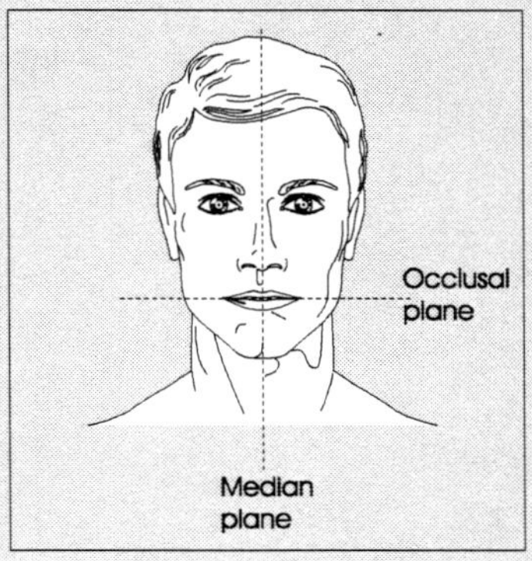

Upper right	Upper left
8,7,6,5,4,3,2,1	1,2,3,4,5,6,7,8
8,7,6,5,4,3,2,1	1,2,3,4,5,6,7,8
Lower right	Lower left

To represent a quadrant we draw the halves of the upright and crossbar that define that quadrant.

5,4 ⏋

Lower right 1st&2nd bicuspid,

⎣1,2,3

Upper left central, lateral, cuspid

The teeth are then designated by numbers for the permanent dentition and letters for the deciduous dentition. The numbers, or letters, start at the central and count up to the third molar. The permanent central is therefore "1", and the permanent third molar "8", the primary central is "a", and the primary second molar is "e". Multiple teeth can be designated by a single quadrant sign: start from the midline in the order of their position in the arch.

FDI

FDI is an abbreviation for *Fédération Dentaire Internationale.* This system is also based on dividing the mouth into quadrants. However, the quadrants are numbered in a clockwise direction. The quadrant numbers are:

upper right - 1st quadrant	*upper left - 2nd quadrant*
lower right - 4th quadrant	*lower left - 3rd quadrant*

The individual teeth are again identified by numbers in each quadrant starting with the central, 1-8.

A specific tooth is referred to by its quadrant number and then its position in the quadrant by the tooth number. The two numbers are separated by a period.

Therefore, the upper right central is called 1.1. Each tooth must be identified individually: 1.1, 1.2, 1.3, etc.

This system works very well in conversation, when this would be pronounced either, tooth one-one, tooth one-point-one or tooth eleven. The correct usage is one-point-one, however all three methods are commonly used.

For the primary dentition, the quadrant number is carried on in a clockwise direction.

upper right - 5th quadrant	*upper left - 6th quadrant*
lower right - 8th quadrant	*lower left - 7th quadrant*

Universal system

The universal is the simplest naming convention. It numbers the teeth from 1 to 32, starting with the upper right third molar and continues in a clockwise direction around the upper arch. The numbering then goes from the upper left third molar (#16) to the lower left third molar (#17) and continues around the lower arch to the lower right third molar (#32).

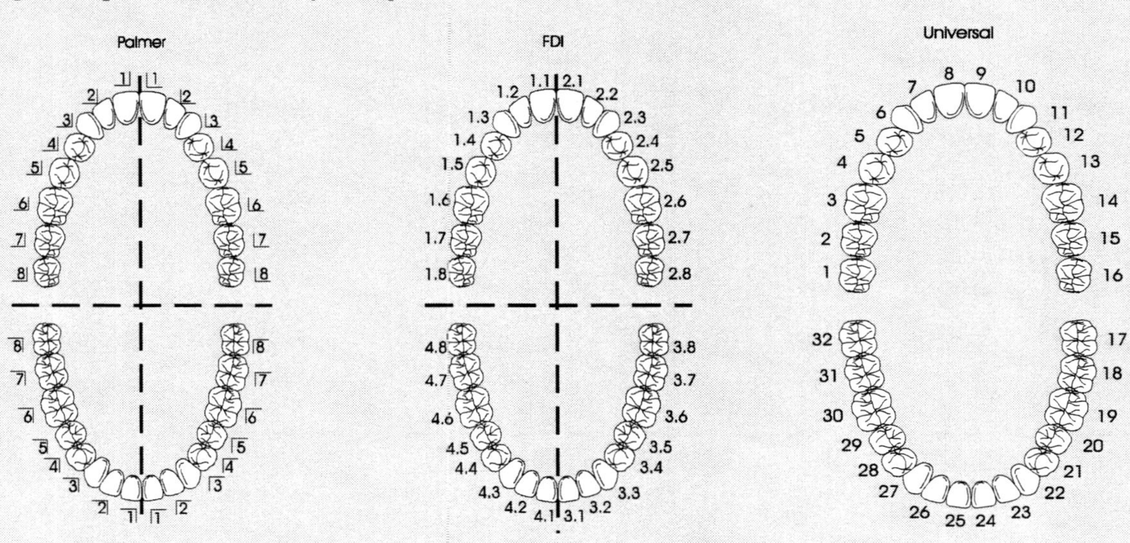

3 Orthodontic materials

"The materials are indifferent, but the use we make of them is not a matter of indifference"
Epictetus
A.D. 50-120

"To repeat what others have said, requires education; to challenge it, requires brains."
Mary Pettibone Poole, A Glass Eye at a Keyhole, 1938

The four major materials that we work with in the orthodontic laboratory are:

1.) Gypsum materials - which are used to produce the working and study models.
2.) Stainless steel - which forms the wires, tubing, and bands used in the appliances.
3.) Solder - which attaches the separate pieces of wire to form the appliances.
4.) Acrylic - which is used to form the acrylic plate.

Gypsum products

There are two specific types of models used in the orthodontic laboratory.

The first type is the working models that are needed to fabricate appliances. These models are very similar to the working models used in any laboratory.

The second type is the study models which are specially trimmed and polished, and are used for diagnostic and record purposes by the dentist.

We will concentrate on the fabrication of a set of orthodontic study models, the more extensive and exacting of the two procedures.

Orthodontic study models

Orthodontic study models — also called diagnostic study models or DSMs — are a set of casts which are trimmed to exacting measurements with geometrically symmetrical bases using anatomical planes of reference for guidelines.

They are used for several purposes:

- to allow the dentist to observe and measure the teeth outside of the mouth for diagnostic purposes.
- to let the patient see their teeth to help the dentist clarify the treatment and its objects to them.
- to act as a permanent, three dimensional record of the patient's pre-, mid- and post-treatment dental relationships.

It is common for a patient to have three sets of DSMs made over the course of orthodontic treatment. These are the pre-treatment set, which is used for diagnosis and case consultation, the mid-treatment set, which is used to verify the patient's progress, and the post-treatment set, which is a permanent record of the final results of the treatment.

These models are stored by the dentist — or patient — for a period of up to several years. They must be aesthetically presentable, well dried and finished, and durable.

Pouring impressions for orthodontic study models

When pouring an impression for an orthodontic study model, as any other impression, you must first ensure that the impression has been properly disinfected. Do not trust anyone else to have performed this for you outside of your laboratory. It is better that an impression be disinfected twice, so that you know it was done once. You must also wear latex gloves any time you handle an impression.

An orthodontic study model is poured using orthodontic stone or orthodontic plaster. Orthodontic stone and orthodontic plaster have both been dyed a brilliant white, and orthodontic plaster is slightly denser and harder than regular plaster.

An orthodontic study model is poured using a base former to ensure that sufficient material is available to properly trim the base. One of the most common mistakes when trimming these models is simply not having enough material to produce a properly formed base.

Always use a vacuum spatulator to mix the orthodontic stone. This will ensure that the stone is dense and hard, and also that there will be no voids in the base which will need to be filled later.

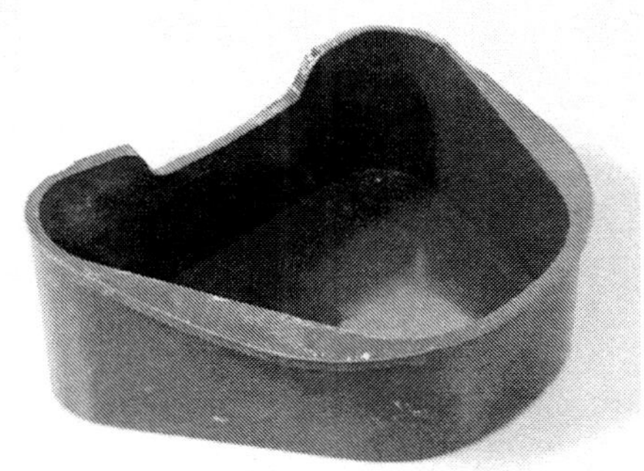

Fig. 3.1 Base former for study model

Measure your water into the vacuum bowl first, then add your stone. Seat the lid on the bowl and mix under vacuum for at least 30 seconds.

First pour the stone into the baseformer, simply place the former on the vibrator and let the stone run into it. Next flow stone into the occlusals and incisal edges of all teeth in the impression, starting from one end and working around to the other. Add stone over this until it reaches the top of the tissue areas, then add some more to overbuild the impression slightly.

Invert the impression onto the stone in the base former. Twist the impression gently to seat the stone mixtures together and then ensure that there are no undercuts produced under the periphery of the impression.

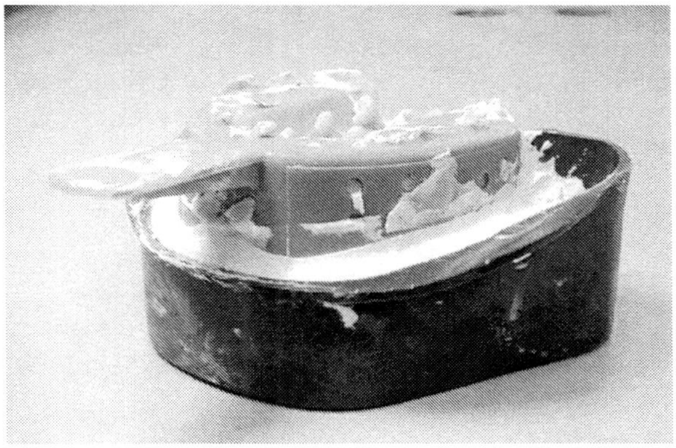

Fig. 3.2 Lower impression in base former, notice the occlusal plane has been oriented approximately parallel to the bench top.

Smooth the periphery of the stone to just above the periphery of the impression to ensure that the impression trays do not become locked into the stone bases. Do the same in the lingual region of a lower impression. This will help to ensure that teeth are not broken as the impression is removed.

Allow the models to set for at least 1 hour before removing the impression. When removing the impression first trim around the periphery with a knife to unlock the tray from any stone that may interfere with its removal. Remove the tray by lifting the posterior of the tray slightly, and then remove it by pulling up and forward (anteriorly and occlusally) on the handle. If the tray will not come away easily, it may be necessary to pry gently at the periphery with a knife to work it off.

Trimming orthodontic study models

Parts of an orthodontic model trimmer

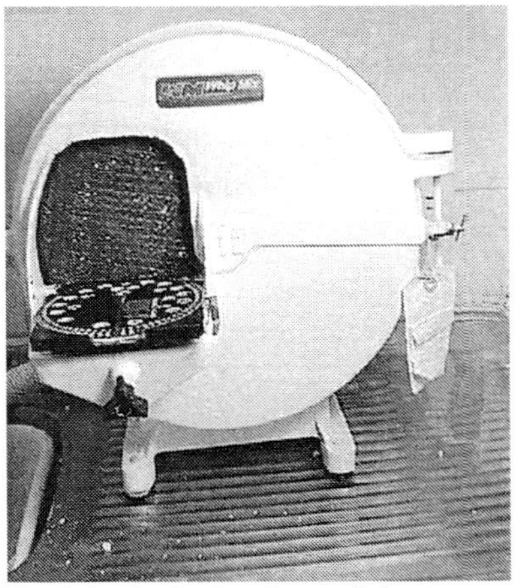

Fig 3.3 Orthodontic model trimmer

An orthodontic model trimmer is different from standard model trimmers found in most laboratories. It has a large 12" diameter trimming wheel, with an enlarged trimming window to accommodate the larger base of an orthodontic model. The trimming table has a movable guide which has stops every 5°, allowing accurate angles to be trimmed. It also includes two trimming guides: a large padded occlusal plane guide, and a small guide for setting the table to different angles.

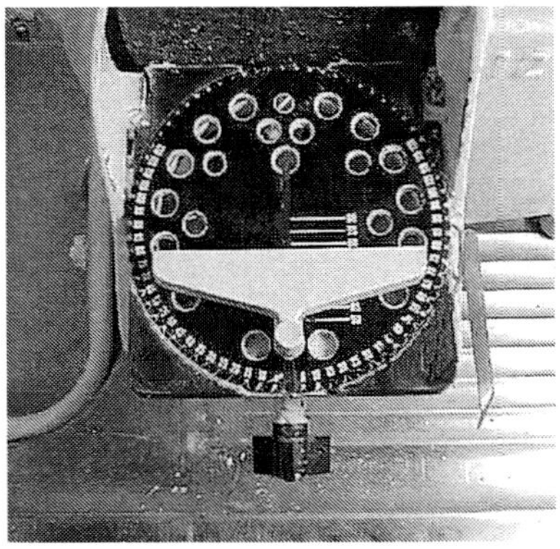

Fig.3.4 Adjustable angle guide

Planes of reference

The basic references for all of the angles and surfaces that are used when trimming orthodontic study models are the occlusal and medial planes.

Occlusal plane

The occlusal plane provides the reference for trimming the top and the bottom of the models. The top of the upper and bottom of the lower are both trimmed parallel to the occlusal plane.

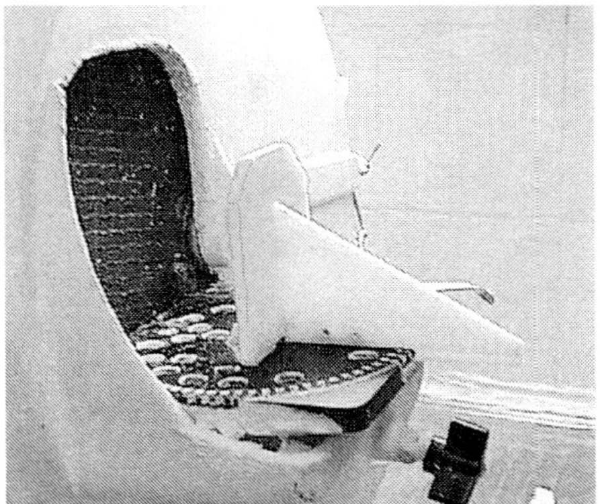

Fig. 3.5 Occlusal plane guide

Medial plane

The medial plane provides the reference for trimming the backs (posterior borders) of the set of models. The backs of the models must be perpendicular to the midline and the occlusal plane.

Orthodontic study models requirements

A set of orthodontic study models has two parts, the anatomical portion and the art base portion. The anatomical portion is that part of the model which includes the teeth and associated tissues. The art base is the material base of the model which supports the anatomical portion and gives the overall shape to the models.

The parts of the art base are:

1.) the posterior border (back)
2.) the heels
3.) the sides (65° and 60°)
4.) the anterior (front).

The requirements for the form of the art base are:

- the top and bottom of the set — in occlusion — are parallel to the occlusal plane.
- all vertical sides of the models are perpendicular to the top and bottom.

the models stand in occlusion when placed on their posterior borders or either posterior heel.

- the overall height of the models in occlusion is between 65-70 mm.

(note: all angles are measured in relation to the posterior border of the models.)

- the sides of the upper model are trimmed to an angle of 65°.
- the sides of the lower model are trimmed to an angle of 60°.
- the heels of both models are trimmed to an angle of 115°.
- the anterior portion of the upper is trimmed to an angle of 25°
- the anterior of the lower forms a smooth arc from the distal of the 3.3 to the distal of the 4.3.

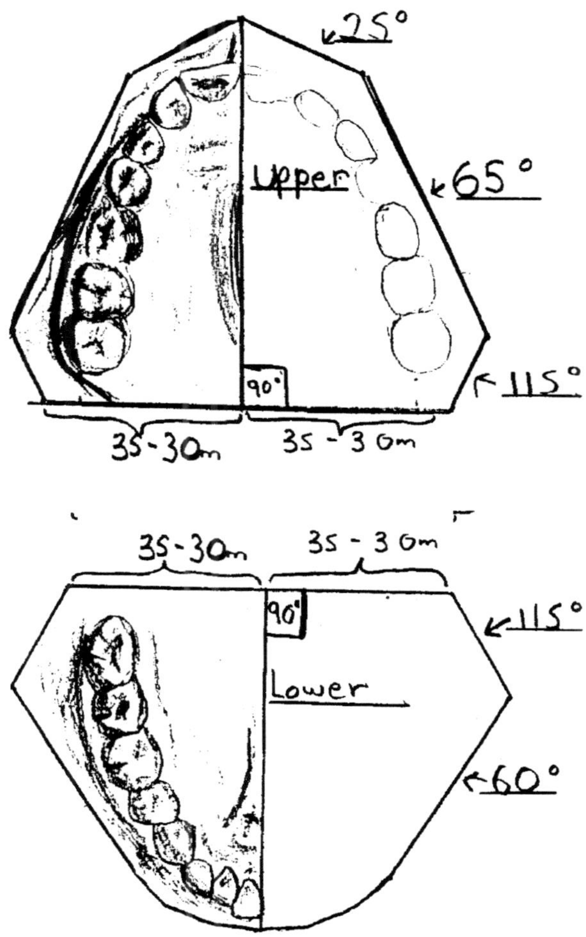

Fig 3.6 Upper and lower base forms

Steps in trimming study models

The first thing that needs to be done is the removal of any bubbles from the occlusal surface of the teeth and checking that the models fit the supplied bite. Cut the bite along the buccal line angles of the lowers so that the teeth can be clearly seen seating.

Start by trimming the top of upper model parallel to the occlusal plane. To do this use the large occlusal plane guide. Place the occlusals of the teeth on the padded surface to check that no other part of the model is interfering with them sitting on the guide. The most common point of interference is the posterior of the model. If a portion of the model interferes, remove it with a knife. On most cases the centrals and bicuspids will contact the plane. The large guide is used at a setting of 0°. Trim the upper model no thinner than 40 mm from occlusal to base at this point.

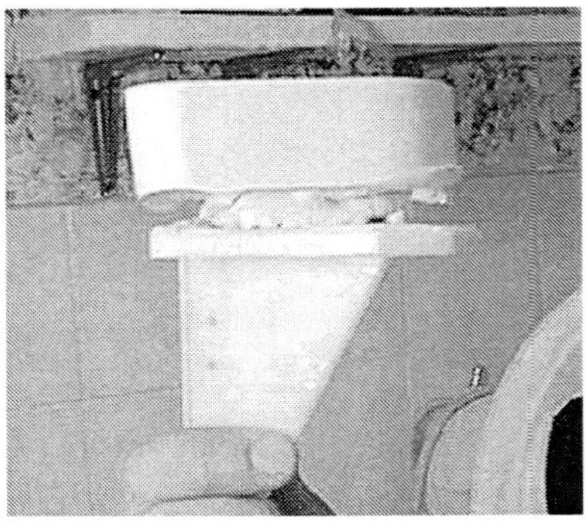

Fig. 3.7 Ensure that the posterior of the model does not interfere with the guide

Using a soft pencil, mark the midline of the model. Two landmarks are used to determine the midline: the mid-palatine fovea and the second pair of rugea. The mid-palatine fovea are two small depression at the junction of the hard and soft palates. Draw the midline as a straight line from a point midway between the fovea to a point midway between the second pair of rugea. In most cases, this line will follow the mid-palatine raphe, also passing over the incisive papilla and between the centrals.

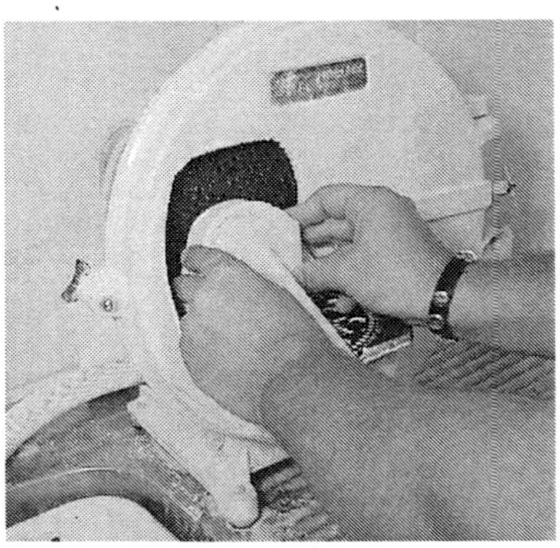

Fig 3.8 Trim top of upper parallel to occlusal plane

Place the upper model with its top on the trimming table. Trim the back (posterior) of the model so that the posterior border is perpendicular to the midline. Test this by placing the model on its back and observing how close the midline is to vertical. Trim the posterior border 2-5 mm from the maxillary tuberosity. Check before trimming too far that this measurement will not involve trimming any teeth on the lower model when the posterior borders of the models are trimmed to equal lengths. If so, leave the upper posterior border longer.

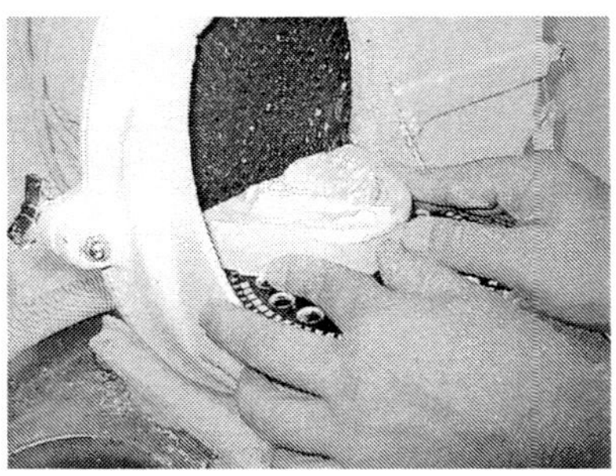

Fig. 3.9 Trim back of upper 90° to midline

Place the upper and lower in occlusion in order to trim the bottom of the lower parallel to the occlusal plane. With the models in occlusion, place the top of the upper against the large guide plane and trim the bottom of

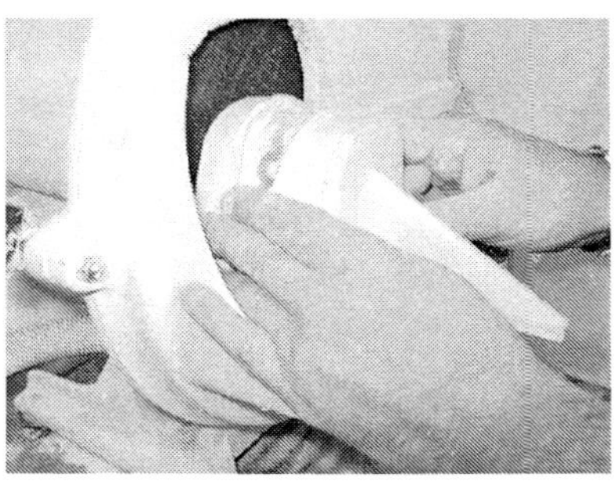

Fig. 3.11 Trim bottom of lower with the models in occlusion

the lower model. Do not trim the lower model to a height of less than 40 mm.

Place the models in occlusion and mark the posterior border of the upper on both heels of the lower model. Trim to within 2 mm of these marks. Pretrimming to this point will result in less trimming time with the models in occlusion, therefore, there is less chance of breaking teeth.

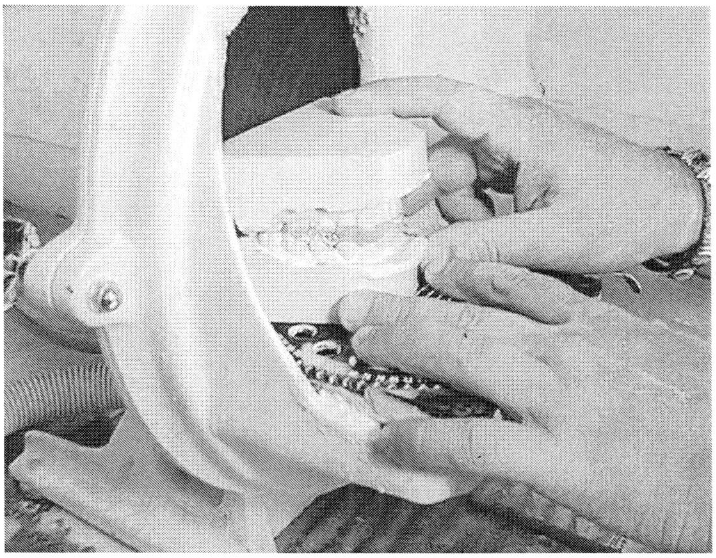

Fig. 3.11 Trim posteriors to equal lengths in occlusion

Place the upper and lower in occlusion and trim until the posterior border of both models match. Do not change the upper's relationship to the midline. The models should now stand in occlusion when placed on their backs.

Trim the sides of upper to 65° by placing the back of the model against the adjustable angle guide. The angle guide is turned until the 65° mark is centered in the front of the table. Trim both sides of the upper to 65°, rotating the table to trim the second side.

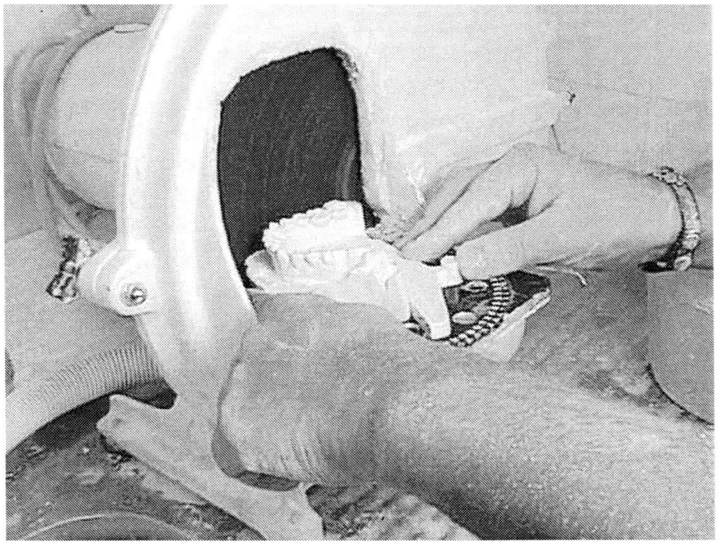

Fig.3.12 Trim side angles. Upper 65°, lower 60°.

When you are first learning to trim orthodontic study models it is useful to place a mark on the art portion of the models 7 mm buccal to the gingiva under the bicuspid region on both sides of both models. Trim the side angles to this point initially. The measurement is somewhat arbitrary, but it will result in the sides of the model starting off close to symmetrical. Starting symmetrical is a big step towards ending symmetrical.

Trim the sides of the lower model to 60°, it is also acceptable to use 55° for the lower sides.

One of the trickiest parts of orthodontic study models to trim accurately is ensuring the symmetry of the back of the model. It must be precisely the same distance from the midline to each side. If you achieve this, the point at the front of the upper model will line up exactly with the midline and the entire model will be symmetrical. If not, then you will find it impossible to get the shape of the rest of the model to balance.

Make a small pencil mark on the posterior border of the upper at the midline. Next, measure the approximate width of the buccal cusp of the most posterior molar. This distance should be between 60-70 mm. For this example we will use 66 mm.

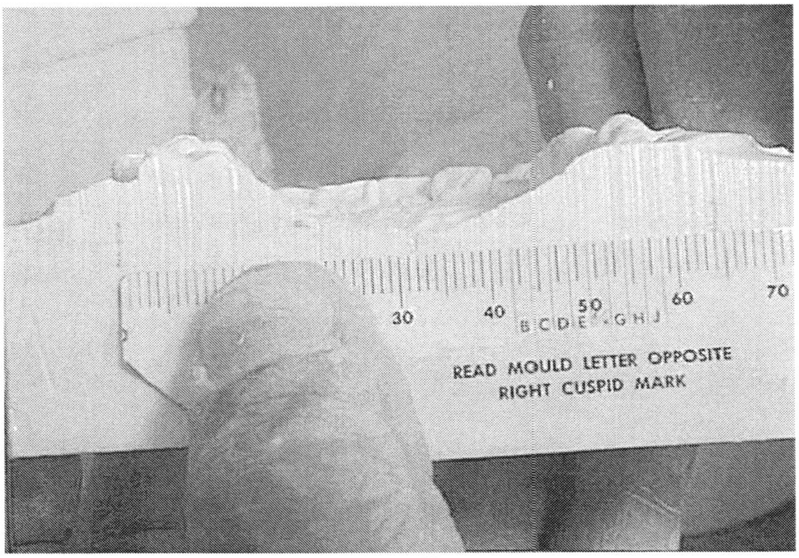

Fig. 3.13 Measuring to trim symetrically on posterior

Divide this measurement by 2 (66÷2=33), and place the ruler on the midline at this measurement, 33 mm. Now mark the back of the model at 0 mm and 66 mm. You have now found symmetrical points about the midline which can be used as guides for trimming the posterior heels.

Place the upper and lower models in occlusion, and put them onto the guide table with the upper on the trimming table. There are two ways to trim the 115° heels. Either place the back of the models on the guide when it is set to 115°, or place the 65° side of the upper against the guide when it is set to 0°.

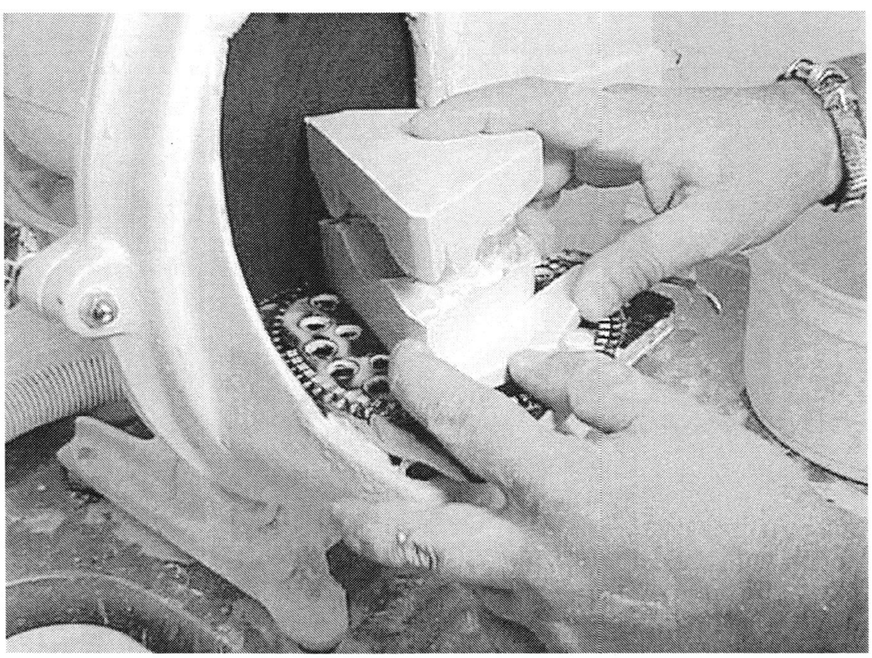

Fig. 3.14 Trim heels together with the models in occlusion

Trim the heels into the symmetrical marks. Measure from the midline to each side and adjust until the distance is equal, to within 0.5 mm or less. All of this trimming must be done with the models in occlusion to ensure that the heels of the upper and lower match. This will allow the models to stand in occlusion when placed on their heels.

Separate the models, and adjust the width of the heels by trimming the

65° angle. The width of the heels should be between 12-20 mm, with the 65° angle being no less than 2-3 mm from the tissue at its closest point. Measure the width on both heels and if they fall within this range (they usually do if the 65° side was measured 7 mm from the tissue), trim the longer heel to match the shorter. Repeat this procedure on both the upper and lower.

Trim the anterior of the upper model to an angle of 25°. The two sides must be of equal length (±0.5 mm) with the point formed by these angles on the midline between the central incisors.

Trim the anterior of the lower model to form an arc from the distal of 3.3 to the distal of 4.3. This arc should approximately match the curve formed by the labial surface of the lower anterior teeth, and come within approximately 3 mm of the labial surface. A good guide to use when trimming this arc is the peripheral roll formed by the lip when the impression was taken.

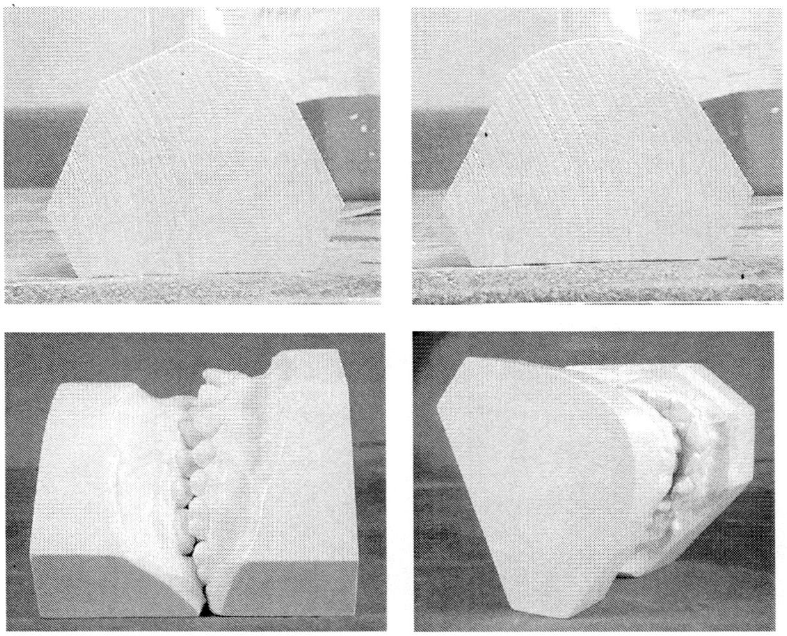

Fig. 3.15 Views of model bases and models standing in occlusion

Trim this arc in one smooth sweep across the model, do not trim in small sections or the arc will be faceted — made up of short straight sections.

The art bases of your models are now complete, and they should be symmetrical. The models should stand in occlusion when placed on their posterior border or heels. Now adjust the overall height of the models to their final dimension.

The overall height in millimeters should be between 65-70 mm.

The models should be proportioned as follows.

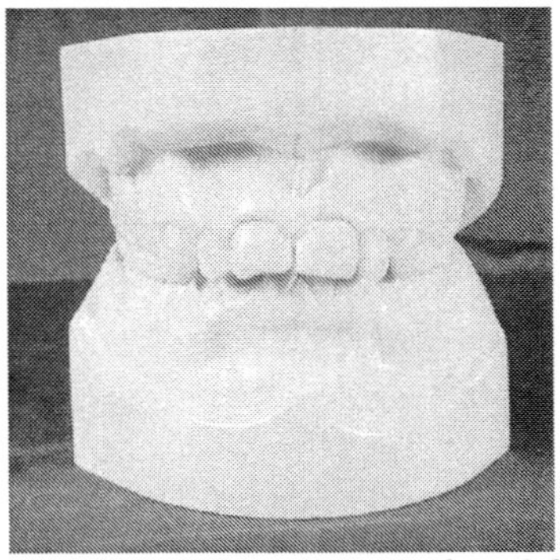

Fig 3.16 Anterior view of models

The bases of the models should form 2/3 of the overall height, with the anatomical portion forming the remaining 1/3. Place the models in occlusion on their posterior borders and adjust them until the two bases are of equal height.

While this is being done, be aware that the overall height must be 65-70 mm.

The trimming of the models is now complete and they are ready for finishing.

Finishing and polishing orthodontic study models

Carefully define the anatomy of the models around the gingiva of the teeth and remove any bubbles on the palate and in the facial sulcus. Trim out the facial sulcus to create a full even peripheral roll with a knife. Trim the art base of the model in curves that go from angle point to angle point of frenum, to be aesthetically pleasing.

Fill any small voids in the model with orthodontic stone. If a vacuum was used to mix the stone, there should be no voids.

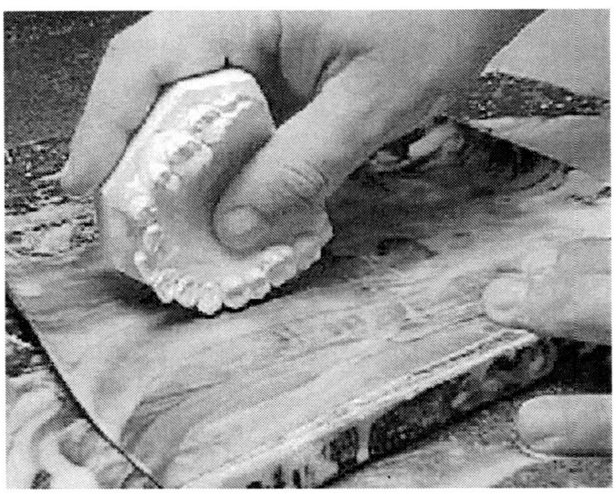

Fig.3.17 Sanding the side (65°) of upper model

Sand the sides, top and bottom of the models smooth. 400 grit wet/dry sandpaper works well for this, as do large whetstones (used to sharpen knives). Lay the wet sandpaper on the bench and smoothly draw each side of the model over it until all striations from the trimming wheel are gone. The bases of the model must be perfectly flat and smooth on all sides.

The models must be completely dry before polishing. Allow the model to dry for two days at room temperature, or use a drying oven for one hour.

We have also found that a microwave oven can be used to dry the models if used on low power for short durations. Dry them for 3 minutes on low power, then open the oven for 2 minutes to allow steam to escape and the heat to equalize throughout the model. Dry for another three minutes on low power and let the model cool for a period. The model is now ready for soaping and polishing. Microwaves tend to create very localized heat. Therefore, if the models are heated too long, or if the heat is not permitted to spread throughout the model, the model will crack.

The polishing solution that is used for orthodontic study models is referred to as "polishing soap" and may be purchased from supply companies premixed.

In the past you could make your own "polishing soap" by mixing "Ivory Snow Laundry Soap" with boiling water, however this product was discontinued in 1993. The new "Ivory Snow Detergent" does not work as a polishing soap but will in fact dissolve the models, as some of us found out to our chagrin.

When the polishing soap develops large chunks of solid matter it is time to replace it. The life span of the material can be three months to a year.

To polish the models, submerge them completely in the polishing soap for 15 minutes. Remove them, rinse lightly under running water and place on a rack or towel to allow excess soap to drain. After 15 minutes, polish the models to a high gloss with a soft towel.

If you soap several sets of models at once, be sure not to mix them up.

The patient's name, the date and the doctor's name should be placed on the back or top of each model. This may be incised into the stone, written on with a marker or placed on a label.

Metals in orthodontics: wire, tubing, bands

Stainless steel

Stainless steel is used in orthodontics to hold removable appliances in the mouth, to form springs to move the teeth and for the manufacture of the bands and brackets in fixed appliances, as well as a multitude of other purposes. With few exceptions, when you work with a metal in orthodontics, that metal is stainless steel.

But what is stainless steel?

Steel is an alloy of iron and carbon containing less than 2% carbon. Stainless steel is steel which contains more than 11% chromium (from 11 to 30% is considered stainless). It can also be alloyed with a number of other metals to produce various desired qualities. The stainless steel which is used in orthodontics is *18-8 stainless steel*, the name indicating that the alloy contains 18% chromium and 8% nickel (also 0.15% carbon).

Chromium is what makes stainless steel stainless. Chromium has a property which is called the *passivating effect.* This is a layer of oxide which is formed on the surface of the alloy when it is exposed to a mild oxidizing agent — such as the oxygen in air. This passive layer is very thin and transparent, but it is also extremely tough and imperious to oxidizing agents. Once this layer is formed, no further oxidation will take place unless the layer is disturbed.

Wire is the most common form in which stainless steel is used in the laboratory, however, it is also supplied as tubing, ribbon (for forming custom bands) and prefabricated bands.

Wire is tempered as dead soft, hard or spring hard and comes in large coils (usually 60 or 500 g.) or straight lengths (14").

The shape of a wire describes its cross-sectional form. Stainless steel round wire can be purchased in widths ranging from 0.25 mm (0.010") to 1.5 mm (0.060") and is measured in millimeters, thousandths of an inch or gauge. The metric system is becoming the standard measurement used. Other shapes of wire and their uses are:

- rectangular — including square, used for springs and final arch wire for bracket cases; identified by its dimensions (e.g..- .018 x .025)
- braided (round and rectangular) — several fine wires braided to create a larger diameter. These are more flexible than solid wires. They are used for initial arch wires for bracket cases.
- half round — used primarily for Akers clasps.

AMERICAN WIRE GAUGE SIZES
(Browne & Sharpe)
TO DECIMAL, INCH & MILLIMETER

GAUGE	INCH	MM.
1	0.289	7.35
2	0.258	6.54
3	0.229	5.83
4	0.204	5.19
5	0.182	4.62
6	0.162	4.12
7	0.144	3.66
8	0.128	3.26
9	0.114	2.91
10	0.102	2.59
11	0.091	2.30
12	0.081	2.05
13	0.072	1.83
14	0.064	1.63
15	0.057	1.45
16	0.051	1.29
17	0.045	1.15
18	0.040	1.02
19	0.036	0.91
20	0.032	0.81
21	0.028	0.72
22	0.025	0.64
23	0.023	0.57
24	0.020	0.51
25	0.018	0.45
26	0.016	0.40
27	0.014	0.36
28	0.013	0.32
29	0.011	0.29
30	0.010	0.25
31	0.009	0.23
32	0.008	0.20
33	0.007	0.18

Fig. 3.18 Wire size chart

Properties of stainless steel

Stainless steel has several properties important to its manipulation in the laboratory.

It is work hardened readily — the more a piece of wire is bent the more its hardness increases. Excessive bending will break a wire due to fatigue. Even when a wire does not break immediately, overworking it with multiple bends will result in the wire becoming unusable in the mouth. Always be aware of how much bending a wire has received. If it has taken too many bends to adapt, throw it away and start a new one. This is always better (and in the long run cheaper) than using a wire which breaks soon after it is placed in the mouth.

Stainless steel is easily soldered when the proper methods are used (see section on soldering). Stainless steel should never be heated to the point that it glows red hot. It is especially sensitive to heat in the range of 700-800° C. This causes two unwanted changes in the alloy.

First, the metal loses its temper and becomes *annealed*. Annealing is a process that softens the wire rendering it useless for orthodontic work. 18-8 stainless steel cannot be effectively heat tempered in the laboratory after annealing has occurred.

Second, the carbon and chromium in the alloy combine and are deposited at the grain boundaries of the metal. This causes the metal to become brittle and its resistance to corrosion is reduced. This condition is known as *"weld decay"*.

Bending wire

The first, and most important, rule of wire bending has to do with cutting the wire. Small off-cuts of wire can be shot off at high speed when they are cut. These ends are extremely sharp and will fly across an entire room if not controlled. It is, therefore, the first rule of orthodontics that when you cut wire, you hold onto both sides of the wire being cut. If the off-cut is too small to hold, you can hold the cutters against your leg (always wear long pants or lab coat) to control the cut piece and ensure it does not hit anyone.

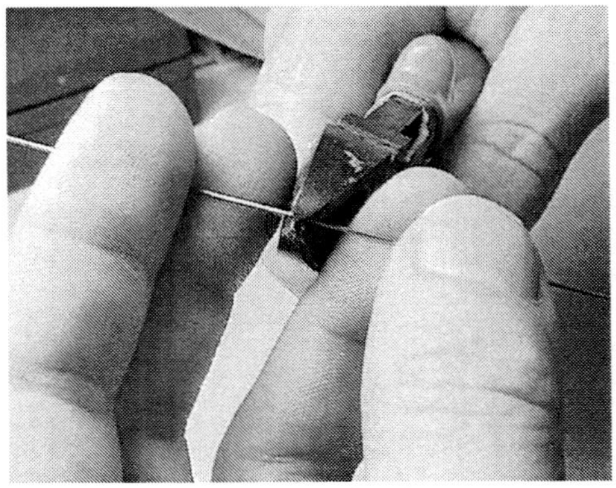

Fig. 3.19 Hold both ends of wire when cutting

Your pliers are used to hold the wire, like a vise. Do not use the pliers to apply the force that bends the wire. The forces are applied with your fingers. Bending the wire with your pliers will result in excessive wear and possible breakage of the pliers. Hold the pliers comfortably in the palm of your hand with your first finger placed between the handles. This grip will allow the maximum control of the pliers when bending.

When using 139 bird's beak pliers, sharp angles of 90° or less should be made on the square beak of the pliers. Loops and bends of more than 90° should be made on the round beak.

To bend a sharp angle, place your finger or thumb on the wire directly against the beak of the plier. Press the wire against the beak with your finger while holding the wire firmly in the pliers.

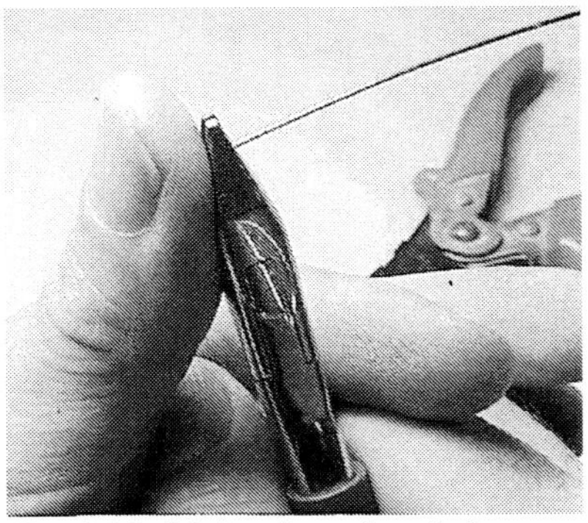

Fig 3.20 Make sharp bends by placing your finger close to the pliers

Bends should only be made at an angle of 90° to the jaws of the pliers. This allows you to make an accurate bend while placing the least amount of pressure on the wire from the pliers. Squeezing the handles excessively hard can result in the jaws nicking the wire. This will be a weak point in the wire (and a stress concentrator) causing the wire to have a shorter serviceable lifespan. A nicked wire should not be used in an appliance.

Large or gentle bends can be made by pressing on the wire farther from the point where it is held by the jaws, or by using only your fingers. To form a gentle curve using your fingers, use one of these two methods. Hold the wire firmly in one hand and form a curve by drawing the thumb of the other hand along the wire. The second method is to place your two middle fingers in the center of the wire and your thumbs near the ends, flex the wire between the thumbs and fingers until the desired curve is achieved. Using your fingers to bend avoids nicks or kinks being placed in the wire. It is also easier to bend the wire on a single plane when bending with your fingers.

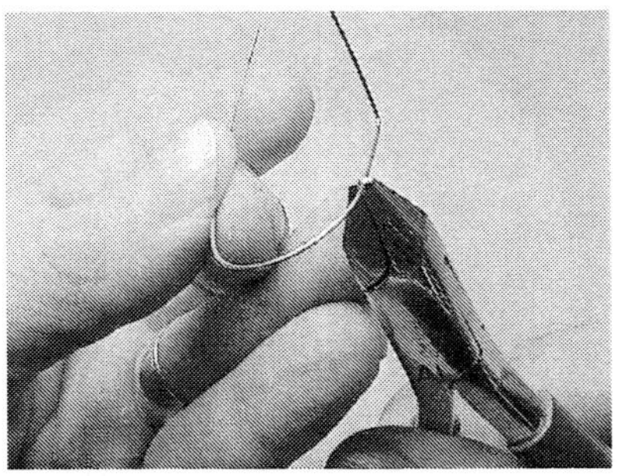

Fig.3.21 Make large curves by holding the wire far from the pliers

If a wire must be level in a single plane, such as an arch wire, check it by placing it on a flat surface (the desktop) and ensuring that the entire wire touches the surface.

When a wire is being bent, one bend is made at a time and then the wire is test fitted against the model. This ensures that the wire will fit precisely. If the wire does not seat properly in its place after a bend, the bend that was just made is obviously the point that needs to be corrected. When fitting a wire to the model, use a soft lead pencil or a fine tip felt marker to mark the next point at which the wire must be bent. After the bend is adjusted, check the wire, adjusting again if necessary, before continuing to the next bend.

If an angle is bent too much, lessen the angle by placing the square beak of the plier inside the angle and pressing gently on the handles.

Bend wire of the size indicated to fit the drawings on the following page. The wire must cover the image and lie flat to the page.

Wire Bending Exercise

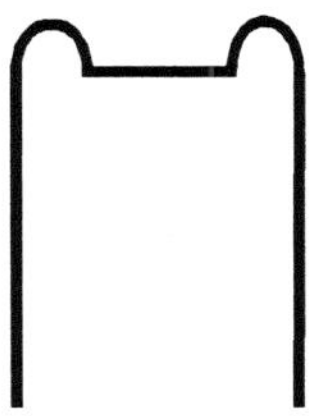

0.7

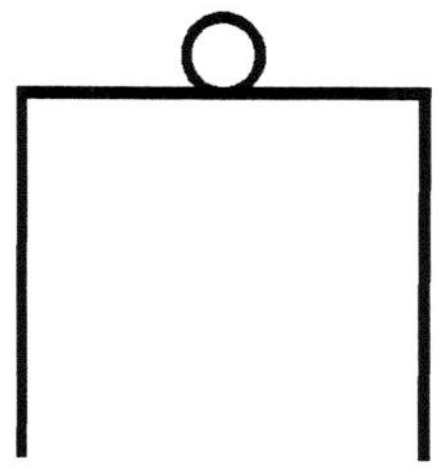

0.7

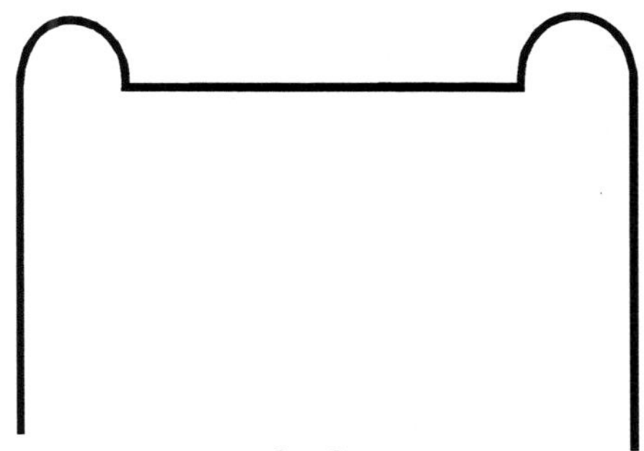

0.8

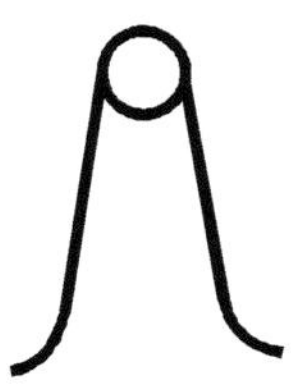

0.7

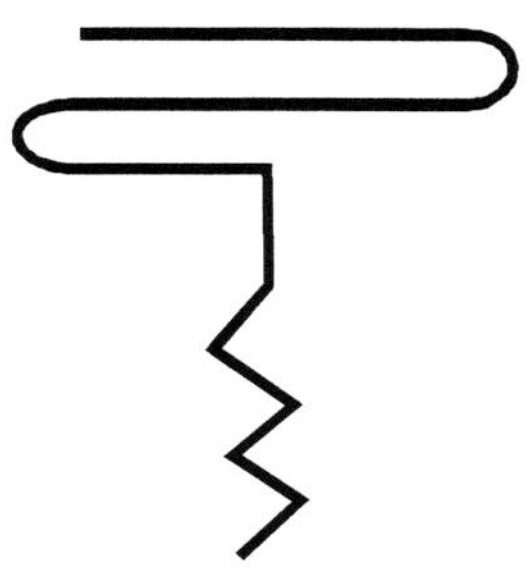

0.7

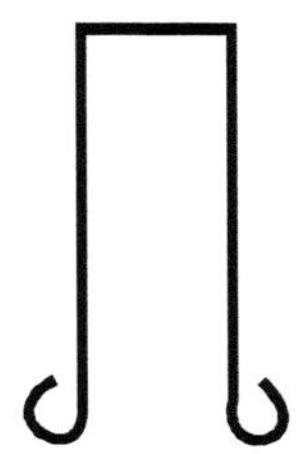

0.5

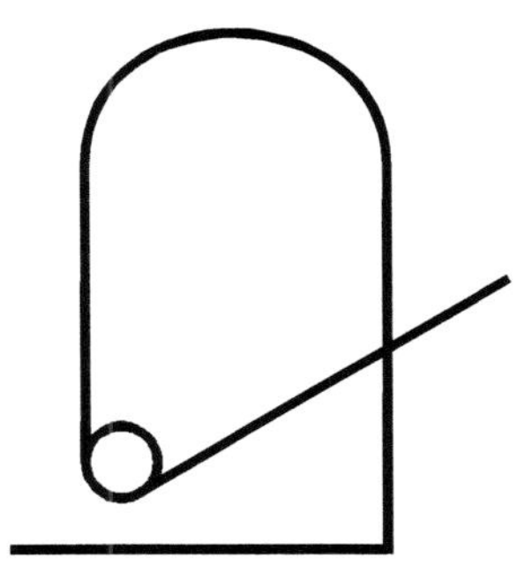

0.7

Use wire size indicated
by number under each shape.
Wire should lie flat on paper
and cover drawing on paper
Secure wire to sheet with one
piece of tape for each shape.

Other wire alloys

Elgiloy

Elgiloy is a cobalt-chromium-nickel alloy originally developed for making watch springs. A normal distribution of these elements would be:

- cobalt 40%
- chromium 20%
- nickel 15%
- as well as Mo, Mn, C, Be and Fe.

Elgiloy exhibits excellent properties for orthodontic use and is supplied in a variety of sizes and tempers. The tempers are colour coded:

- red — spring hard
- green — semi-spring hard
- yellow — hard
- blue — soft (not dead soft).

Elgiloy is formulated to work harden during bending, with a reasonable amount of bending the wire finishes at the desired temper. Elgiloy can also be easily tempered in the laboratory using a furnace or by passing a current through the wire with a spot welder.

Nickel-Titanium

Nickel titanium wire is used primarily in the arches for straight wire brackets. It has the unique ability to maintain its form even through extreme deformation. You can literally tie the wire in a knot, and when you release it will return to its original shape as though nothing has happened. No other wire has this ability.

It can also exert a steady, gentle force almost without regard for the amount of deformation (bending) induced in the wire. Other wires exert different levels of force depending on how much deformation is present at any time. The more the wire is bent, the greater the force. As the tooth moves, the wire bends less and exerts less force. Therefore, most springs or arches tend to exert too heavy a force at the beginning and too light a force at the end. Nickel-Titanium can also be referred to as NiTi. NiTi wires exert the same amount of force on the tooth through its entire range of movement. This allows the tooth to move faster and without damage.

NiTi also has the property that when it is chilled it becomes more malleable (easier to bend), but when the temperature is raised it once again tries to assume its original shape. Some manufacturers refer to this as thermal activation.

So why isn't NiTi used for every spring we make rather than just performed arch wires? Because NiTi wants to return to its original shape, it is extremely difficult to bend. It can be bent by applying heat to the wire during bending, however, hand forming is still difficult. The expense of the wire also precludes its use in common appliances.

Tubing

Tubes are used as insertion points for removable components, and for their ability to allow components to move while attached to an appliance. Tubes are made from stainless steel and are named — and measured — by the inside diameter of their opening. Most tubes are still referred to in imperial sizes (inches).

Extra-oral attachments — such as headgear — are placed into tubes either attached to a removable appliance or welded to bands. These tubes are .045" so that the facebow will fit snugly into the tubes. Many appliances use tubes to allow active components to move within the appliance. Such uses call for the tube to be slightly larger than the wire used. This lets the wire move without binding. Auto Hawleys use tubes of .020-.024" and wires from .012" round wire to .010x.020" square wire. Band coil space regainers use tubes of .036" for wires of .032" (0.8 mm).

Band material

Bands may be purchased premanufactured or be custom fabricated in the laboratory. Band material is made of a thin ribbon-like stainless steel.

Premanufactured bands come in a wide range of sizes, with or without prewelded attachments. These bands are formed and sized to be specific to different teeth and different quadrants. They are made for incisors, cuspids, bicuspids, first molars and second molars. To have a complete inventory of bands for all these teeth in all four quadrants can be an expensive proposition.

Band materials is supplied in 8' rolls which can be cut to length for individual bands. This material is measured by its height and thickness, the two most common sizes being:

- .180x.005" — used for molar bands
- .150x.004" — used for bicuspid bands.

It is advisable to have this material because there will always be a tooth that does not fit a premanufactured band. For instructions on making a band with band material see the section on fixed appliances.

Metal joining: solder, flux, soldering and spot welding

When fabricating orthodontic appliances it is frequently necessary to join metal components. There are two methods of joining commonly used: soldering and spot welding.

Soldering is the joining of two pieces of metal by melting an alloy of a lower melting point between them. Soldering joins mainly through mechanical bonding of microscopic irregularities on the surfaces and is dependent on the wetting of the surface of the metals. There is evidence, however, of metallic bonds being formed.

Spot welding is the direct fusing of the two pieces of metal being joined. There is no intermediary metal in a spot weld joint.

Solder

Soldering of orthodontic appliances is an easily accomplished task with practice and when using the proper materials and procedures. The solder used is a silver solder, chosen for its strength and the ability to solder the stainless steel without damaging the alloy (when used properly). The solder does not have the tarnish resistance of a gold solder, however, for the limited lifespan of an orthodontic appliance its resistance is sufficient.

A solder must have certain definite qualities.

It must have a defined melting temperature to allow quick identification of the point at which the solder has melted and flowed onto the joint. It must flow at a temperature which does not result in damage to the wire being soldered. It must be able to resist the hostile environment of the mouth, without introducing dangerous materials into the patient. It must be economical to manufacture and use.

Silver solder is an alloy of copper and zinc to which silver is added. The silver acts to reduce the melting temperature and increase the tarnish resistance. An approximate formula for such a commercially available solder might be:

- silver 56%
- copper 22%
- zinc 17%
- tin 5%. (composition of Dentaurum silver solder).

Silver solder for orthodontics is supplied in the form of a wire. Thinner sizes are preferable as the solder will melt more easily, 0.5-0.6 mm works well.

Flux

Flux is the first step in a successful solder joint.

Flux is the white paste which is applied to clean the metal which is to be soldered and protect it from oxidation. Ideally a flux should have these properties:

- it must have a melting point lower than that of the solder.

while it is melting the flux should not effloresce or pull away from the surface being soldered.

- it should spread evenly over the work surface after melting.
- it must be able to dissolve metallic oxides.
- it should be easy to remove after soldering is complete.

The flux used with stainless steel is a potassium fluoride flux. An average flux would contain these:

- Potassium fluoride — 50% — to remove the passive layer
- Boric acid — 34% — to lower the melting point, inhibit efflorescence of the borax glass
- Borax glass — 8% — improves flow of flux, dissolves oxides, removes easily from work
- Sodium carbonate — 8% — lowers melting point and increases fluidity.

Orthodontic flux is mixed with water and can be rewetted if it dries out. It should be applied to the joint to be soldered before heating has commenced. Orthodontic flux performs several important functions in the soldering process:

- it acts to protect the hot metal of the solder joint from oxidizing and removes oxides already on the metal.
- it removes the passive layer on the surface of the metal so that the solder can bond.
- it acts as a temperature indicator to tell us when the joint is hot enough to accept the solder.

As the flux and metal are heated the flux undergoes several changes in appearance. First, the flux bubbles as the mixing water is boiled off. Second, the flux acquires a hard, porous white surface. Third, the flux melts and flows as the borax glass fuses, and it spreads over the work surface. The flux now has a clear, glass-like appearance.

When the flux acquires this clear, glass-like appearance the metal has reached the temperature at which it can accept the solder. Solder the joint. When the solder has cooled, the flux is a hard, clear glass. It is easily broken off with a knife or pliers. Any flux that does not break off can be removed with a steel bur. Do not use a stone as the flux will quickly fill in the abrasive surface.

If the flux has a greenish tinge, the joint has been overheated and the flux will be difficult to remove.

Soldering

Silver solder can be applied using several soldering methods. It can be soldered using a flame, either the compressed air and gas flame of an orthodontic blowpipe, or the flame from a hand held butane torch. It can also be soldered using an electric current — as applied from a spot welder — to generate heat.

When a flame is used for soldering it is important that the soldering take place in the reducing zone of the flame. This is just off of the tip of the inner bright blue cone of the flame. This is also the hottest part of the flame.

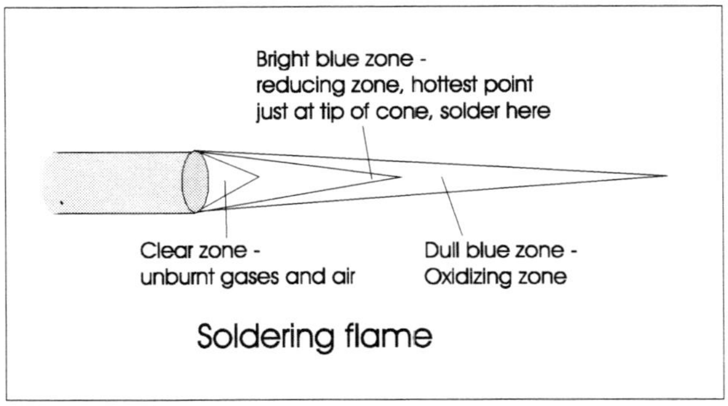

Fig. 3.22 Soldering flame

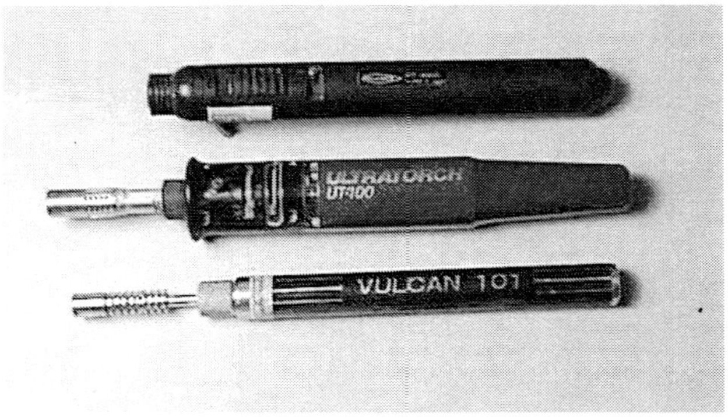

Fig. 3.23 Several handheld butane torches used to solder silver

Once a coloured oxide film has begun to form on the surface of the stainless steel, solder will not adhere. You must apply the proper flux to the metal before heating begins (see previous section).

Solder will not flow to cold metal, the metal must be warmed to the correct temperature before the solder will flow onto it, approximately 900° F. Trying to apply solder to cold metal will result in the solder melting and forming an ever larger ball at the tip of the solder wire. Heat the metal to the correct temperature — as indicated by the flux (see previous section) — before applying the solder.

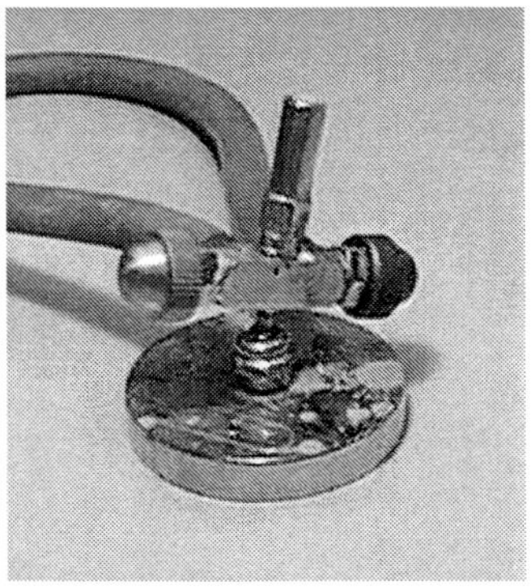

Fig. 3.24 Orthodontic blowpipe for soldering, burns compressed air and natrual gas.

When the metal is at the correct temperature the solder will first soften to a plastic condition and then flow onto the joint. Lay a length of the wire across the joint at a time, rather than pushing the point of the wire into the joint. This is a faster, yet more controlled method of applying solder.

Continue applying solder until the appropriate amount has accumulated on the joint. Ideally

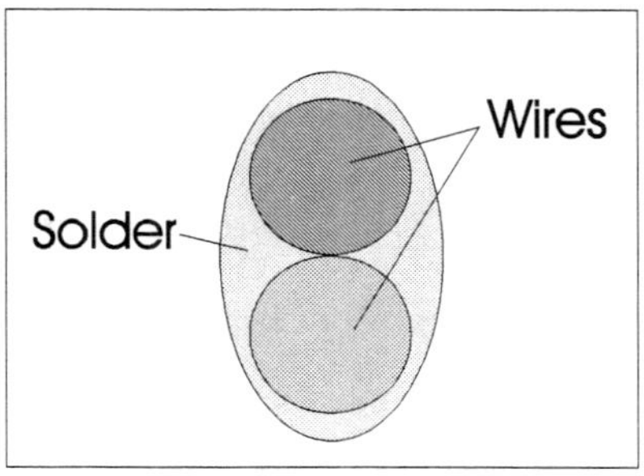

Fig. 3.25 Solder joint (cross-section view), solder completely encases wires.

the wires involved in the solder joint should be completely encased in the solder. This is not strictly necessary from the point of view of the mechanics of the solder joint, however, it is something of a traditional sign of a good solder joint and adds to the strength of the joint.

When sufficient solder is deposited, remove the solder wire and continue heating. The solder's flow point is indicated by the formation of a bright, mirror-like surface under the flux covering. When this is reached the solder flows and smooths itself evenly on the joint. Remove the heat from the joint, let it cool for a few seconds, then quench the joint in water.

In this molten state the solder can be moved about the joint in two ways, by heat and gravity. The solder will move towards the heat of the flame (or contact with electro-soldering). Therefore, you cannot push the solder to the position that you want. You must instead heat the area that you want the solder to flow to and the solder will be drawn towards the heat. Gravity can be used to assist in this by ensuring that the solder is moving downhill. Do not maintain the solder in this molten state too long, or the solder and the wire will become overheated.

Be careful to never overheat the joint when soldering. This is not only to be avoided for the damage that occurs to the stainless steel, as previously discussed, but also because prolonged heating of the solder after it has melted and flowed will result in the lower melting components of the solder boiling off. This changes the composition of the solder, weakening it and results in trapped gas bubbles when the heat is removed, also weakening the joint.

If the joint is extremely overheated the flux will draw off of areas of the wire or band and the wire will oxidize. This is a heavy black oxide layer that the solder will not flow over. In instances that the temper of the material is not critical, the joint can be resoldered, however, this oxide layer must be completely removed by trimming or pumicing first.

An overheated joint will almost certainly contain porosity. Such porosity will not usually be evident until the joint is trimmed. The porosity can be removed by applying flux to the joint liberally, coating the entire joint. Reheat the solder gently. The flux will lift any trimming debris out of the voids, allowing the solder to flow together and the voids to disappear.

Trimming and polishing a solder joint

The objective of a good soldering job is that when the soldering is finished, no trimming should be necessary. There is almost always a small amount of trimming to be performed, however, there should never be a large amount of trimming needed.

Trimming of silver solder is much the same as trimming any metal in the dental laboratory. Silver has the advantage of being a relatively soft metal, which means that it can be effectively trimmed with steel burs. Any other abrasive that is commonly used in the laboratory will also work: stones, carbides, aluminium oxide disks, etc. You must be careful during trimming not to remove too much solder or thin the diameter of the wire. This will weaken the joint and the appliance.

After trimming, the surface should be smoothed with a soft rubber wheel to remove striations. A light pumicing is also effective in smoothing the surface.

Polishing of the joint is done with chromium oxide (green stick compound). It can be used on a buff, chamois, or a felt wheel.

Spot welding

Spot welding is a method of attaching two pieces of stainless steel by passing an electric current through them. A high-voltage, low-amperage current creates a very localized heat source between the two pieces. The surfaces of the metal in contact melt and fuse together in a very localized area. Pressure on the pieces improves the strength of the joint. Several welds should be made for each joint, and several joints should be made on each piece.

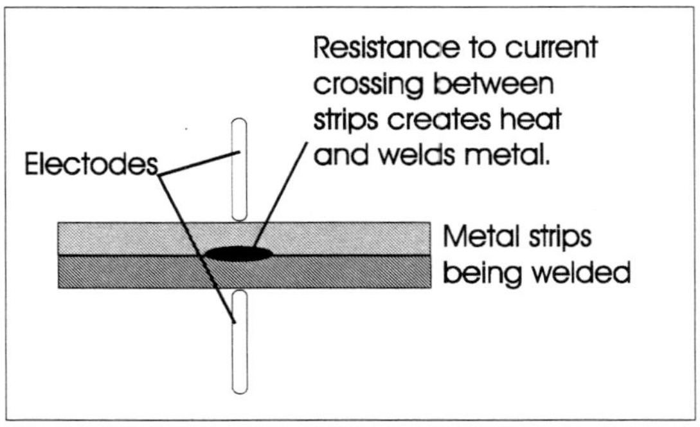

Fig. 3.26 Joint created by spot welding

Spot welding can be used to attach components by itself or as a tack weld to hold them for soldering. Wires which are welded and then soldered have extremely strong joints.

Large wires are welded using high power; thinner wires are welded with lower settings so as not to damage them.

Acrylic

Polymethyl methacrylate acrylic (PMMA) is the material used to form the acrylic plate of an orthodontic appliance. It is the same basic material as the acrylics used in other areas of the dental laboratory.

PMMA is used in the laboratory most commonly in the form of a powder and a liquid. These are both composed of the same type of molecules, with some minor chemical additions to each to help in the setting reaction. This setting reaction is called *"polymerization"*. Polymerization is a chemical reaction that results in the joining of many small moleclues of the same type to form one large molecule. The basic unit in this chemical is a single molecule of the material which is called a "*mer*".

The names of the powder and liquid that are used when working with acrylic now come into context. The powder is the polymer. *Poly* means many, therefore this material is many mers. It is composed of short chains of mer molecules.

The liquid is the monomer. *Mono* means one, therefore the liquid is made of single mer units.

The usual method of application in orthodontics is called the sprinkle or salt and pepper technique. A detailed description of acrylic processing and finishing with this method is presented in the section on *Basic techniques.*

The polymerization reaction begins when the polymer and monomer are mixed. The monomer must wet every crystal of polymer. In the sprinkle technique that means that there must be no spots of dry powder left during application. The polymer contains a chemical which starts the polymerization reaction. This chemical is known as the *"initiator"* and is usually benzoyl peroxide. The initiator requires something to help it start the reaction. In the heat cure acrylics used in denture bases this additional ingredient is heat. The acrylic that is used in orthodontics contains a chemical in the monomer known as an *"activator"*. This activator begins the polymerization process when it reacts with the initiator in the polymer. Because heat is not needed to start the reaction these types of acrylics are referred to as cold-cure, self-curing or autopolymerizing acrylics.

The polymerization process has three different stages. The first stage is the *"induction stage"*. This is the stage at which the initiator is activated and becomes a highly reactive molecule called a *"free radical"*. These free radicals quickly attach themselves to a monomer molecule and in doing so open a bond on the monomer which lets it bond to another monomer molecule.

Once the reaction has started it continues with little resistance. This is called the *"propagation stage"*. Propagation continues until the free radicals have all reacted. This point is called *"termination"*, when the reaction can no longer continue.

This process creates long chains of molecules which give the acrylic its strength. These chains have a coiled shape, and the mass of the acrylic can be thought of as resembling a bowl of spagetti. If an additional chemical called a *"crosslinking agent"* is present, then the chains are also linked together across themselves giving greater strength to the acrylic.

Orthodontic acrylics can also be used as a dough by simply mixing the polymer and monomer in a mixing bowl and then applying the mixture to the model while it is in a moldable state.

In most industrial applications PMMA is formed by molding under heat and pressure. In the dental laboratory some prosthesis are fabricated in this manner by using a *"vacuum former"*. This method can be referred to as *"thermoforming"*. Acrylic used for thermoforming is supplied in *"blanks"* to fit vacuum former machines. PMMA is a thermoplastic material, meaning that is softens under heat. A large heating element of the vacuum former softens the material. It is then pressed to the shape of the model by atmospheric pressure when the vacuum removes the air between the model and the acrylic blank.

"PRESS ON. Nothing in the world can take the place of persistence. Talent will not; nothing in the world is more common than unsuccessful men with talent. Genius will not; unrewarded genius is a proverb. Education will not; the world is full of educated derelicts. Persistance and determination alone are omnipotent."
Calvin Coolidge

"Sometimes a winner is just a dreamer who never gave up."
Unknown

Tools and equipment

"I am always doing that which I can not do, in order that I may learn how to do it."
Pablo Picasso
1881-1973

"If you would thoroughly know anything, teach it to others."
Tryon Edwards (1809 - 1894)

4

I always run into the same response when I tell technicians that I do ortho. They say "How can you stand all that wire bending; it drives me crazy".

The symbol of ortho technicians has got to be their pliers. The pliers we use are at the heart of our wire bending, and good pliers can make the difference between a well bent wire and an exercise in frustration.

There are innumerable different designs that you can buy, from the simple to the exotic, but there are several common factors that will define good pliers.

There are two common types of pliers: stainless steel pliers and tungsten carbide inserts pliers.

Stainless Steel

Stainless steel pliers range from very low to high quality. The price of the pliers is generally a good determinant of how long they will last. Some cheap pliers will wear beyond use in a matter of days, while a good pair can last for years. Stainless steel pliers are not as durable as the inset pliers for daily wire bending, however, they are not as brittle and do not rust.

Tungsten carbide inserts

In order to improve the wear resistance of pliers, manufacturers will make the bending surface of the plier from a harder material. This is called an insert which is then braised or soldered onto a stainless steel handle.

The metal used in the insert is commonly called tungsten carbide, however, in most pliers today it is actually a tool steel. The tungsten carbide inserts are extremely brittle and will break if dropped. The tungsten carbide is also vulnerable to rusting and should not be exposed to moisture for any period of time.

The tool steel inserts have almost as good wear resistance as the tungsten carbide but are less likely to break and more resistant to rust.

Generally an insert plier will be of better quality and last longer than a stainless steel for not appreciably more money.

I always recommend that people buy good insert pliers of the types that they will use everyday and cheap steel pliers that they can feel free to modify for special purposes.

Types of pliers

139 (bird's beak)

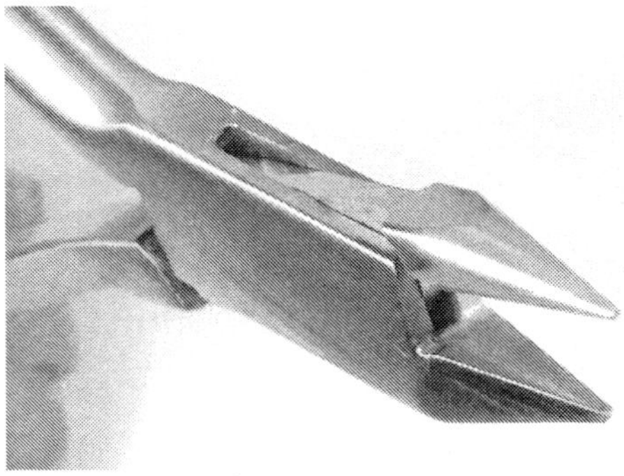

Pliers courtesy of Orthopli

Fig. 4.1 139 pliers

The 139 bird's beak pliers are the best design of plier for general use. If you own only one pair of pliers this is the kind that you should have.

The 139 has 1 round beak and 1 square beak. This configuration allows you to easily produce both sharp angles and rounded bends. The 139 has generally short beaks, allowing them to be used on larger wires without damaging the pliers.

You must be careful not to exert excessive pressure on the pliers when bending with the tip. The round beak has less surface area on the wire and can create a nick fairly easily.

Adams (square jaw)

The Adams' plier was designed by Dr. Adams to bend his (what else) Adams clasp. It is a plier with 2 square jaws, by his original definition, each jaw terminating in a 1 mm square tip. Today you can get Adams' style pliers in a number of sizes to bend wires from light to very heavy. The large Adams pliers are particularly useful for torquing bends. The wire is held tightly between the jaws and then rotated about its long axis.

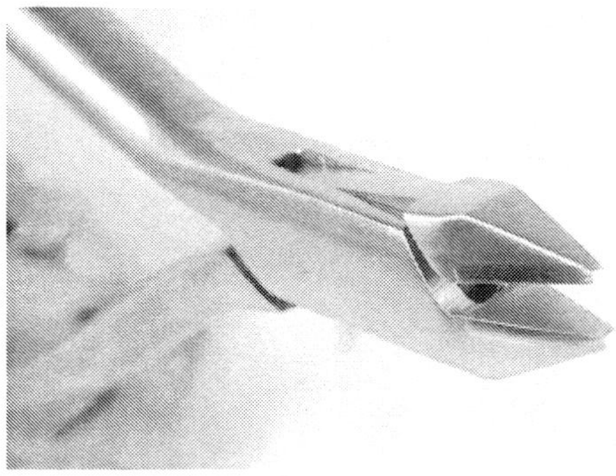

Pliers courtesy of Orthopli

Fig. 4.2 Adams pliers

3 prong

3 prong pliers have two jaws on one side and one on the other. The single jaw rests between the two jaws of the opposite side. When the handle of the plier is squeezed, the single center jaw presses the wire against the two outer jaws to form the bend. They are used to make controlled adjustment to the wire in a specific place. These pliers are particularly useful for final adjustment of bent wires, and bends in limited space.

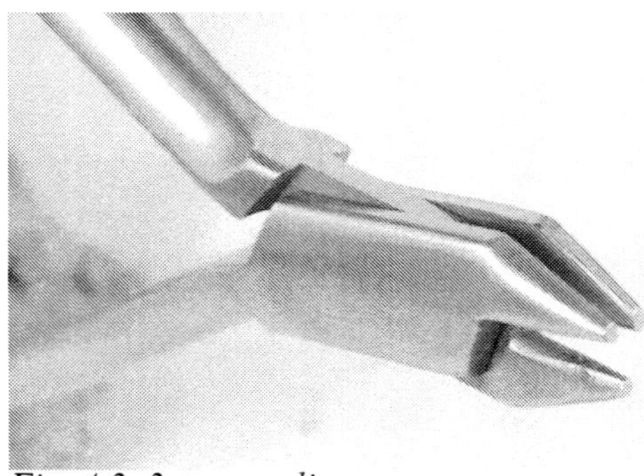

Pliers courtesy of Orthopli

Fig. 4.3 3-prong pliers

3 prong pliers will leave nicks on the wire if used too aggressively. Some people use these pliers for almost all of their bending, however, because of the danger of nicks, I use them only sparingly, generally for final adjustment.

Spring pliers (loop forming pliers)

There are several different pliers that may be used in bending springs. Some are specifically designed to do this, some are more general usage designs. A 139 will serve as an adequate spring plier if necessary.

Several of the designs use a concave beak fitted to a stepped round beak. The stepping on the round beak allows you to form loops of various uniform sizes. This design works well, but as with the 3 prong pliers, you must be careful not to press too hard or the concave beak will nick the wire.

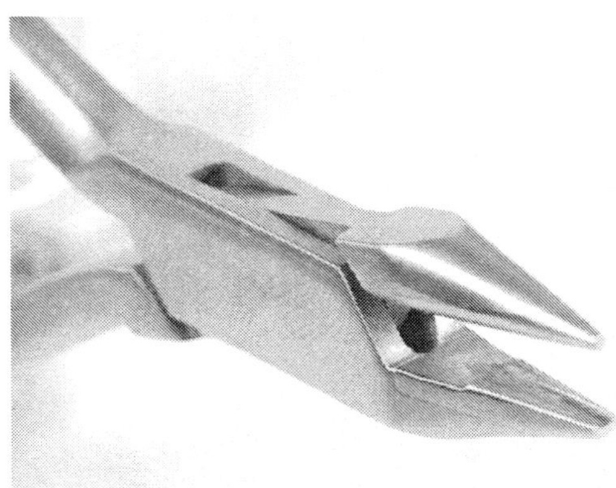

Pliers courtesy of Orthopli

Fig. 4.4 Loop forming pliers

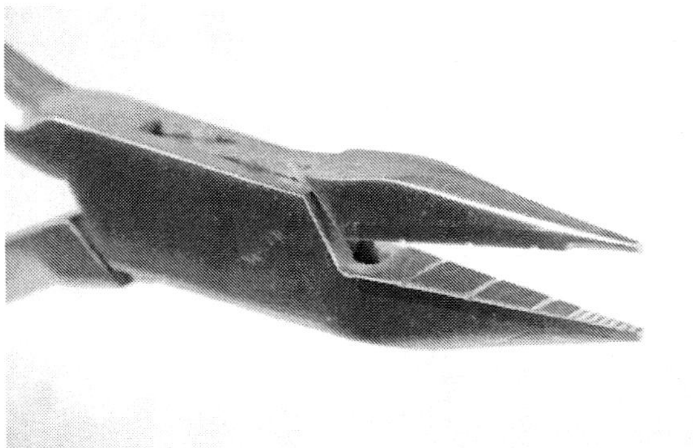

Pliers courtesy of Orthopli

Fig. 4.5 Jarabek pliers

The type of pliers that I use for spring and loop bending is called a jarabek. One jaw has a round tapered tip leading to a flat surface with spaced grooves. The opposing jaw has a flat serrated tip leading to a flat area with grooves matching its opposition. The fine tip allows for small, tight helixes, while the flat areas are good for adjusting fine wires.

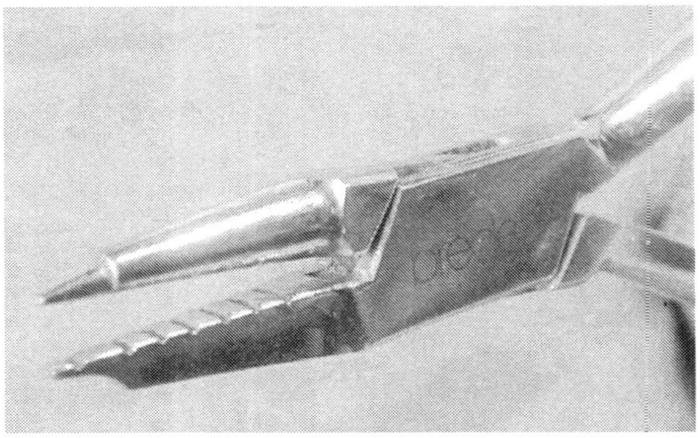

Fig. 4.6 Labial bow pliers

Labial bow pliers

Labial bow pliers are a pair of speciality pliers that I find exceedingly useful if you do ortho full-time. They have a large tapered round beak with a series of grooves on the opposing flat beak. They let you quickly bend uniform loops in a variety of sizes. The heavy beaks allow you to bend large wires easily. A similar plier is known as the "Three Barrel" plier.

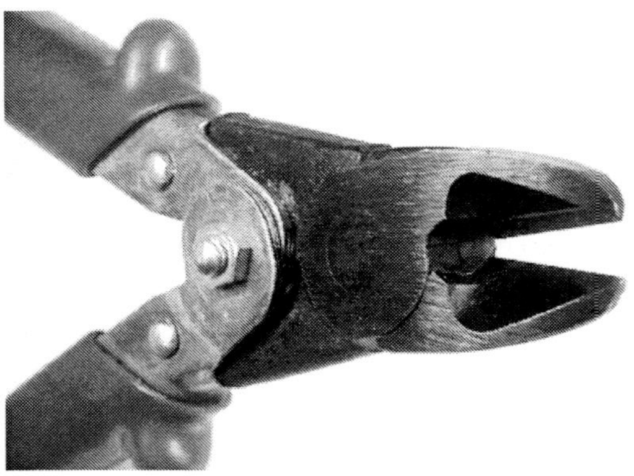

Pliers courtesy of Orthopli

Fig. 4.7 Hardened wire cutters

Wire cutters

Good wire cutters are essential for ortho. You can go to the hardware store and buy $10 wire cutters, but they will not have a hardened tip and will not cut some materials easily. You can use them, but if you use proper cutters you won't go back.

Spatula and carvers (handtools)

There are numerous designs of carvers and spatulas available from supply houses. These are some examples of types generally used:

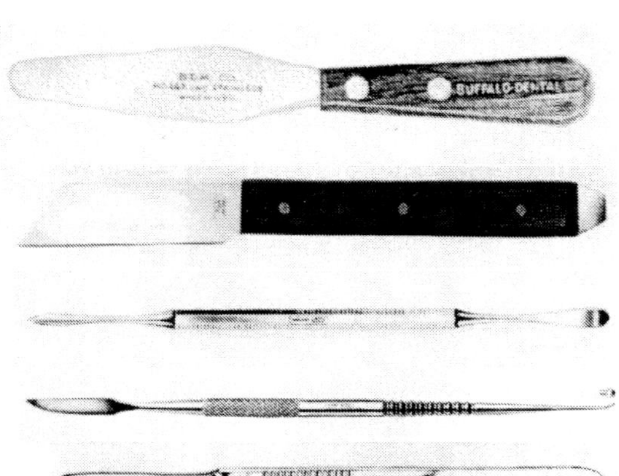

Courtesy of Cental Dental®

Fig. 4.8 Hand tools

plaster spatula andplaster knife

#7 wax spatula

hylin, Le Cron or Zahle type carver

scalpel.

Equipment

Orthodontic model trimmer

The orthodontic model trimmer is different from the trimmer you will generally find in a lab; it is also about twice the price. The wheel is 12" instead of 10" to accommodate the larger bases of the ortho models. It is also fitted with a rotating trimming table which is locked at marked intervals of 5 degrees. The trimming table has a guide aligned with 0 degrees that accepts two trimming guides. One guide is for angle cuts in conjunction with rotating the table, and the other is a flat plane to be used in trimming the base of models parallel to the occlusal plane.

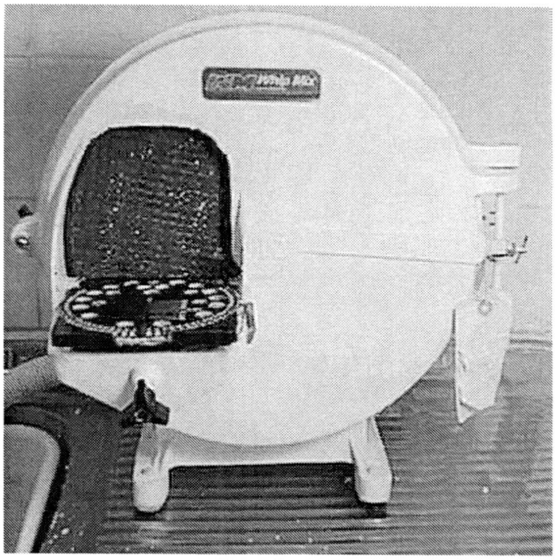

Fig. 4.9 Orthodontic model trimmer

Pressure pot

The pressure pot has an attachment to allow compressed air to be introduced into the pot for curing acrylic. The pressure to be used is 20 psi, the safety release on most pots will vent at 25 psi.

Your pressure pot should be a commercially available model, purchased from a dental supply house. It is possible to jury-rig your own pressure pot from consumer parts. I strongly advise against it. The pressure pot has the potential to be one of the most dangerous pieces of equipment in the lab. If there should be an accident, your insurance could be voided by a home made pot.

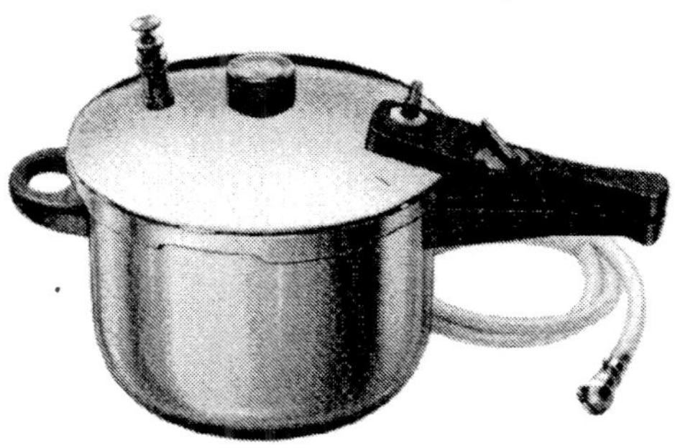

Fig. 4.10 Pressure pot

Courtesy of SNF-Forsestadent®

Bench lathe

The bench lathe is used for reducing large areas of acrylic. It can have a manual chuck that must be stopped to change the bur, or an automatic chuck with a clutch called a quick chuck.

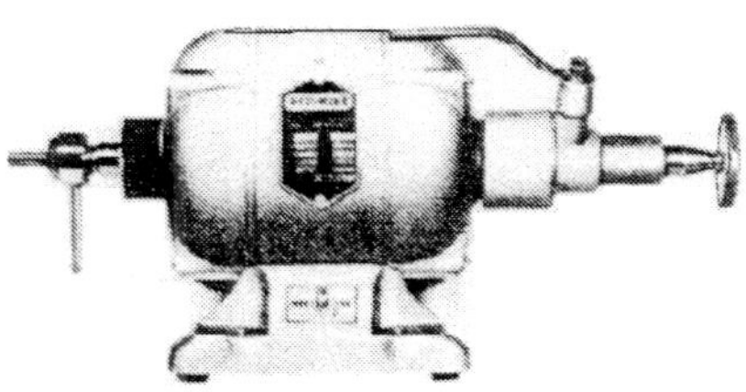

Fig. 4.11 Bench lathe with Quick Chuck

Courtesy of Cental Dental®

Handpiece

There are many different models of handpieces available. They are used for precision trimming and polishing of small items.

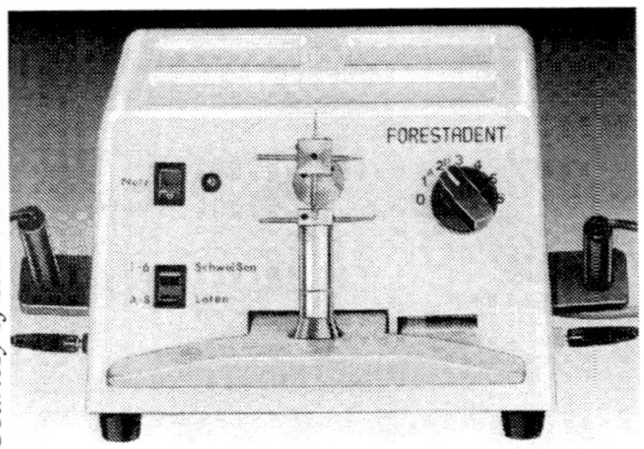

Courtesy of SNF-Forsestadent®

Fig. 4.12 Spot welder

Spot welder

The spot welder is an indispensable piece of equipment in an ortho lab. It is used to attach accessories to bands, or to tack weld wires to hold them is place for soldering.

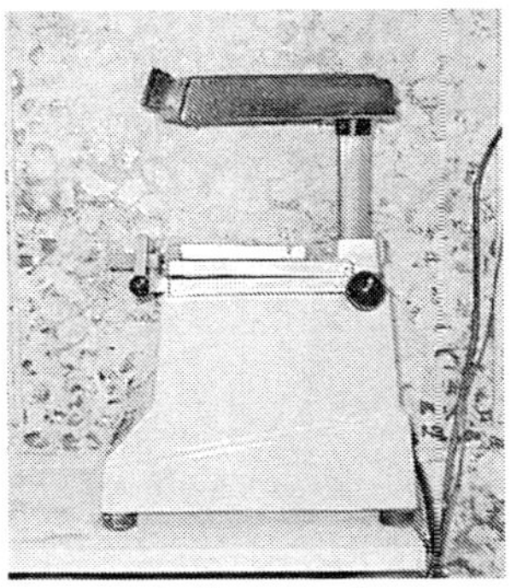

Fig. 4.13 Vacuum former

Vacuum former

The vacuum former is used to form thermoplastic materials about a model. Air is removed from between the model and the hot material, and then air pressure forms the material. This can be used with a variety of appliances from mouthguards to nightguards to retainers. Some similar devices work by injecting compressed air on the side of the material opposite the model, forming it to the model. This type is more accurate, but also much more expensive.

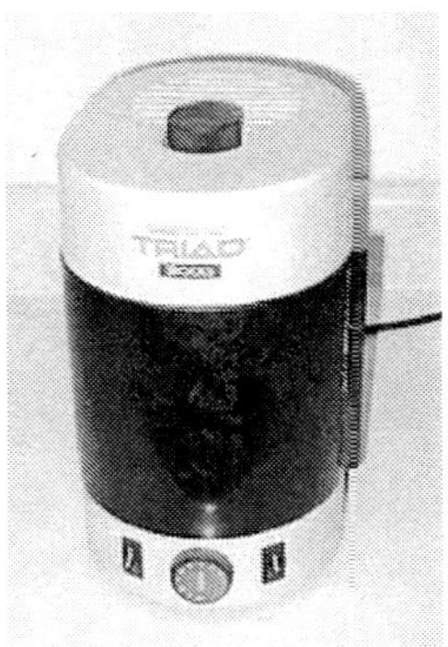

Fig. 4.14 Light cure oven

Light cure oven

Light or photo cure materials are cured by exposure to bright or ultraviolet light. This material can be used for custom impression trays, retainers, or block out for bleaching trays.

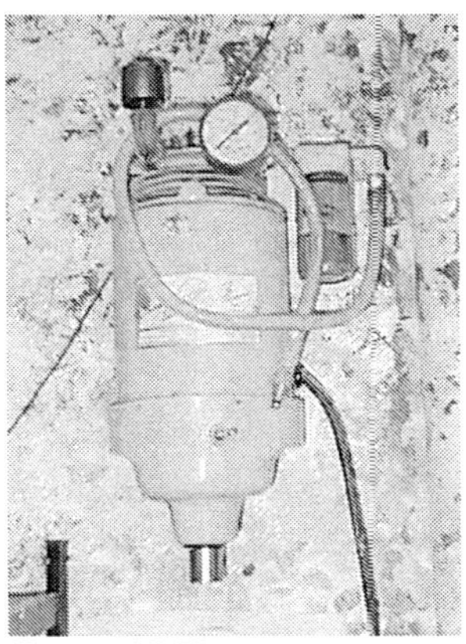

Fig. 4.15 Vacuum spatulator

Vacuum spatulator

The vacuum spatulator mixes gypsum materials under vacuum. This increases the density of the stone — making it stronger — while eliminating voids in the model.

"When the only tool you have is a hammer, you tend to treat everything as if it were a nail."
Abraham Maslow

"One only needs two tools in life: WD-40 to make things go, and duct tape to make them stop."
G. Weilacher

5 Basic appliances and fabrication techniques

"Only those who have the patience to do simple things perfectly ever acquire the skill to do difficult things easily"
Author Unknown

"In theory, there is no difference between theory and practice; In practice, there is."
Chuck Reid

There are many different types of removable appliances used in orthodontics. Some appliances are designed to accomplish one specific objective, while others have the flexibility to be used in a number of situations. The same appliance can be known by different names in different parts of the country, different cities, even in different offices on the same street.

All appliances have certain basic requirements that they must meet. In broad terms, any oral prosthetic must meet these conditions. In order of importance for orthodontic appliances, they should be:

- functional,
- comfortable,
- aesthetic.

An orthodontic appliance must be functional; this means that it must be capable of efficiently performing the task for which it was designed. An appliance that cannot perform its function is worthless.

An appliance should be as comfortable as possible for the patient to wear. This requirement is subservient to the function of the appliance. In other words, a comfortable appliance that is not functional is useless, but we do our best to make a functional appliance comfortable. The appliance will not work if the patient doesn't wear it because it is uncomfortable. Unfortunately, this is not a goal which can always be met. Some designs will be uncomfortable no matter what, and with these the patient's commitment to the treatment is important for success.

As much as is possible, we make the appliance aesthetically pleasing and unobtrusive in the patient's mouth. Again, this is less important than the proceeding requirements. Some appliances, such as headgear, will always be large, uncomfortable and ugly; but they work. That is the overriding concern.

Classifications

Orthodontic appliances can be classified in a number of different ways. When we look at how appliances are used in the mouth, we can break them into:

- passive,
- active,
- functional (myofunctional).

When we use the criteria of how the appliance is held (retained) in the mouth, we can divide them into:

- removable,
- fixed.

Classification by appliance usage

Passive

A passive appliance is one that does not exert force when in the mouth. The purpose of such an appliance is to maintain the mouth in the state that exists at the time of the appliance's fabrication. Simply, it is to hold the teeth in place, inhibiting any movement (revision from - and make sure that they don't move).

Active

Active appliances are designed to accomplish certain movements by the placement of forces upon the teeth. The forces are exerted by discreet components on the appliances and can act on single teeth or groups of teeth. The forces exerted by active appliances are generated within the appliances and exerted upon the specific oral structures to be corrected.

Functional

Functional appliances use the muscles of mastication and the oral cavity to create conditions which will encourage the growth or change of the oro-facial complex. These appliances generally do not exert a force themselves, i.e. they do not use a spring or screw to push on anything, instead they use the positioning and stretching of the muscles to produce the forces that are required. The changes that then occur are not so much the movement of teeth, but changes to the supporting structures. Functional appliances are also referred to as orthopedic appliances.

My definition of a functional appliance is "an appliance which effects changes to the oro-facial complex through the redirection or elimination of the affects of muscle forces on the TMJ, alveolar ridges and the teeth."

Classification by insertion

Removable

A removable appliance is just that, it is removable from the mouth, by the patient, at any time. What holds the appliance in the mouth when it is in function are clasps or another disengagable retentive mechanism (i.e. suction or acrylic engaging undercuts).

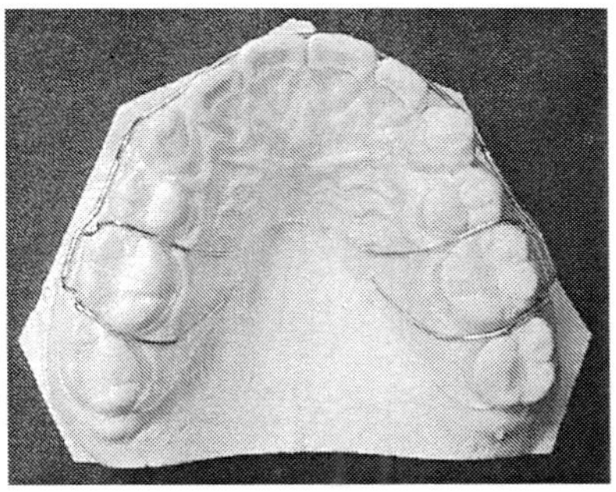

Fig. 5.1 Removable appliance - hawley retainer

Fixed

Fixed appliances are those which cannot be removed, after insertion, without damaging or destroying the appliance. There are several methods of retention that may be used with these types of appliances. The type of fixed appliances that are most commonly fabricated in the dental laboratory use stainless steel bands as the method of retention. Stainless steel bands are small rings of stainless steel which are adapted to fit tightly around a tooth, and then held into the mouth with cement. Components are then soldered to the bands to provide the functionality

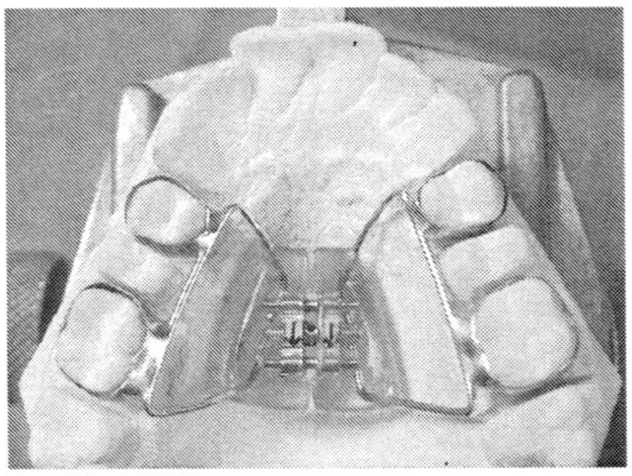

Fig. 5.2 Fixed appliance - Rapid Palatal Expander

of the appliance (arches, springs, brackets, etc.). Some other types of fixed appliances are those which use a small mesh retentive pad (brackets) or a similar bonding point for direct bonding to the tooth, and those in which an acrylic pad is bonded over large areas of the teeth.

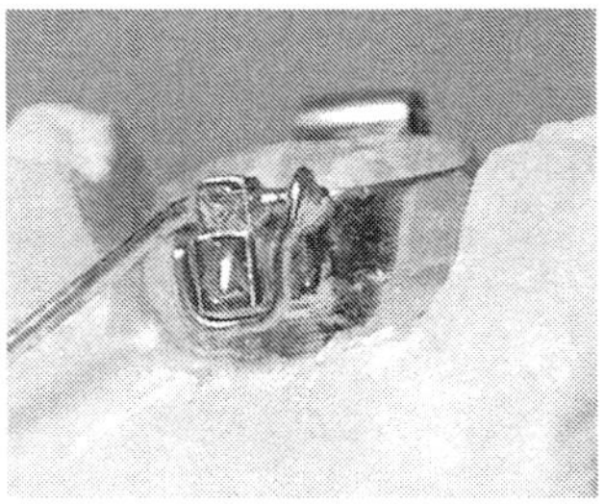

Fig. 5.3 Fixed/ Removable attachment

A subset of the fixed appliances are the fixed/removable. These are appliances which rely on cemented bands for retention, but include an attachment, which allows the body of the appliance to be removed from the mouth without damage. This allows easier and more accurate adjustment of the appliance outside the mouth.

Anatomy of an ortho appliance

Most appliances are just a collection of components arranged together to perform specific functions. The basic functions that these components can perform are:

- retention,
- force application,
- tooth control,
- stabilizing body and anchorage.

Retention is the name that we give to the method of attachment of the appliance in the mouth. As we have already noted, appliances can be fixed into the mouth or removable. A fixed appliance uses bonding or cement to attach the appliance to the teeth. A removable appliance uses clasps to create retention.

The force application aspect of an active appliance is that part of the appliance which moves the teeth. This may be a spring, elastic,

Retention?

What is retention?

Retention is the generic term that we use to identify what holds an appliance — or denture, or partial — in the mouth. It is the mechanism through which the appliance resists the dislodging forces that act upon it. Dislodging forces can be anything from the active forces exerted by a spring or screw to the piece of gum that the patient is chewing.

So how does retention work?

We can gain retention in a number of ways. When we talk about retention in a full denture, that retentive force is gained by the close fit of the denture base to the tissue and the suction that is created by the capillary action of the saliva that is in a thin layer between them. This suction retention can be very powerful, it is similar to what happens when you put a drop of water between two glass microscope slides, but it only works when you have a thin even layer of water. That is why it is so important that a denture base fit the patient exactly, there is little adjustment and no polishing done to the tissue side of a denture.

An ortho appliance or partial denture acts differently. These have no suction seal. In order to have a suction seal you must have that continuous close fitting border, which neither a partial or ortho appliance have.

Remember the rubber stick'em darts that you had as a kid? They would adhere so tightly to the window that if you tried to pull it off by the stick, the stick would pop off. But if you slid your fingernail under the edge of the rubber suction cup, you broke the seal and the dart would fall right off. Partials and

Continued . . .

retention continued

ortho appliances are simply missing that seal, even though some people will tell you it is there.

Then what keeps them in the mouth?

They rely on mechanical retention that is created by placing part of the appliance in an undercut.

What is an undercut?

An undercut in that portion of the tooth that is cervical to the greatest circumference of the clinical crown of the tooth.

If you've ever walked along a meandering stream, you've probably seen an undercut. The outside bank of the stream has an overhang where the water has carried away the earth but left the grass above it. This is an undercut bank.

I like to use a basketball to explain how we use an undercut to retain an appliance in the mouth.

Put a basketball on the table with the centreline horizontal. The centreline is now the widest part of the ball, everything above curves in to the top and everything below curves in to the bottom.

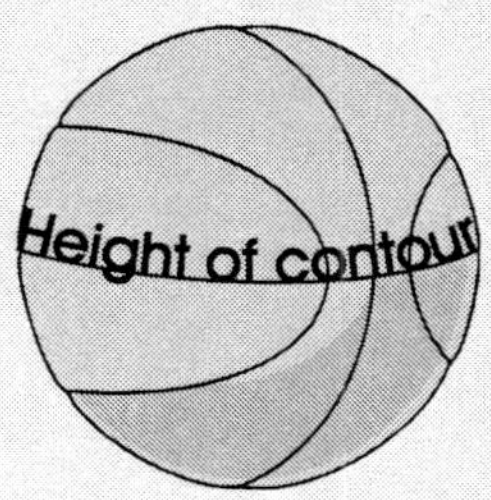

This is your "greatest circumference", also called the height of contour or survey line.

To lift the ball off the table we could place two sticks under this line and lift. Its important to note that we need two sticks, with only one the ball would just roll away. The second stick steadies it, or provides a reciprocating force (reciprocation).

To make the basketball act like

Continued . . .

an expansion screw or anything used to place a force on the teeth. No matter how fancy the component is, there are only two ways that we can direct a force in order to move a tooth. We can either push a tooth, or pull it. Simple as that, it is just the application of this simple force that can be complex.

Some components serve the function of acting to control the position or movement of the teeth. The most common example of this is the Hawley arch. When used in a retainer, it holds the teeth in position to stabilize them. When used in conjunction with an active component, a spring pushing from the lingual of a tooth, it acts to limit or control the amount of movement that the spring can perform.

What I call the "body" of an appliance is what holds all the disparate components together. In an acrylic removable appliance this would be the acrylic plate. In a fixed lingual arch, this would be the arch wire. As well as serving as the base to which all other components are attached, the body of an appliance can act as anchorage and retention.

Removable orthodontic appliance fabrication

The basic Hawley retainer

Dr. C.A. Hawley introduced his retainer design in 1919. Since then it has become the standard for orthodontic designs. A great number of removable appliance designs are derived from the Hawley retainer, both upper and lower. The basic Hawley retainer has two Adams clasps on the 6's, a Hawley arch from canine to canine, and an acrylic plate.

This design can be modified to accomplish an infinite number of objectives. The fabrication of the Hawley retainer also involves most of the skills used for any removable appliance and is, therefore, a good starting point for anyone learning laboratory techniques.

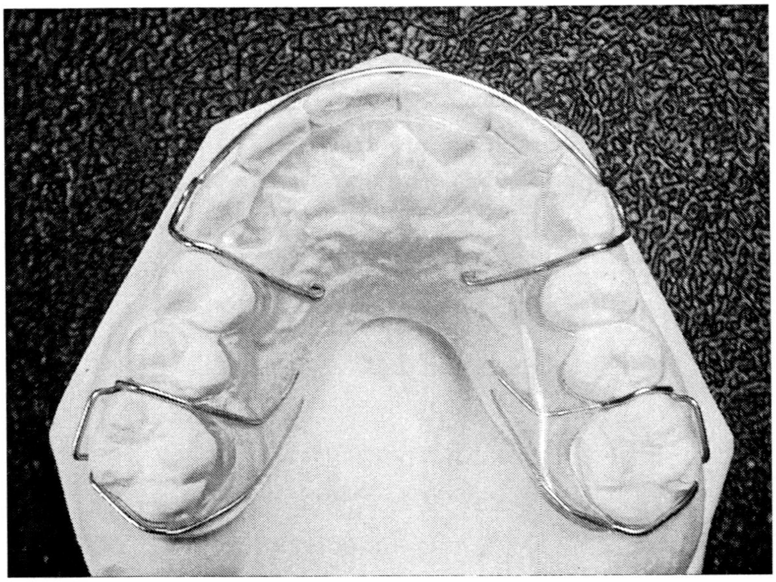

Fig. 5.4 Basic Hawley retainer

As a retainer, the Hawley is used in the final phase of orthodontic treatment to help stabilize the teeth in their corrected positions. It acts as a passive appliance — not exerting a force — it constrains the teeth from being able to move back to their original positions (relapse). A fairly standard prescription for wearing a Hawley is six months to one year of full time wear, and then another year of night time wear. The patient's instructions will depend upon the dentist's preferences.

In this age of adult orthodontics, retention times are getting longer, as it takes longer for bone to stabilize in an older patient.

The basic Adams clasp

The first step in making a Hawley retainer is to bend the Adams clasps.

The Adams clasp is the most commonly used clasp for orthodontic appliances. It is usu-

retention continued

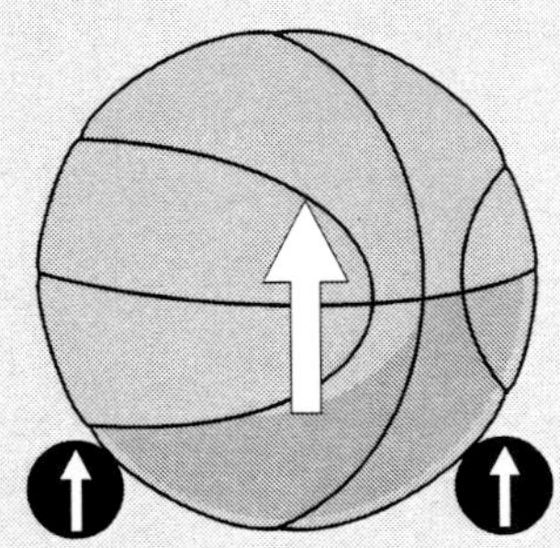

a tooth, we would have to nail it to the table. The sticks in the undercut would now act to hold whatever they were attached to the table, against any force that tried to lift it. This is the way that a trailer hitch works.

The mechanism that the sticks represent is a clasp, and the difference of this model to a clasp, is that the clasp is designed to allow the appliance to be taken in and out of the mouth, yet provide sufficient retention to keep it in the mouth when it's supposed to be there.

The secret to this is the flexibility that is built into our clasp arms. They have the ability to flex over the widest part of the tooth and spring back to settle against the tooth in the undercut. When a force then tries to dislodge the appliance the clasp is pulled occlusally, where it is forced to bend as it stretches over the height of contour of the tooth. As long as the force dislodging the appliance is less than the force needed to stretch the clasp, the appliance will stay in the mouth. Adding additional clasps

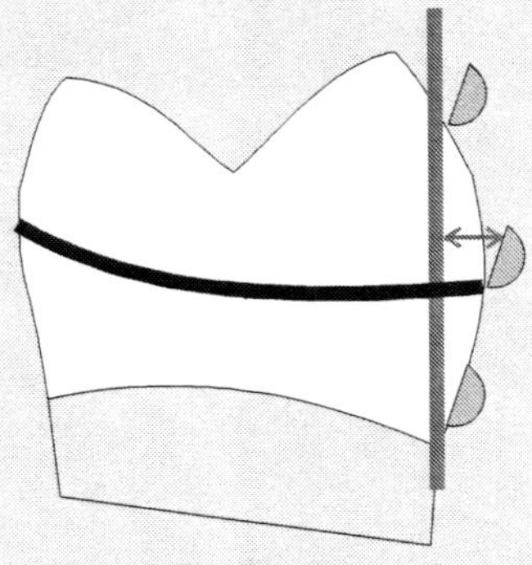

increases the retention of an appliance.

A properly designed and constructed clasp is always passive — meaning it exerts no force on the tooth — except when the appliance is being dislodged.

A clasp must always have two "arms", whether they are wire or the acrylic body of the appliance to the lingual of the tooth. Only one of the arms is in the undercut. This is called the retentive arm. The other arm is kept above the height of contour and is called the reciprocal arm. Its purpose is to steady

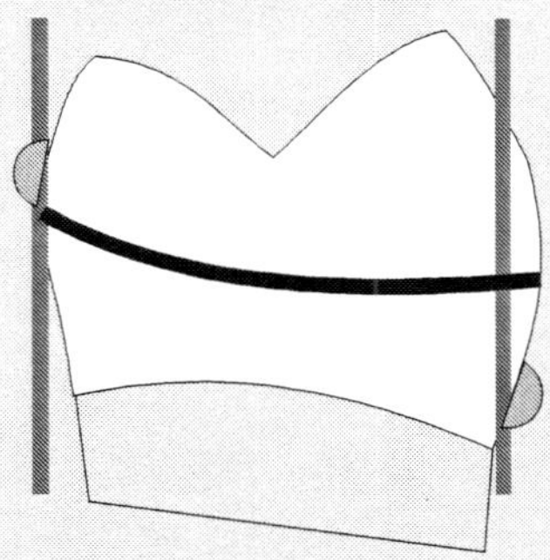

the tooth against the lingualizing pressure of the clasp when it engages the undercut to resist dislodgement. A clasp that does not have reciprocation is really a spring.

ally placed on the first permanent molars, however, it can also be used on the other molars (both maxillary and mandibular), the bicuspids, primary molars, and even on the centrals. The bicuspids are the second most common positioning for these clasps.

There are several reasons for its popularity.

First, the Adams clasp is extremely retentive, which allows it to offset the dislodging forces of active orthodontic components in an appliance. It engages undercuts on the mesio-buccal and disto-buccal line angles of the teeth it clasps. Because the Adams is a continuous clasp encircling the tooth, the wire segments from acrylic attachment point to undercut is quite short. This stiffens the clasp and dictates that a larger force is needed to unseat the clasp.

The Adams is also a sub-gingival clasp. The design of the Adams is such that the retentive elements of the clasp can engage an undercut on a tooth which is not fully erupted. A significant number of orthodontic patient's are young and have teeth (at the time of treatment) with little or no undercuts. The ability of the Adams to go beneath the gingiva to engage an undercut without damaging the tissue is very useful.

The Adams clasp presents us with a design that can be adapted to a variety of functions. It is easy to modify an Adams by attaching other components to the buccal bar, such as auxiliary clasps, springs or arches. This gives us great flexibility in designing an appliance incorporating Adams clasps.

Anatomy of the Adams clasp

The parts of an Adams clasp are:

- the retentive eyelets or arrowheads
- the buccal bar or bridge
- the mesial and distal arms
- the retentive tags.

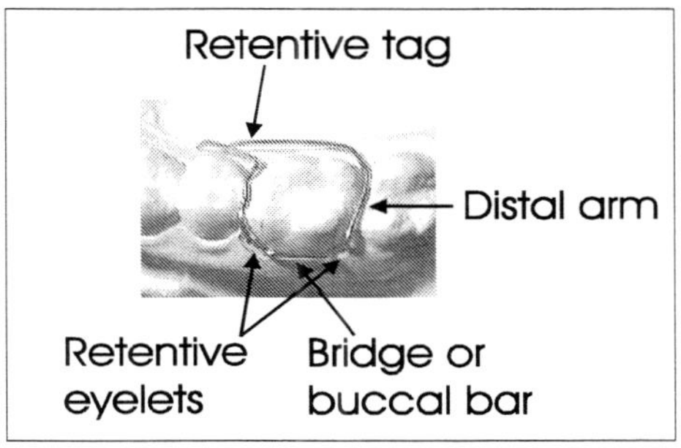

Fig 5.5 Anatomy of an Adams

Bending the Adams clasp

To begin bending an Adams clasp we must make the subgingival preparations that will provide access to the retentive area used by the clasp.

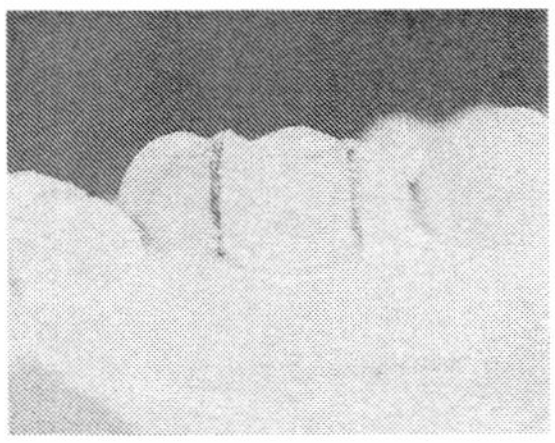

Fig. 5.6 Lines drawn from cusp tips

Lines are drawn from the cusp tips to the gingiva, parallel to the long axis of the tooth. The undercuts that we will utilize are located to the mesial of the mesial line and distal to the distal line. Each preparation will extend from the line approximately 3 mm along the gingival margin.

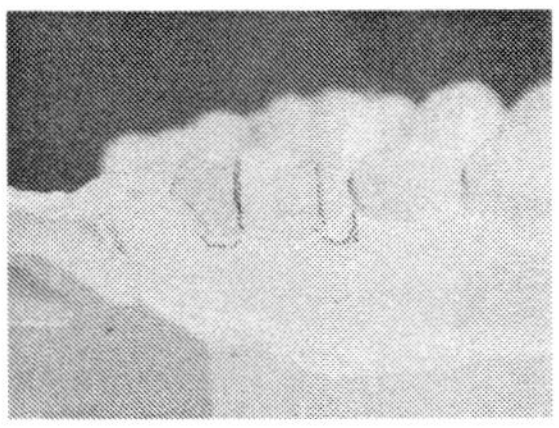

Fig. 5.7 Clasp preparations

The preparations should be made with an instrument that does not have an exceedingly pointed tip (e.g. a scalpel). A pointed tip will produce a square preparation which makes it difficult to seat the clasp in with repeatable accuracy. An instrument with a more rounded blade (e.g. a #7 wax spatula) will produce a rounded preparation which allows easy seating of the clasp. The preparation should have a depth of 1-1.5 mm at its deepest point, where the retentive eyelets will be. The mesial and distal of the preparation should then taper smoothly toward the gingival margin from this point. A large square preparation is not necessary.

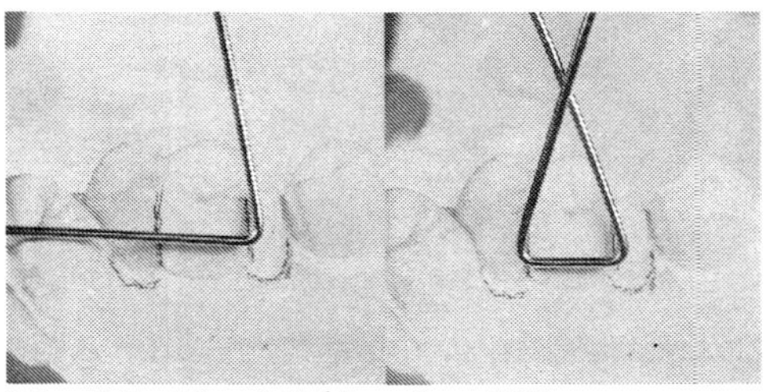

Fig. 5.8 1st and 2nd bends ≈ 70°

Start bending with a piece of 0.7 mm wire 5-8 cm long. The first bend is made approximately 5 mm from the center of the wire. This bend will form an angle of approximately 70°.

The second bend is made 0.5 mm past the line on the opposite side of the tooth from the first bend. It is also made to a 70° angle. The wire should now have a triangular shape.

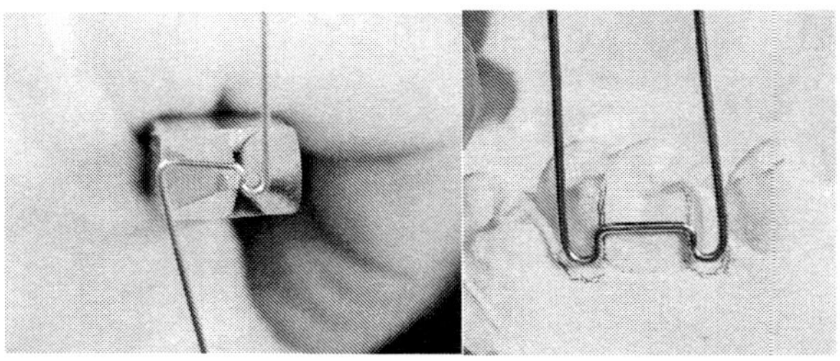

Fig. 5.9 Forming retentive eyelets

Grasp the wire with the square jaw of your 139 pliers on the inside of the angle and the tip of the round jaw on the outside, then bend the wire 180° around the round jaw. This small loop can be called the arrowhead or eyelet of the clasp. Repeat on the other side of the wire. These eyelets are the retentive elements of your clasp. They are the only portion of the Adams clasp which should contact the buccal surface of the tooth.

Grasp each eyelet in your pliers so that the jaws of the pliers hold both sides of the eyelet. Bend each eyelet to form a 45° angle with the bridge (or bar) of the clasp. The two eyelets should then form an angle of almost 90° between themselves.

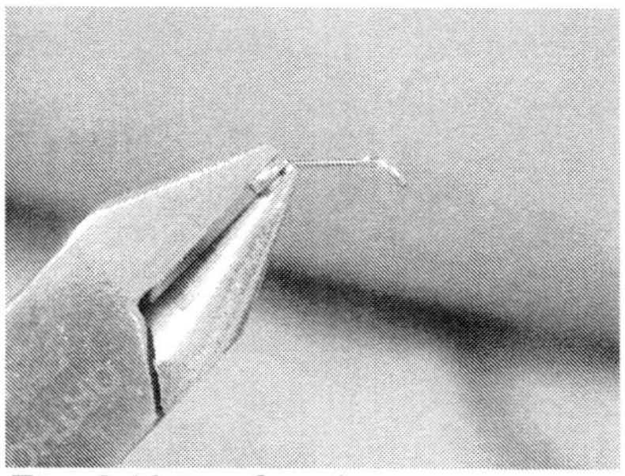

Fig. 5.10 Bend eyelets 45° to bar

The rough clasp is now ready to test fit against the tooth. Place the eyelets into your preparations and hold the tag ends of your wire so that the eyelets form a 45° angle with the buccal surface of the tooth. The buccal bar of the clasp should be 1 mm from the buccal surface of the tooth. The eyelets are now adjusted until they are flush against the tooth at the point of contact — at the bottom of the loop in the center of your preparation. This positioning of the eyelets is important because it is what allows the clasp to engage undercuts subgingivally without displacing the tissue in an exceedingly damaging manner. When the eyelets are adjusted properly they slide between the tooth and the tissue easily.

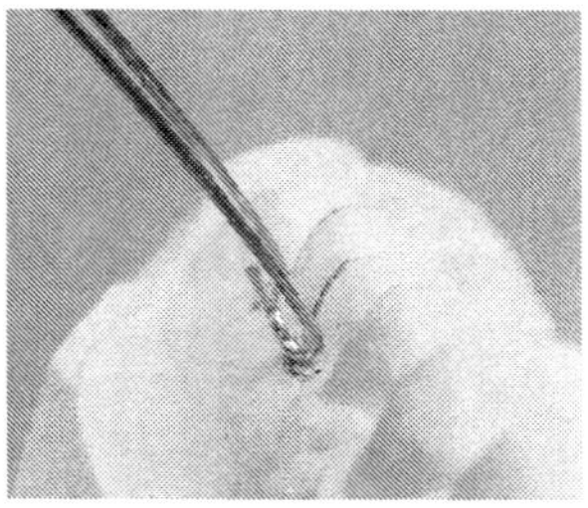

Fig. 5.11 Eyelets 45° to the bucccal surface

The method that I have just described for making the eyelets is different than the one originally described by Adams. In his method, the pliers used to form the eyelets are the square jawed Adams pliers with the 1 mm square tips. This method works well, however, I find that most people prefer to use the 139 plier method to obtain consistently sized eyelets.

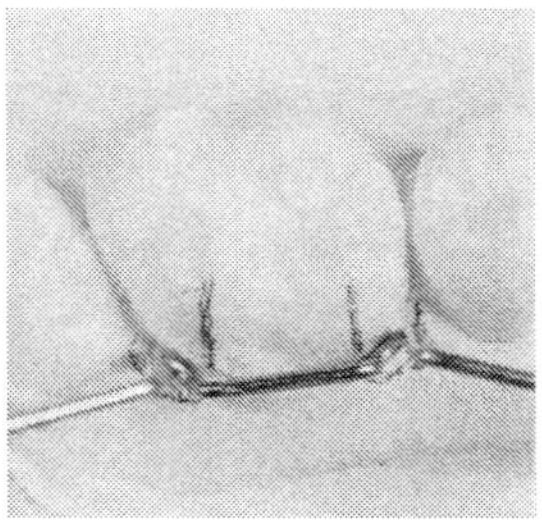

Fig. 5.12 Eyelets closely fitting tooth in preparations

Place the round beak of the 139 inside the now bent eyelet, with the square jaw to the outside of the wire. Bend the wire 90° over the square jaw. The two sides of the eyelet should be the same height. Repeat this on the other eyelet. You have now completed the buccal portion of the Adams clasp.

The remaining unbent wire will now form the mesial and distal arms, and retentive tags for your clasp.

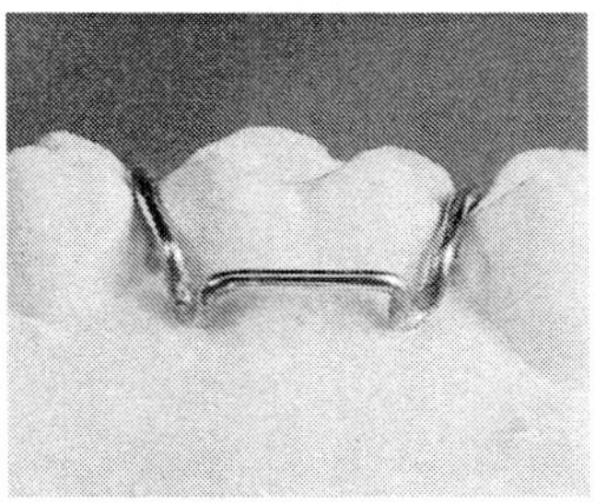

Fig. 5.13 Completed eyelets

Work with only one arm of the clasp at a time. Trying to work on both sides at once will generally lead to a clasp which does not quite fit properly. I always find it easier to start with the mesial arm. Adjust the mesial arm so that it goes straight from the mesial eyelet to the mesial embrasure. The wire should lay passively in the embrasure when both eyelets are seated in their preparations. Mark the wire at the

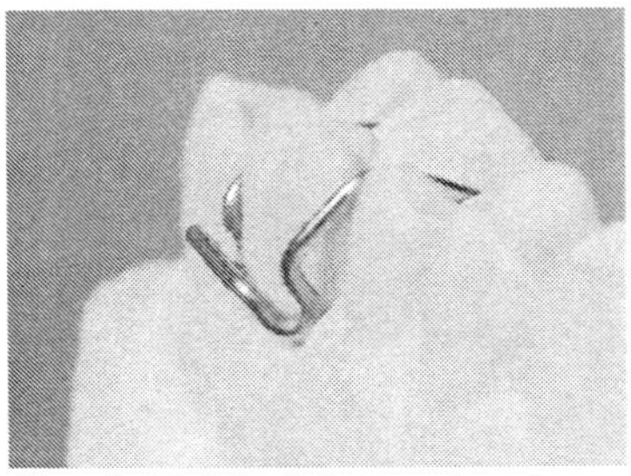

Fig. 5.14 *Mesial arm closely adapted through embrasure*

point at which it passes over the embrasure and bend it down until it lays in the occlusal embrasure. Adapt the wire tightly through the embrasure. The wire must be well adapted in this region to ensure that there are no functional interferences created.

Where the wire passes from the occlusal embrasure to the lingual embrasure, it is bent down into the lingual embrasure and adapted to conform with the palate. 1 mm of relief is left between the wire and the palatal tissues. This ensures that the wire will be completely surrounded by the acrylic, creating strong retention of the clasp to the appliance.

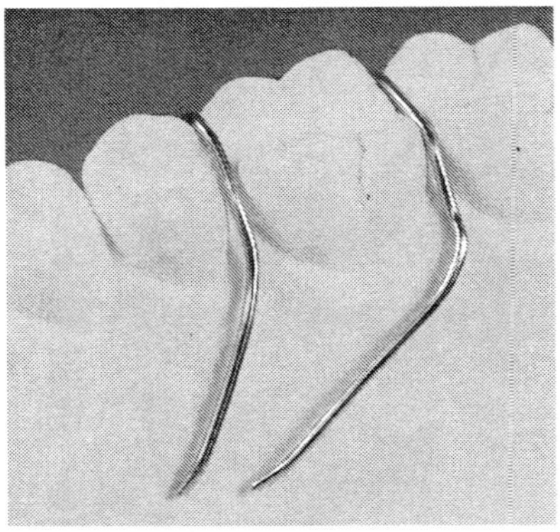

Fig. 5.15 *Retentive arms bisect the lingual embrasures*

The wire should bisect the lingual embrasure, not being placed too close to either of the lingual tooth surfaces that it passes between. I always prefer to bend tags in the posterior region with a slight curve to the anterior. I find that this produces an aesthetically pleasing clasp and appliance, as well as keeping the tags of my wires out of any area where I might need to reduce the acrylic.

The tag is finished off with a "retentive tag". This helps to ensure that the clasp stays embedded in the acrylic without moving. On a two arm clasp, such as an Adams, the design of the retentive tag used is not of paramount importance. The tags must remain 1 mm off of the palatal tissue to ensure that they are completely encased in acrylic. The double arms ensure that the wire will stay stable and well attached. This point is much more important on single arm clasps, such as the ball or circumferential clasp.

The common designs used for retentive tags are:

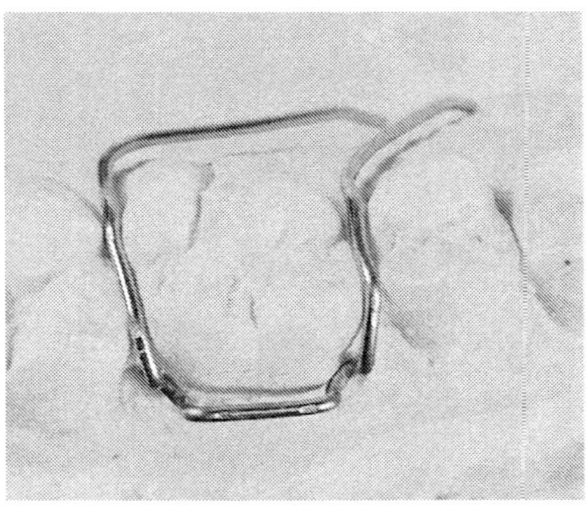

Fig. 5.16 *1 mm of relief between retentive tags and tissue*

• Curly Q - the end of the wire is bent into a closed end loop;

• Zig-Zag - a number of 90° bends are made in the end of the wire, generally 4 or 5;

• 90° tag - a 90° bend is made parallel to the palatal tissue;

• Dog leg - the terminal 1-2 mm of wire are bent down until to contact and rest lightly on the palatal tissue. This dog leg will act as a spacer holding the tags of the clasp off of the tissue during the sprinkling of the acrylic. It also acts as the third leg of a triangle to stabilize the clasp while you bend the distal arm. The tip of the wire that rests on the tissue will be completely surrounded by acrylic during sprinkling. This is my preferred tag for the adams clasp.

The mesial arm of the clasp is now completed; repeat these steps on the distal arm.

When your clasp is completed, I suggest that you immediately attach it to the model by placing a drop of wax on one or both of the eyelets. There is nothing more frustrating than losing a finished wire, and for some designs you must stabilize the clasp so that you can bend auxiliary components that will be attached to it.

The basic Hawley arch

The Hawley arch is the second component in the Hawley retainer. It is the wire that you see running across a person's smile when they are wearing a retainer.

The Hawley arch is a common feature in many appliance designs. As with the Adams clasp, one reason for this is the versatility of the arch.

The function of the Hawley on a retainer is to control the teeth, to make sure that there is no unwanted movement after the end of treatment. The retainer can do this because the teeth are held between the arch wire passing across their buccal surface and the acrylic plate that is closely adapted to their lingual surface. They have nowhere to move.

A second function of the Hawley becomes apparent when it is used in conjunction with an active component which is pushing on the lingual of a tooth. The tooth will continue to move as long as there is sufficient force from the lingual component unless there is an obstacle to the buccal to restrain it. The Hawley arch can provide this control stop. The arch is bent to pass on the buccal of the tooth in the position where the buccal of the tooth should come to rest. The tooth, when it hits the wire, can advance no further.

Another common use of the Hawley arch is as an attachment for components which place a lingualizing force on the facial surface of a tooth. Springs can be soldered to a Hawley arch which can be used to move a tooth to the lingual. The arch itself may be used to lingualize the anteriors by slightly tightening the Wilson loops.

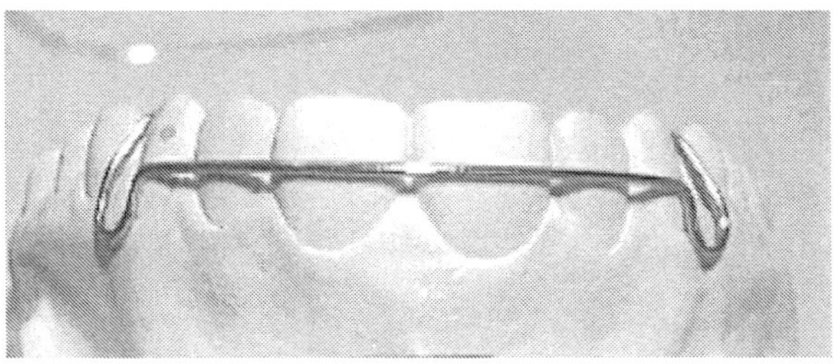

Fig. 5.17 Hawley arch - labial view

The basic Hawley is bent to run from the distal of the 3 to the distal of the 3 (cuspid to cuspid), where it then passes through the cuspid/1st bicuspid (cuspid-first bicuspid) embrasures to attach to the acrylic plate. The arch wire should lay across the widest point of the buccal surface of the teeth, just occlusal to the interdental papilla, where it can exert the greatest control over the teeth.

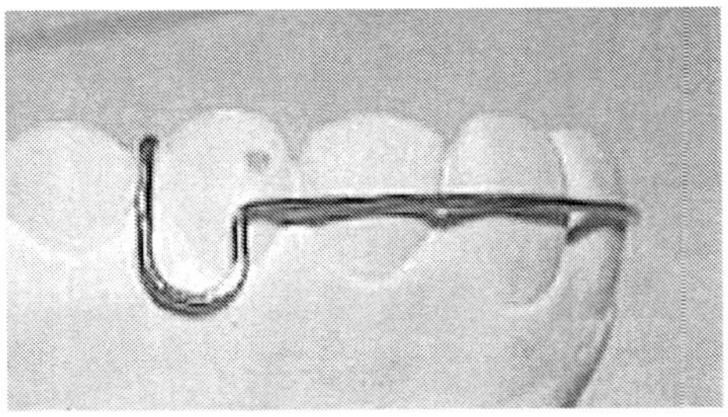

Fig. 5.18 Wilson loop

At the junction of the mesial and middle thirds of the cuspids, the wire bends 90° towards the gingival and then forms a 180° loop. This makes a semi-circle which comes back up to the occlusal and then passes through the cuspid/1st bicuspid embrasure. This loop is known as the Wilson loop. The Wilson loops give flexibility to the arch wire, as well as providing adjustment points for the arch.

Most arch wires bear a passing resemblance to the Hawley arch, and are bent in a similar manner. Other arch designs will be discussed later.

Bending the Hawley

The Hawley arch is fabricated with 0.8 or 0.9 mm hard wire. 0.8 wire is used when the arch is used as a retainer or as a lingualizing element. 0.9 wire is used when the arch will have components soldered to it.

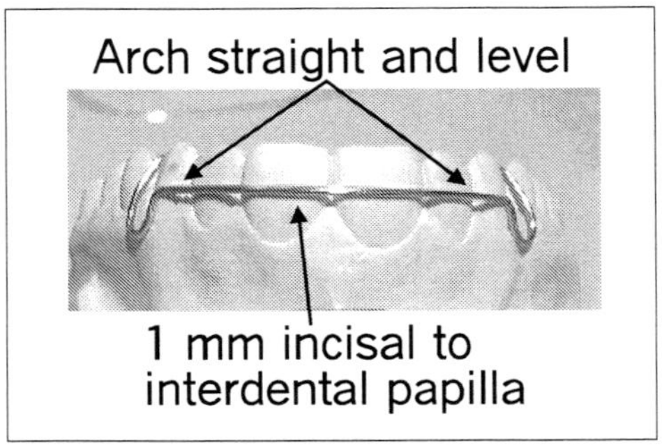

Fig. 5.19 Labial view

The labial section of the arch wire passes across the labial surface of the incisors at the widest portion of the teeth (just incisal to the interdental papilla). The wire must be straight and level with the incisal edges of the anterior teeth. It should have no wows or kinks in it when viewed from the labial. A labial arch should form a smooth arc — as symmetrical as possible while conforming to the curve of the labial surfaces of the teeth.

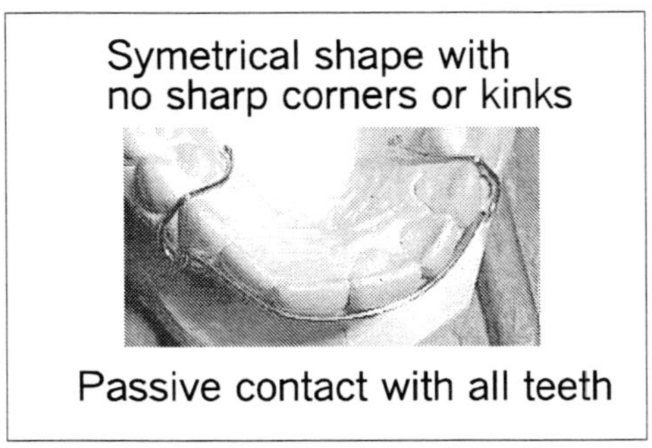

Fig. 5.20 Incisal view

The wire rests in passive contact with the labial surface of all incisor teeth. This means that it touches the labial surface of each tooth, but places no pressure on the tooth. This is one of the most difficult skills to master when learning to bend any arch wire. It is important because a wire that is off of the teeth has no control of them. Conversely, a wire that is too tight to the labial surfaces becomes a spring, dislodging the anterior of the appliance.

At the junction of the mesial and middle thirds of the cuspids, the wire contacts these teeth and then makes a 90° bend towards the gingiva. The wire passes down over the tissue for 6-8 mm and then describes a 180° bend with the distal arm of the loop parallel to the mesial arm. This loop is the width of the cuspid from the contact point to the distal embrasure between the cuspid/1st bicuspid — generally about 6 mm.

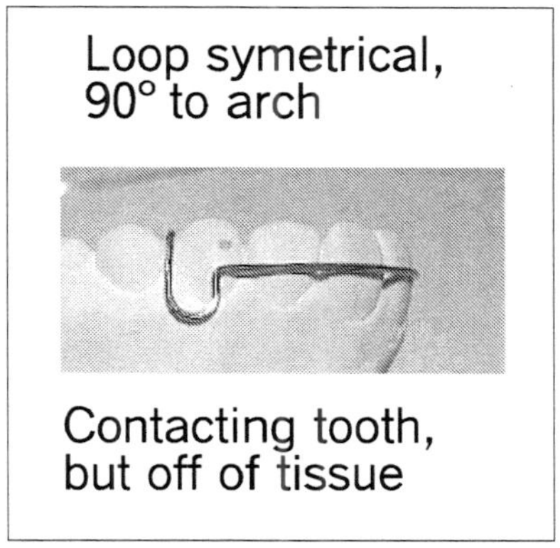

Fig. 5.21 Saggital view - Wilson loop

The loop is referred to as the Wilson loop. The Wilson loop passes over the tissue with 1 mm relief. There must be no tissue impingement (contact with the tissue).

A tip that can help you create this 1 mm of relief while you are learning to bend the Hawley, is to place two pieces of medical adhesive tape over the tissue in the cuspid region. It is usually easier to bend a wire to a surface than to bend it off of a surface. You can now bend the wire to conform to the tape. When the tape is removed your wire will have 1 mm of relief from the tissue.

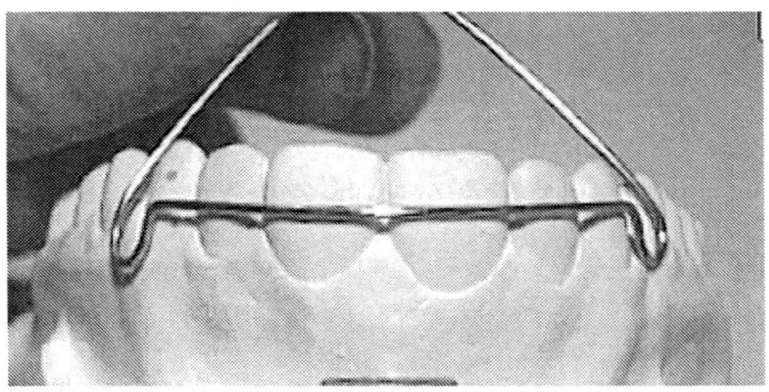

Fig. 5.22 Contour distal arm of Wilson loop to tissue

The distal arm of the Wilson loop continues to follow the contour of the tissue until it passes tightly through the embrasure between the cuspid/1st bicuspid. The wire must pass in tight contact with the occlusal of the teeth through this embrasure, in order that no functional interferences will be created.

The arms are then contoured to the palate, leaving a 1 mm relief for acrylic to encase the tag wires. I bend the tags of the Hawley arch slightly to the distal so that my tags end lingual to the 4's or 5's. This is because the palate in this region is usually relatively flat, making this a simple bend to finish. If the tag is bent to the anterior (lingual to the incisors), you will be bending your wire to fit a compound curve (curving in two directions at

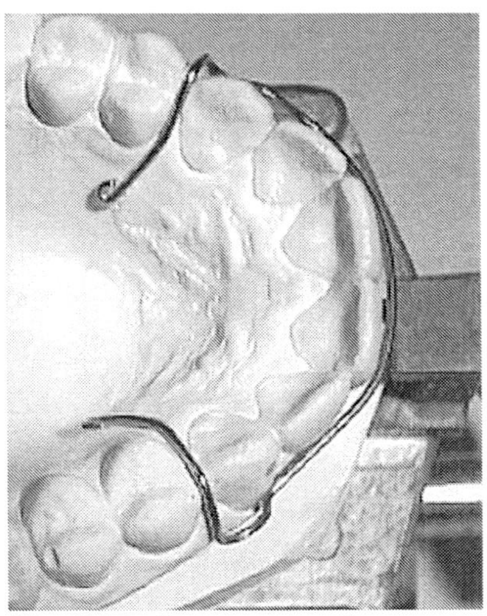

Fig. 5.23 Contour retentive tags to palate

once). This is a much more difficult bend to make.

The tags will now end in a retentive element similar to the ones described for the Adams. My preferred tag for the Hawley is the curly-q. There is no particular reason for this other than that is what I was taught.

Forming the arch from the center out

There are two basic methods that may be used to form the Hawley arch. You can either start in the middle of the wire and bend towards each end, or you can start at one end and bend to the opposite end.

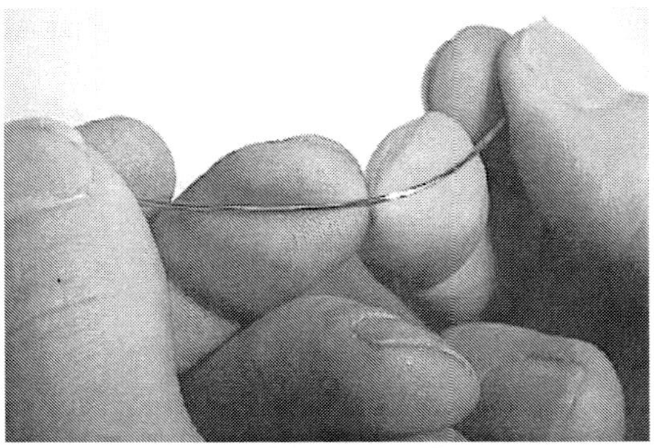

Fig. 5.24 Form arch shape with fingers

To start in the middle of the wire, first form a general arch shape with your fingers and adjust it until it matches the contour of the labial surfaces of the incisors and contacts the cuspids at the junction of the mesial and middle third.

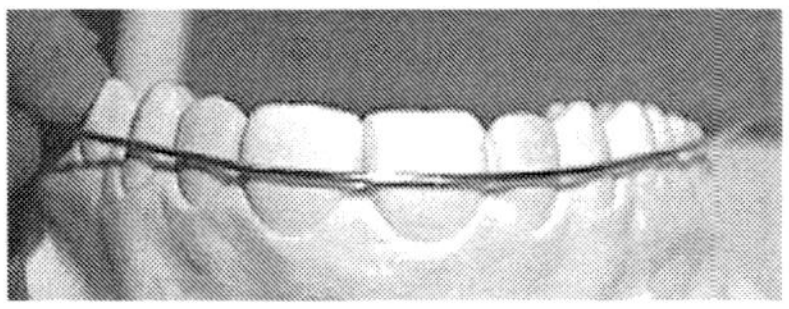

Fig. 5.25 Arch positioning

Mark the wire at these points on the cuspids, marking both sides at the same time. Grasp the wire in the pliers to make the 90° bend at these points.

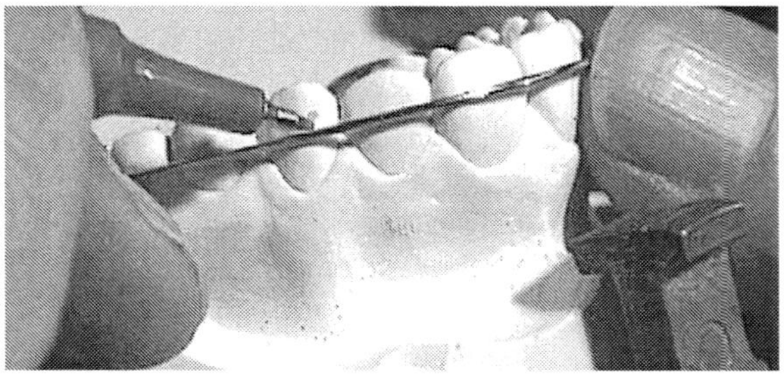

Fig. 5.26 Mark 90° bend for Wilson loops

In order to create the necessary relief for the wire over the tissue, place the wire in the pliers so that the arch is parallel to the jaws of the pliers. Now rotate the wire until the arch makes an angle of approximately 10° above the line of the jaws of the pliers. Bend the wire down 90°.

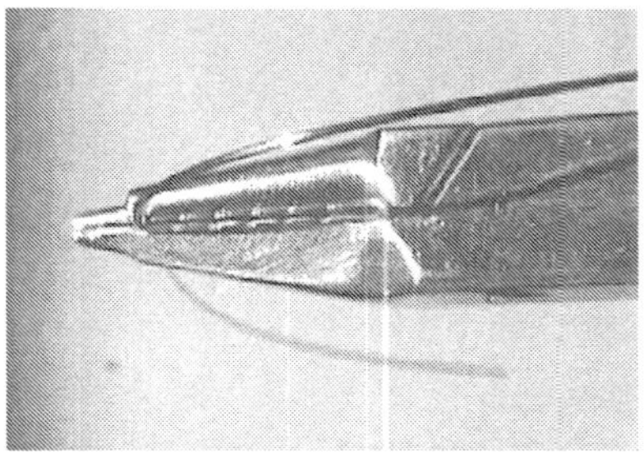

Fig. 5.27 Rotate wire 10° occlusally in pliers before bending.

At this point check that the wire is going in the right direction to form the necessary relief. Place the arch on the bench with the tag ends pointing up. The tag ends should be pointing slightly out from the vertical. It is easiest to see this close to the 90° bend. If the wire is not going slightly out, it is easy to adjust it at this time. Grasp the arch with the pliers hard up against the 90° bend and rotate the tags outward slightly. If you have flat jaw pliers use them for this task. Now check the arch on the table top again.

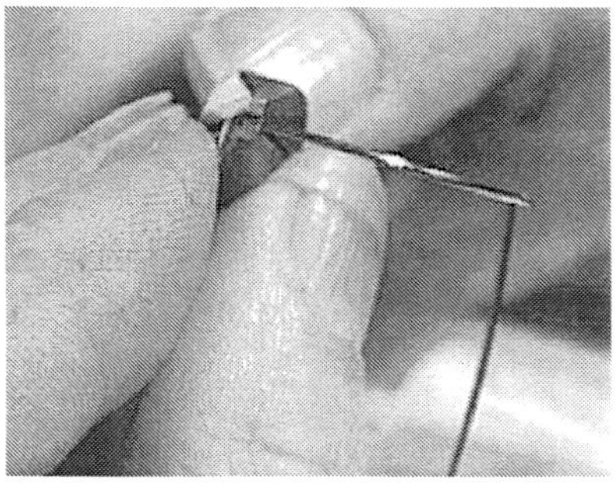

Fig. 5.28 Adjust loops outward if necessary, using large Adams pliers to hold the wire at the 90° angle and twist labially

Use a large section of the round beak on the 139 pliers to create the wide curve of the Wilson loop. Most cuspids are approximately the same width, so once you find the area on your pliers that creates the correct sized loop, you may wish to mark it. A simple fine felt tip marker can accomplish this without damage to your pliers. You can also cut a slight groove into the square jaw of your pliers at the proper size; just be sure never to groove the round beak. Labial bow pliers or three barrel style pliers come with grooves that let you create specific sizes of loops. If you are bending wire full time, I would recommend one of these pliers be in your toolkit.

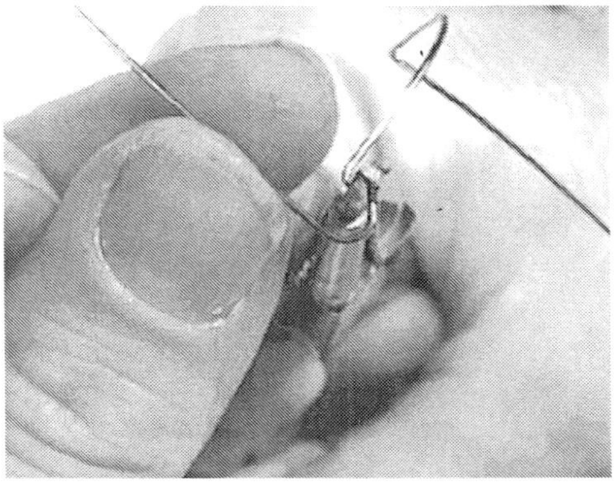

Fig. 5.29 Form the Wilson loops with a wide section of the round beak of the 139 pliers

To prevent tilting of the labial portion of the arch when contouring the wire over the embrasure, place the wire in its correct position on the teeth and then mark the level at which it is to be bent at both embrasures at the same time.

Finish the wire in the palate.

Forming the arch from one end

To begin the Hawley arch from one side, start by bending the large arc of the Wilson loop. Bend the 90° angle to the mesial of the Wilson loop, and contour the distal arm of the wire over the embrasure. With this as your staring point, contour the wire across the labial surfaces of the incisors in the same manner as already described, resting passively on the labial surfaces of the anteriors. Finish the arch with the other Wilson loop and retentive tag.

The basic acrylic plate

The acrylic plate forms the base of a removable appliance, the substructure to which everything else is attached. The acrylic plate is the connector, retention, anchorage, bite opener, and even active element, usually all at the same time. I refer to the acrylic plate as the "body" of the appliance. The basics of the PMMA acrylic that comprise the plate have been discussed previously, so we will now look at fabricating the plate for a simple Hawley retainer.

The processing of the acrylic is the last major step in fabricating any removable appliance. The models are first prepared, the wires are then bent and waxed into place on the models, any wax blockout or special preparations are made, and then the acrylic is processed, trimmed and polished.

Sprinkle method

The most common method of processing an orthodontic appliance is referred to as the sprinkling, or salt and pepper method. This involves dispensing the monomer (liquid) and polymer (powder) directly onto the working model and mixing them there. No premixing of the materials is done. This method has the advantage of saving time. There is no wax up, flasking, or boil out to perform. It is also accurate and an economical use of materials when done correctly. The sprinkle method shall be covered in detail later in this section.

Modelling technique

Another method used in orthodontics is the modelling technique, or dough method. This is similar to the method used when performing a cold cure repair on a denture. The monomer and polymer are mixed in a bowl and allowed to set to a doughy consistency. A small amount is removed in a fluid state and allowed to run under the wires on the model to ensure there are no voids under them. The dough is removed from the bowl when it no longer sticks to your hands. Placing a thin coating of Vaseline on your fingers will ease handling of the material. Too much Vaseline can interfere with the polymerization process.

The acrylic is then placed on the model and adapted to the desired shape and thickness. Excess acrylic may be removed with a knife, and the periphery trimmed to shape at the same time.

With the present questions and concerns being raised as to the health issues of working with PMMA, I find it difficult to recommend this method of acrylic application. If you do use the modelling technique to fabricate your acrylic plates, I strongly suggest that you wear gloves at all times when working with the acrylic.

Acrylic plates — general requirements

There are several basic requirements that the design of the acrylic plate must meet.

It should be obvious that the plate must be closely adapted to the palatal tissues, seating snugly without rocking.

The thickness of the plate should be uniform. 2-3 mm is an average thickness in most cases. In some circumstances — such as when covering a component such as an expansion screw — areas of the plate may need to be thicker.

Lingual and posterior borders

The best general outline for a maxillary plate is a *horseshoe palate*. This design provides good support, while providing improved patient comfort. The width of the acrylic in the posterior regions should be approximately 10-15 mm. The plate should extend to the lingual of the most distal tooth.

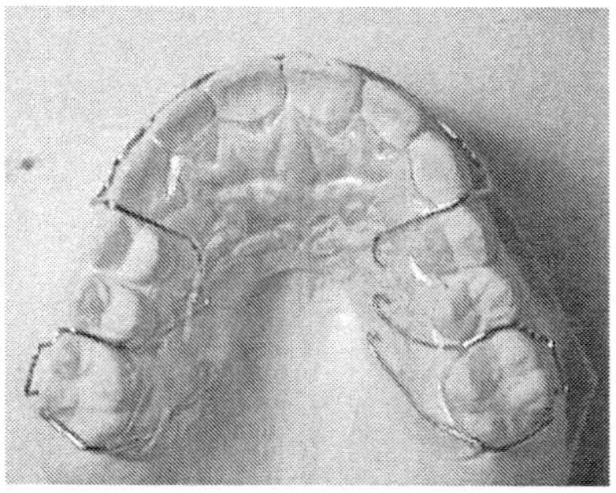

Fig 5.30 Horseshoe palate, see colour photo Page 5-29

It is not necessary in most appliances to cover the entire palate. In terms of construction details, a full palate uses more material, takes more time and is more difficult to trim and polish correctly. If expansion screws are to be added to an appliance the palatal region of the horseshoe must be filled in to prevent the screw from being positioned too far anteriorly.

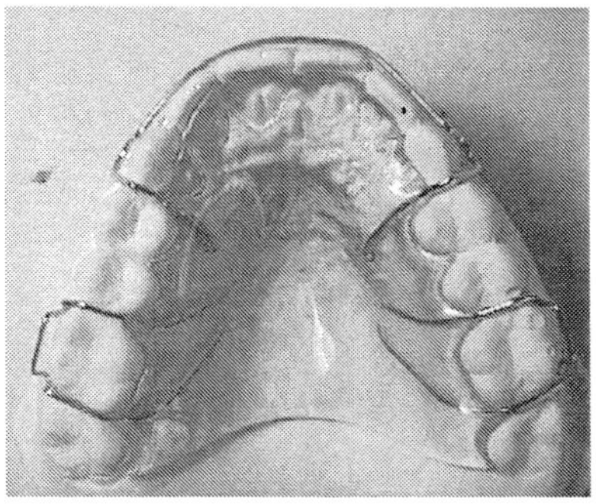

Fig. 5.31 Full palate, see colour photo Page 5-29

A mandibular plate extends 10-12 mm apically from the gingival margin, dependent on the depth of the lingual sulcus. Unlike a denture base, we do not wish to carry the acrylic all the way down into the sulcus, and, as will be discussed, we do not want to engage any undercuts that will make insertion difficult or painful for the patient.

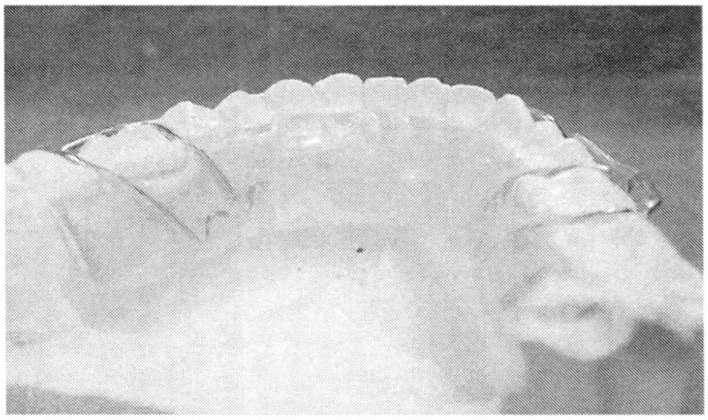

Fig. 5.32 Mandibular lingual border. Note that the acrylic does not extend into soft tissue undercuts and is free of the lingual frenum. See colour photo Page 5-29

The anterior portion of the mandibular plate must be designed as not to impinge upon the lingual frenum. This dictates in many cases an anterior height of only 5-7 mm, which makes the mandibular plate more flexible and more prone to breakage than the upper. This may necessitate some additional thickening of the plate in the anterior region for appliances with an exceptionally short anterior height

The borders of both the upper and lower should be smooth and rounded. Do not bevel or feather the borders down to a sharp knife edge.

Occlusal borders

The posterior occlusal design of a basic acrylic plate is the same for the mandible and maxilla.

In the posterior, the acrylic extends ½ -$^2/_3$'s of the height of the clinical crown, terminating occlusal to the height of contour. This is in the middle to occlusal third of the teeth. The least tooth coverage that can provide effective support for the appliance is generally the most comfortable for the patient. The border must be occlusal to the height of the contour to provide a degree of support and ensure close adaptation to the lingual of the teeth.

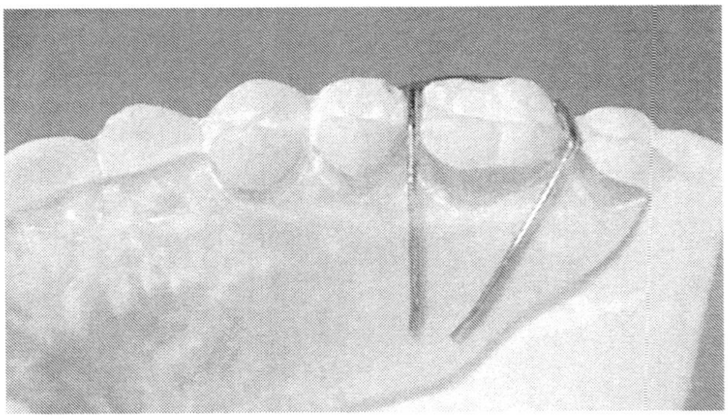

Fig. 5.33 Lingual occlusal acrylic borders. Note that the acrylic is scalloped in the posterior and flat in the anterior. See colour photo Page 5-29

The occlusal border should be slightly scalloped in the posterior, slightly higher in the interdental septa (to cover the interdental papilla) and slightly lower in the center of each posterior tooth. The acrylic septa should extend all the way into the interdental embrasure to provide continuous contact with the lingual surfaces of the posterior teeth. These acrylic septa are generally 1-2 mm in length and should be carefully trimmed to remove excessively sharp edges.

On an upper appliance, the occlusal border of the appliance must not interfere with the lingual cusps of the lower posteriors.

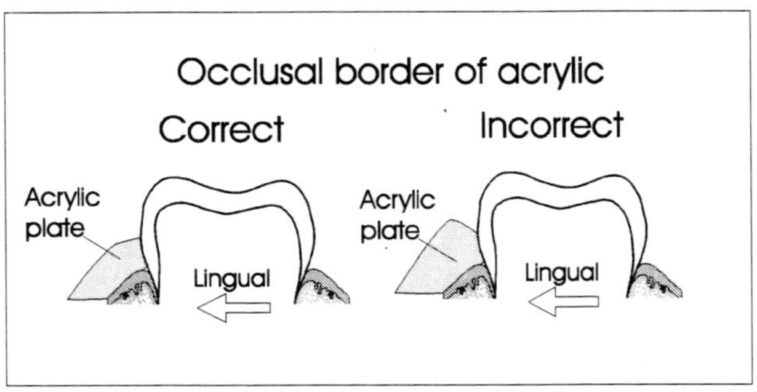

Fig. 5.34 Posterior occlusal border. Note that there should not be a "trench" formed by the acrylic at it's junction with the teeth.

The occlusal border of the acrylic should meet the lingual of the posteriors with a slight taper to the occlusal. Some technicians prefer to finish this border at a right angle to the lingual surface, however, it should never have a taper to the gingival. A gingival taper to this border will create a trench around the linguals of the posterior teeth which is a food trap and uncomfortable for the patient.

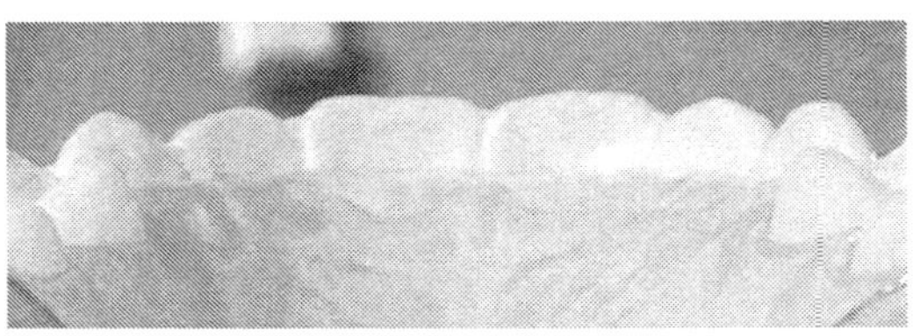

Fig. 5.35 The acrylic meets the lingual of the anterior teeth with no scalloping, it forms a smooth flat surface. See colour photo Page 5-29

In the anterior, the basic design for mandible and maxilla are again very similar. From the distal of the 3 to distal of the 3 the acrylic should form a smooth flat surface parallel to the occlusal plane. The height of the acrylic should be just incisal to the cingulum of all anteriors, and the acrylic should conform snugly to the interdental embrasures. The acrylic on the lower may come as close as 2 mm to the incisal, however, on the upper this must be avoided to eliminate accidental opening of the bite.

Acrylic processing — step by step

Wax up and block out

The first step is to ensure that all wire elements are waxed securely to the models in their correct positions. Clasps and arches are fixed to the model by wax placed on the facial portion of the wire. Do not wax the tag to the palate as you would with a partial denture.

In more complex cases, you would also include any springs, expansion screws, hooks, etc. that are part of the appliance. The specifics of these components will be discussed later.

Block out is an important part of the wax up procedure. Improperly blocked out appliances will be difficult to remove from the cast, difficult to place in the mouth and will frequently be the cause of broken teeth on the master model. Some cases will require extensive block out, while others require none. When blocking out, use a fairly soft wax with little or no dye colouring. Pink baseplate wax or white utility wax work well. Dark red boxing or beading wax, or crown & bridge waxes should be avoided. The dyes can leak out of the wax during polymerization staining the acrylic.

On the maxilla, areas to observe when evaluating block out are:

Teeth with moderate to severe undercuts.

Lingual undercuts are the most prevalent, particularly on the posterior lingual surfaces of adult patients. Younger patients seldom have deep undercuts in these regions. Also on adult patients, inspect the interproximal areas of the anterior teeth. Receding interdental papilla can expose troublesome undercuts here. Fill these undercuts with wax without overbuilding your blockout. A small amount of undercut helps to retain the appliance. If the clinician indicates that the tooth is periodontally involved, block out all undercuts to relieve stress on the tooth.

Wide interproximal embrasures or diestemas.

Diestemas will allow the acrylic to flow to the facial surface of the teeth, and cure in a facial undercut region. This is particularly bothersome on anterior teeth. Watch for laterals and cuspids that are labially displaced or not fully erupted A deep or wide embrasure will let acrylic lock in around the tooth, resulting in broken teeth.

Proximal surface undercuts.

When a tooth is missing from the arch, be sure to check for any undercuts on the proximal surface of the tooth adjacent to the edentulous region. It is best to block these undercuts out before bending any wire elements on such a tooth. A wire placed in this undercut will cause unnecessary difficulties later.

Soft tissue undercuts in rugea area.

Any excessively deep, narrow fissures in the rugea, or undercuts created by the rugea may be blocked out with a light wash of wax. Acrylic in these areas will add nothing to the appliance, and can cause discomfort for the patient.

On the mandible, areas to observe when evaluating blockout are:

Soft tissue undercuts.

Undercuts in the soft tissue of the posterior region of the mandible, the retromylohiod fossa, can be severe. While these undercuts can be utilized in a denture for retention, with orthodontic appliances we avoid these areas.

Lingual sulcus.

When working on lower removable appliances, I always place at least a thin layer of wax in the lingual sulcus before sprinkling the case. When the impression reaches all the way into the sulcus I simply fill the peripheral roll with wax. We seldom wish the appliance to intrude on this region in any case. Even a very thin layer — less than 1 mm— provides an area in which to insert a knife blade in order to remove the appliance after processing. The removal is then much easier and the model is not scored by the knife.

These steps must be completed before soaking the model. Once the model is wetted wax will not stick to it.

Soaking the model

The soaking of the model is the next step. This accomplishes two tasks; soaking removes all air from the model thus eliminating concerns of air bubbles rising from the model to perforate the acrylic during curing. Any gypsum model has small voids between the gypsum crystals that are filled with air when the model is dry. If you submerge a dry model in water, you will see small bubbles rising from the model. An improperly soaked model will have similar bubbles trying to escape when the model is placed into the pressure pot to cure. If they come up through the acrylic while it is still soft, they will leave holes in the acrylic plate.

Soaking also helps by acting as a separator. If the voids between gypsum crystals at the surface of the model are filled with water, the monomer will not be able to enter the surface layer of stone and polymerize there. This is what causes the whitish, rough tissue surface on acrylic plates when the model is improperly soaked and separated.

The best way to soak any model is to place it standing on its posterior surface in water that covers no more than 2/3's of the model. This method gives any air inside the model an easy exit. Water is drawn up the model through capillary action. As the water advances, the model changes colour. When the entire model has darkened uniformly, you can be assured that the model is completely wetted.

This method also has the advantage that not all of the model is submerged in the water, and we have a timing method to indicate when the model is completely soaked. Gypsum will dissolve in water at room temperature, and whenever we soak a model, a small amount of surface is removed from the model. To avoid this we should soak models in a clear slurry — a saturated gypsum solution made by immersing a piece of gypsum in water for 24 hours — and submerge portions of the model not involved in the appliance.

If you don't believe that the surface of the model dissolves, try this; cover portions of some teeth with wax and then drop the model into water. In a couple of hours, boil off the wax and see if there is any difference. There will be.

Acrylic separator

Acrylic separator (tinfoil substitute) is now painted onto the model. For orthodontic purposes the separator may be diluted up to 50% with water. The separator may be painted liberally about the model, covering all surfaces that will receive acrylic, as well as all adjacent surfaces. Excess separator is then removed by directing a stream of compressed air at the model.

***Important**: ensure that excess separator is removed from beneath any wire tags on the palate.*

Sprinkling acrylic

Of bottles and powder-liquid ratios

With wires attached, block out complete, and model soaked and separated, you are now ready to proceed with sprinkling the acrylic. The sprinkle method is accomplished with the monomer and polymer being alternately dispensed from separate bottles onto the model.

An 8 oz. pliable squeeze bottle is acceptable for the polymer. A smaller 2 oz. bottle is my preference for dispensing the monomer. Some technicians prefer 4-6 oz. goose neck dispensers.

The bottle used for the monomer must be pliable and have a small delivery hole to provide accurate control of the monomer application on a single drop basis. Monomer application is one of the most important determinants of a well fabricated acrylic plate.

Inaccurate application of monomer can lead to:

- excessive shrinkage of the acrylic — monomer shrinks upon polymerization a great deal more than polymer. The greater the amount of monomer, the greater the shrinkage.
- an excessively thick palatal region — an excess of monomer increases the flow of the monomer-polymer mixture. Most of today's acrylics are designed to acquire a rubbery consistency within a short time of mixing. This is to help in keeping the acrylic in the area where it is sprinkled. Older acrylics would become liquid and flow about the model, forcing the addition of extra polymer to stabilize them. Adding an excess of monomer to a good acrylic will cause the mixture to run to the deepest point of the model, typically the palate. This means that you use extra material, extra time to apply it, and extra time to trim it. The excess monomer will also cause undue shrinkage, probably ruining the appliance.
- inadequate thickness at the gingival margin — same basic problem as the previous point, as the acrylic flows into the palate there is a shortage at the gingival margin.
- patches of dry acrylic — inadequate monomer will leave patches of dry, white powder inside the acrylic plate. This can also be a result of application technique, trapping polymer where the monomer cannot soak into it.
- large air bubbles — this is caused by a combination of poor polymer and monomer application. A too thick layer of polymer that has monomer sprinkled on its surface too quickly will trap the air which is between the grains of polymer. The monomer must be applied so that it has sufficient time to soak through the powder before more is added. If the monomer is dripped too quickly over the surface of deep powder, the surface goes rubber before the air can escape causing the air to form the bubbles. Another cause of large air pockets is air that was trapped inside the model rising into the acrylic when it is placed into the water of the pressure pot.

The sprinkle technique

A number of sources suggest that you should first apply monomer to the model. I prefer to sprinkle polymer first. Applying monomer first is a technique from a time when you had to add polymer to soak up the monomer and stabilize the mixture. The acrylics that are formulated for orthodontics today have

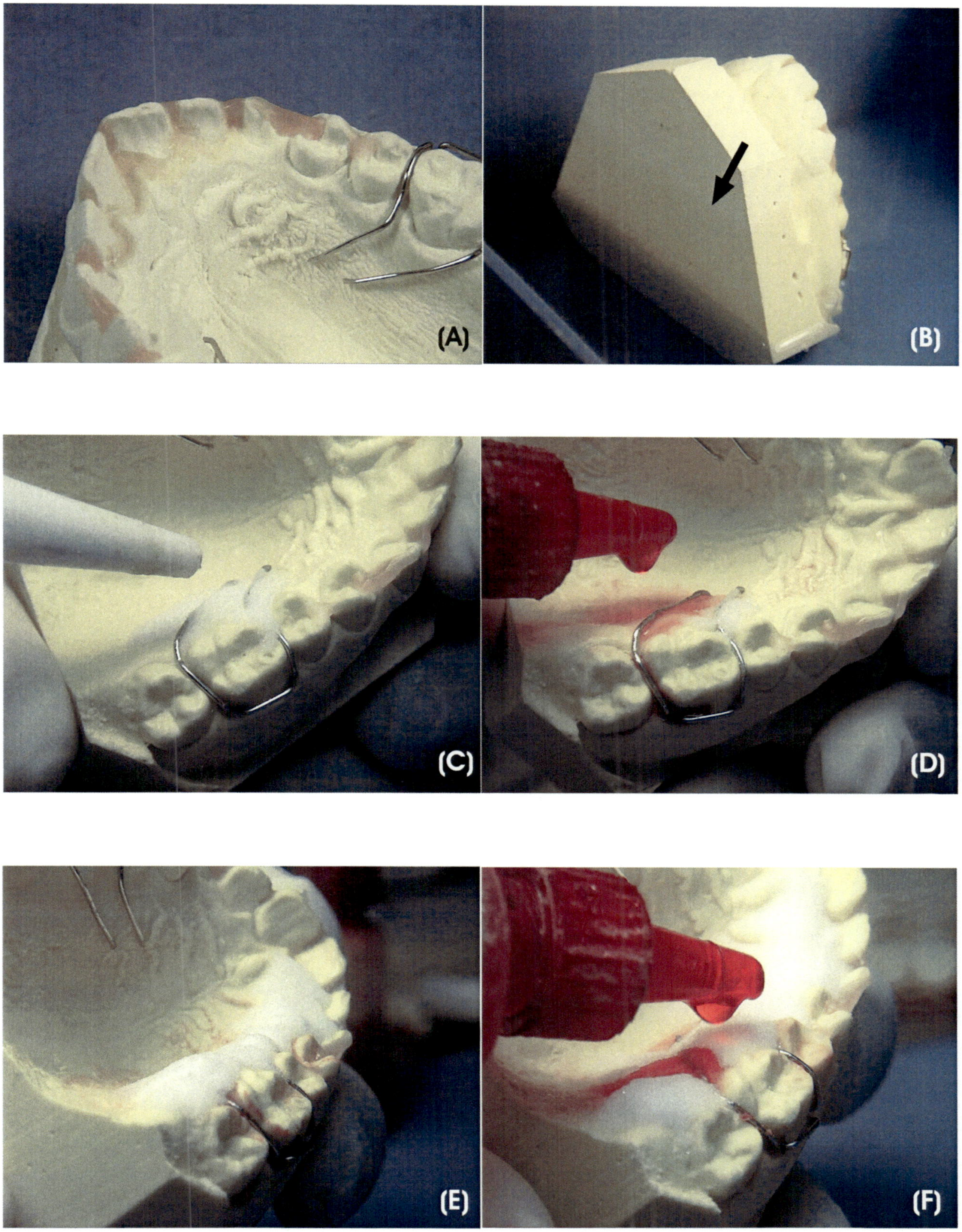

(A) Diastemas and undercuts blocked out with wax. **(B)** Model soaking by capillary action. Note line of darkened stone to which water has soaked (arrow). **(C)&(D)** Sprinkle acrylic under wires to ensure that no air is trapped beneath them. **(E)** Build 3 mm of thickness of acrylic along lingual gingival margins to act as a guide for the thickness of the acrylic palate. **(F)** Drip monomer (liquid), one drop at a time to wet polymer (powder).

plastisizers incorporated into them to stabilize the mix. Some acrylics will stiffen in as little as 30 seconds.

This acrylic gives you good control over its placement and thickness. It is not, therefore, necessary to overbuild the appliance greatly. You must allow some excess for trimming and polishing purposes, however, a small amount should suffice.

Applying monomer first can cause the monomer to penetrate the surface of the stone model, even on a separated model. This will result in a rough, cloudy tissue surface on the appliance.

The order of areas in which to apply acrylic for a simple palate is:

1.) one posterior quadrant
2.) the anterior region
3.) the second posterior quadrant.

Hold the model at an angle with the posterior toward the palm of your hand. The model should be positioned so that the lateral wall of the palate is flat to the bench top. This will help to control the flow of the acrylic as it is applied. Holding the base of the model flat will result in the acrylic immediately running to the palatal midline.

Starting in one posterior quadrant, first sprinkle a small amount of powder under all the wires in the area. This is to ensure that the wires are completely encased in the acrylic plate. If this is not accomplished, the wires will be exposed to the palatal surface, an irritant if not corrected, and a weakness in the appliance.

A single drop of monomer on each of the wire areas will wet the powder under the wires.

Add acrylic in depths of approximately 1 mm at a time. The powder may be added over a large area at one time, however, it should not be added in great depth. Too deep an addition of powder can lead to air being trapped and causing voids when the liquid is dripped on top of it.

The easiest way to obtain an even thickness of acrylic is to build a line of proper thickness and use that to gauge the thickness of the rest of the acrylic. Adding acrylic along the gingival margins is an excellent place to judge the thickness of your palate.

Add a line of powder 1 mm deep from the distal of the most posterior tooth to the mesial of the first bicuspid.

Starting at either the mesial or distal, drip monomer one drop at a time onto the line of powder. When you add a drop, give it a moment to soak into the powder before adding the next drop. The next drop should be placed at the point where the powder stopped being wetted by the previous drop. In this

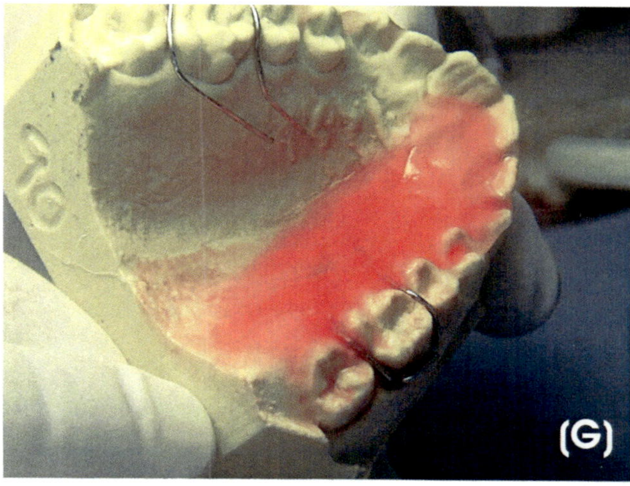

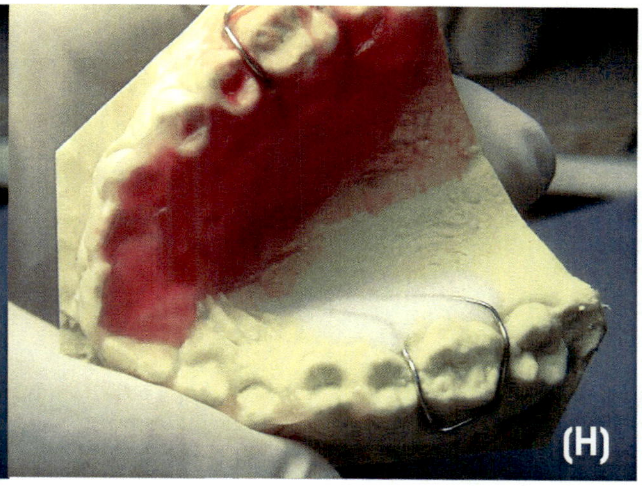

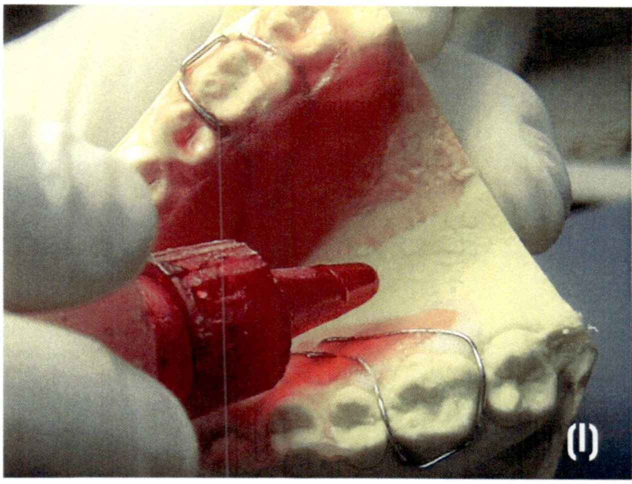

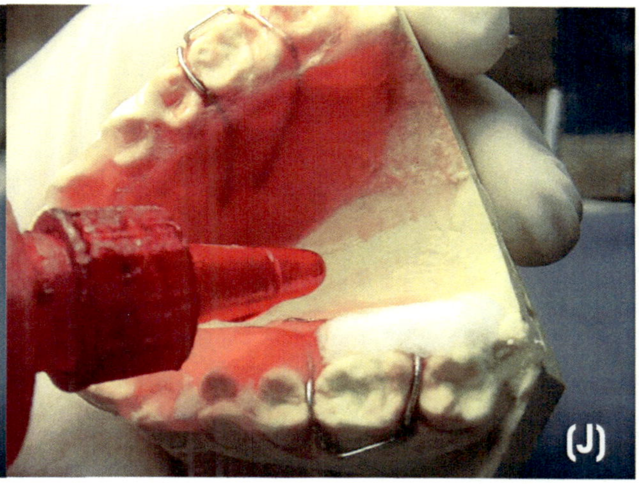

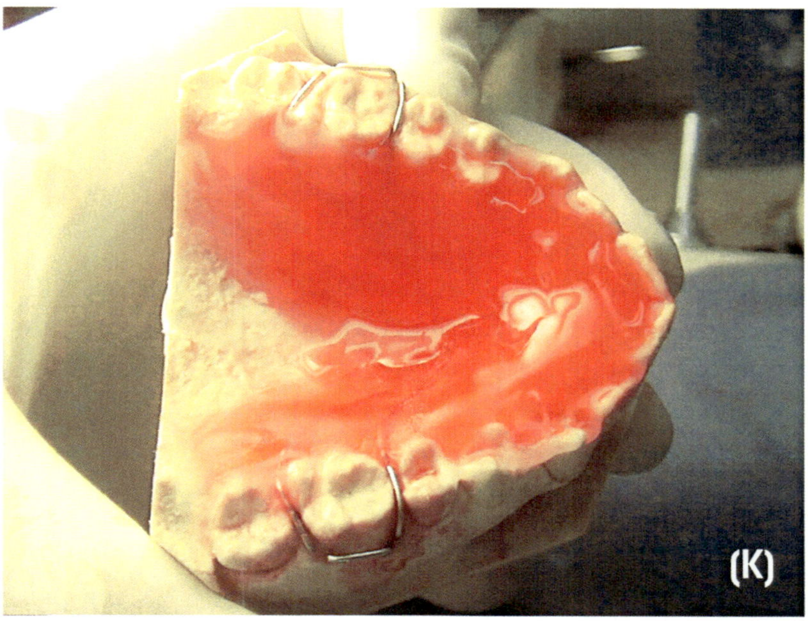

(G) Once gingival area is adequate thickness, fill in from gingival margin to midline. First quadrant now completed.
(H)&(I) Turn model to sprinkle second quadrant, starting by placing acrylic under wires as on other side.
(J) Build acrylic to 3mm thickness along gingival margin. Continue sprinkling palate on second side in same manner as first side.
(K) Completed sprinkled acrylic palate is now ready to place into a pressure pot at 20-25 psi.

manner wet all the powder that you have added. Try to avoid dripping monomer in unconnected spots. This can lead to small areas of dry powder between the wetted area. These are difficult to wet properly without causing air to be trapped.

Repeat this process until there is a line of wetted acrylic 3-4 mm deep along the gingival margins of the teeth. Now start adding acrylic down into the palate — 1 mm deep at a time — using the line you have made to gauge your thickness. You should now have a semicircular form of wetted acrylic, straight across the gingival margins and curving down into the palate.

Begin to add acrylic in the anterior region, the steps being the same as for the posterior. Be sure to bring the acrylic up over the cingulums of the teeth, and add enough to be able to level this area when trimming.

The final quadrant is sprinkled in the same manner as the others. When you are finished, add acrylic to any lines that have formed at the junctions of the areas that are sprinkled.

When you have succeeded in sprinkling a palate several times, you may want to sprinkle in only two steps, sprinkling one entire quadrant and then the other. It is faster, but takes more practice and control.

The amount of working time that you have with the acrylic varies from brand to brand; it is generally in the range of 5-8 minutes. This gives you time to finish without panicking; however, you do not have a great deal of time to fool around once you have started to sprinkle. If you have made a major mistake and know that the acrylic is not going to be acceptable, let the acrylic turn rubbery and then stick an instrument into it and pull it off. It should come off without disturbing your wires. This is much easier than trying to remove it when it is liquid, or removing your wires from the hardened acrylic.

Under pressure (polymerizing in the pressure pot)

The sprinkled appliance is now placed into the pressure pot for polymerization.

The purpose of the pressure pot is to produce acrylic which is dense and porosity free. Acrylic that has polymerized under water pressure is stronger for this reason. The lack of small porosity also makes the acrylic easier for the patient to keep clean. Curing acrylic under air pressure can cause air solution in the monomer on the surface of the uncured mixture, weakening the acrylic.

The pressure pot should be approximately half filled with warm water. The acrylic being cured must be completely submerged. The heat of the water will speed the setting reaction. Do not use water that is too hot; this can cause some warpage of the acrylic plate due to thermal expansion and contraction. The water should be a temperature into which you can comfortably immerse your hand.

The sprinkled model should be placed in the pressure pot under 25 psi for 10-15 minutes. To test whether the acrylic is ready for removal, simply press your fingernail lightly into the surface. If the surface yields, polymerization is not yet complete.

When the model is removed from the pressure pot, the appliance should be removed immediately. This is the easiest time to remove the appliance without damaging the teeth on the model. If the model is allowed to dry, removal becomes more difficult and teeth will frequently break.

Wax that was used to hold wires into place or block out regions of the model should now be removed by pouring boiling water over the appliance. Place the appliance occlusal down in a strainer to accomplish this. Do not subject the appliance to prolonged exposure to boiling water, as this will soften the acrylic and can cause distortion. The wax on buccal surfaces may be boiled off while the appliance is still on the model, but you must be careful allowing the acrylic to cool and stiffen before removing it from the model, or there could be distortion.

Trimming the acrylic plate

The process of trimming takes the mass of cured acrylic and turns it into a comfortable, functional appliance. The tools used to trim will vary from technician. The ones that I am going to discuss will allow quick, efficient production of the finished plate; however, they are by no means the only way to do it. The general difference in trimming preferences is that technicians trained in North America like to use both a bench lathe and handpiece for trimming. European trained technicians prefer just the handpiece.

The basic design requirements of the acrylic plate have been discussed earlier in this section, so I we'll go straight to the trimming procedure.

When you are trimming your first few appliances, you may find it helpful to outline the finished periphery with a pencil before you start. When you are inexperienced at trimming any type of prosthesis, it is very easy to lose your end point after you trim off your starting point. A few seconds with a pencil can eliminate this problem. First review your prescription. Start your line at the most posterior tooth in one quadrant. Bring it to the most posterior tooth in the other quadrant following the prescribed palatal design, horseshoe or full palate.

A horseshoe palatal should have posterior segments 10-15 mm wide, and be slightly wider over the midline. A full palate should start at the most posterior tooth in one quadrant and have slight anterior curve to the midline. It should then curve posteriorly across the palate to the most posterior tooth of the other quadrant.

Now mark the height of the acrylic on the lingual surfaces of the teeth. Draw on the surface that will contact the tooth. In the posterior, make a mark in the center of each tooth, half way between the gingival margin and the occlusal. Connect these marks by drawing a line from the acrylic septa over the interdental papilla to the mark in the center of each tooth. This should give you a sweeping scalloped outline to the posterior segment. In the anterior, draw a line — straight and level — from cuspid to cuspid. This line should be just incisal to the interdental papilla.

Mark a lower plate in a similar manner making your lingual periphery 10-12 mm wide, although this can be deeper if the patient has a deep lingual sulcus. If the patient has large soft tissue undercuts, it is advisable to cut the lingual periphery as short as possible. This will increase the patient's comfort by decreasing the likelihood of interference in the undercut region.

A large stone in the bench lathe is used to form the outline of the acrylic plate. Hold the appliance with the tissue side up towards the stone. Start on the midline cutting into the correct depth. Draw the edge of the stone along your line toward the posterior on one side, using both the edge and the side of the wheel to cut. Return to the midline and repeat on the other side.

Turn the appliance over so that the occlusal is towards the stone and begin trimming around the teeth.

CAUTION: Do not touch the wires with the large stone!

Trim one tooth at a time starting in the posterior. Hold the appliance so that the stone is trimming parallel to the occlusal plane. Use the corner of the stone to cut to the line in the center of each tooth. Draw the stone sideways in a rising curve to the interdental papilla. Repeat for each tooth.

In the anterior, again hold the appliance so that the stone is trimming parallel to the occlusal plane. Using the edge of the stone, which should be flat, trim the acrylic flat and level from cuspid to cuspid following your line.

Now use the stone to reduce any palatal areas of the appliance that are excessively thick.

The basic form of your appliance is now complete.

A large egg bur can now be used to smooth together the areas shaped by the stone. If you do not have a handpiece, the egg bur can complete the smoothing and shaping; however, a handpiece does a better job of finishing details.

A carbide taper bur in the handpiece can be used to finish all the surfaces of the plate. Use it to give the palatal — or lingual on a lower — periphery an even thickness all around. Smooth and refine the acrylic to the linguals of all the teeth, giving the anterior section its flat surface. The acrylic septa in the

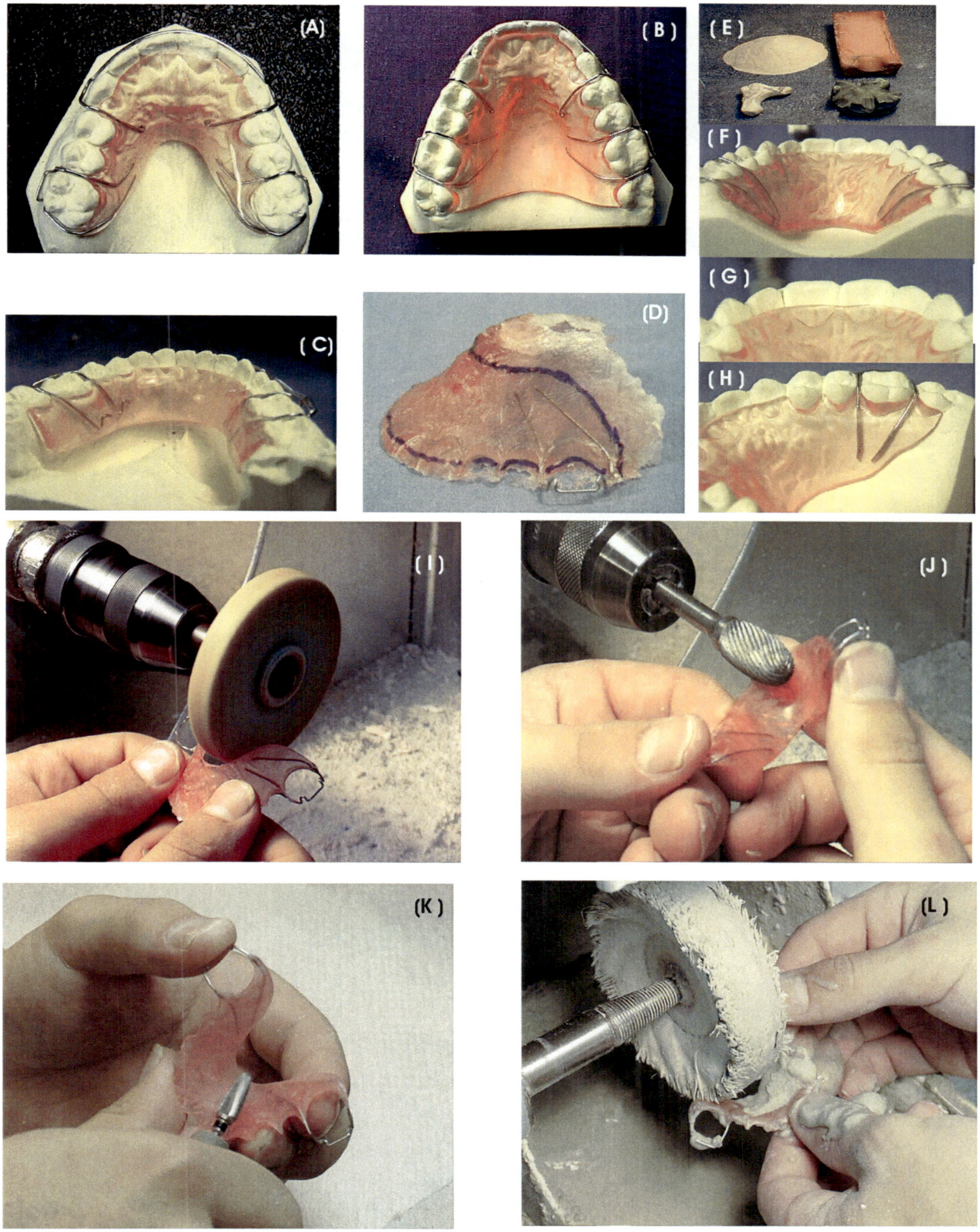

(A) Hawley retainer with horseshoe palate. **(B)** Hawley Retainer with full palate. **(C)** Mandibular lingual borders do not extend to sulcus for patients comfort and to avoid excessive undercuts. **(D)** Draw outline of intended shape on acrylic with a pencil before beginning trimming. **(E)** Polishing materials, clockwise from upper left; Pumice, Tripoli, Chromium Oxide, Highshine. **(F&G)** Anterior Acrylic flat just incisal to the cingulums. **(H)** Posterior acrylic is scalloped at approximately ½ lingual height of the teeth. **(I)** Use large Fastcut stone for initial shaping and gross reduction. **(J)** Large egg bur smooths and blends surface. **(K)** Handpiece is used to add fine detail and smooth. **(L)** Polishing starts with pumice, followed with tripoli, then High shine, Chromium Oxide shines metals.

interproximal embrasures can be trimmed with a scalpel to a 1-2 mm length.

A final smoothing before polishing can be accomplished with an emery cloth in a split mandrel. Running this over the surface of the acrylic blends any irregularities together and removes large scratches. The smoother the acrylic is before polishing, the easier to acquire an acceptable finished surface.

Polishing acrylic

Polishing is used as an inaccurate generic term in this instance. Polishing involves the use of steadily finer abrasive materials that cut finer and finer grooves in a material to produce a smooth shiny surface. To polish acrylic, the materials we use are: pumice, tripoli, and highshine. These materials are applied to buff wheels and used in a bench lathe.

The buffs

The buffs are described by their diameter and the number of layers of cotton muslin they contain. An effective buff is the 4-32, four inches in diameter and 32 layers.

Before polishing can begin, you must prepare your buffs. This is done by spinning the buff on the lathe at low speed and pressing the back of a knife or plaster spatula blade against it. Loose threads from the buff will fly off. Remove the buff from the lathe and pass it over a lighter or Bunsen flame. The ends of the loose threads from the buff will quickly burn away. Wet the buff to extinguish the embers, then repeat this sequence twice more. If you do not prepare your buff before using it to polish, the loose threads will catch in the wires of your appliance and distort them.

Pumice

Pumice is the first abrasive used. Pumice is composed of crushed volcanic pumice stone, however, sometimes sand is used instead. It comes in various grades and removes the large scratches left by the trimming burs in the acrylic. The pumice is used from a tray that is placed under the buff wheel. Mix the pumice with water to produce a mud and apply this to the appliance. You must remember that it is the pumice and not the wheel that does the polishing. If you try to polish the acrylic with insufficient pumice, the friction created by the spinning wheel will create enough heat to put a burn mark in the acrylic.

We mix the pumice with water for two reasons:

to keep the acrylic cool,

to make the dry, dusty material easy to use.

Lightly buff all of the lingual surfaces of the plate using the pumice. Turn and move the appliance so that the pumice is applied from all directions. Do not pumice the tissue surface of the appliance.

When all areas have been smoothed, wash the pumice off of the appliance and inspect it. If any rough areas remain, pumice them again.

Tripoli

The pumice will leave small striations in the acrylic surface because it is a fairly coarse abrasive. The next material to use is the tripoli. Tripoli is referred to as a low shine. It is a fine abrasive that can remove the scratches of the pumice before the final polish. Tripoli is supplied in one pound bars which are applied to a dry buff by holding the bar against the wheel. Use the tripoli in much the same manner as the pumice, buffing all lingual surfaces of the appliance. The tripoli will leave a smooth dull shine on the acrylic when finished. If any rough areas become apparent, return to the pumice to remove them.

The acrylic is now ready to highshine.

Highshine (Polishing)

The highshine step is the only true polishing act in the "polishing" procedure. Polishing does not involve abrasion of the material being polished. Instead, polishing fills in the fine scratches and produces a smooth and shiny surface. Highshine comes in a number of brand names and is generally packaged in bars or sticks.

Highshine is applied from a dry buff. When using highshine polish do not place too much highshine on the buff. An excess buildup of highshine will result in a dull surface on your appliance.

Do not try to overpolish with highshine. Run the buff over the entire surface once. If an area will not shine after you have run the buff over it, it needs more pumice or Tripoli. Pressing with the highshine or shining it repeatedly will not help; it will only waste time. I routinely apply highshine lightly to the tissue of my appliance. An orthodontic appliance does not benefit from "suction adhesion" as does a denture, and the slightly smooth, lightly polished tissue surface makes it easier for the patient to keep the appliance clean.

As the last step in the polishing procedure, the wire work of the appliance should be polished. An excellent shine can be imparted to the stainless steel with the use of chromium oxide on a chamois buff or felt wheel. Polishing at high speed provides the best results. Chromium oxide is also referred to as "green stick", and comes in a one pound cylinder of a bright green colour.

When polishing the metal with the chromium oxide, take care not to buff the acrylic. The metal polish will leave black marks on the acrylic surface.

When the appliance has a satisfactory sheen, it may be placed into an ultrasonic cleaner — filled with a cleaning solution — for several minutes. The ultrasonic will help to remove any debris from the polishing procedure by vibrating it out. The appliance should now be washed in clean water with soap and a soft brush. Disinfect the appliance with a spray disinfectant; place it on the model. It is now ready for delivery to the patient.

Check list

Before sending out any finished appliance, you should check each and every element of the appliance against its design requirements, and the overall appliance against its prescription.

For the basic Hawley elements check these items:

Adams clasp

- the clasps are on the correct teeth
- the clasps are retentive (the retentive eyelets are touching the teeth)
- the retentive eyelets are not impinging on the tissue (45° to buccal bar)
- the buccal bar is 1 mm off the buccal surface of the tooth
- the arms are contoured tightly through the occlusal embrasures
- there are no occlusal interferences
- the tags are long enough to provide retention
- the tags have 1 mm of relief from the palatal tissues
- there are adequate retentive elements at the terminal arms of the clasps.

Hawley arch

- the labial bar of the arch is straight and level with the incisal edges
- the labial bar is placed 1 mm incisal to the interdental papilla, in the region of the interproximal contact on older patient's
- the labial bar contacts the labial surface of all teeth passively
- the Wilson loop begins at the junction of the mesial and middle third of the cuspids, and contacts the teeth at this point
- the mesial arm of the Wilson loop is 90° to the buccal bar
- the mesial and distal arms of the Wilson loop are parallel
- the Wilson loop does not impinge on the tissue
- the distal arm of the Wilson loop passes tightly through the cuspid/1st bicuspid embrasure
- the tags have 1 mm of relief from the palatal tissues
- the tags are long enough to provide retention

- there are adequate retentive elements at the terminal arms of the clasps.

Acrylic plate

- acrylic design matches the prescription (horseshoe, full palate, etc.)
- the acrylic is dense and free from porosity
- the acrylic is well adapted to the teeth and tissues
- no wire is exposed on the tissue surface
- the acrylic is polished to a smooth fine finish with a highshine.

"Kaizen"
Japanese, meaning "a small improvement each day."

"All things are difficult before they are easy."
Thomas Fuller

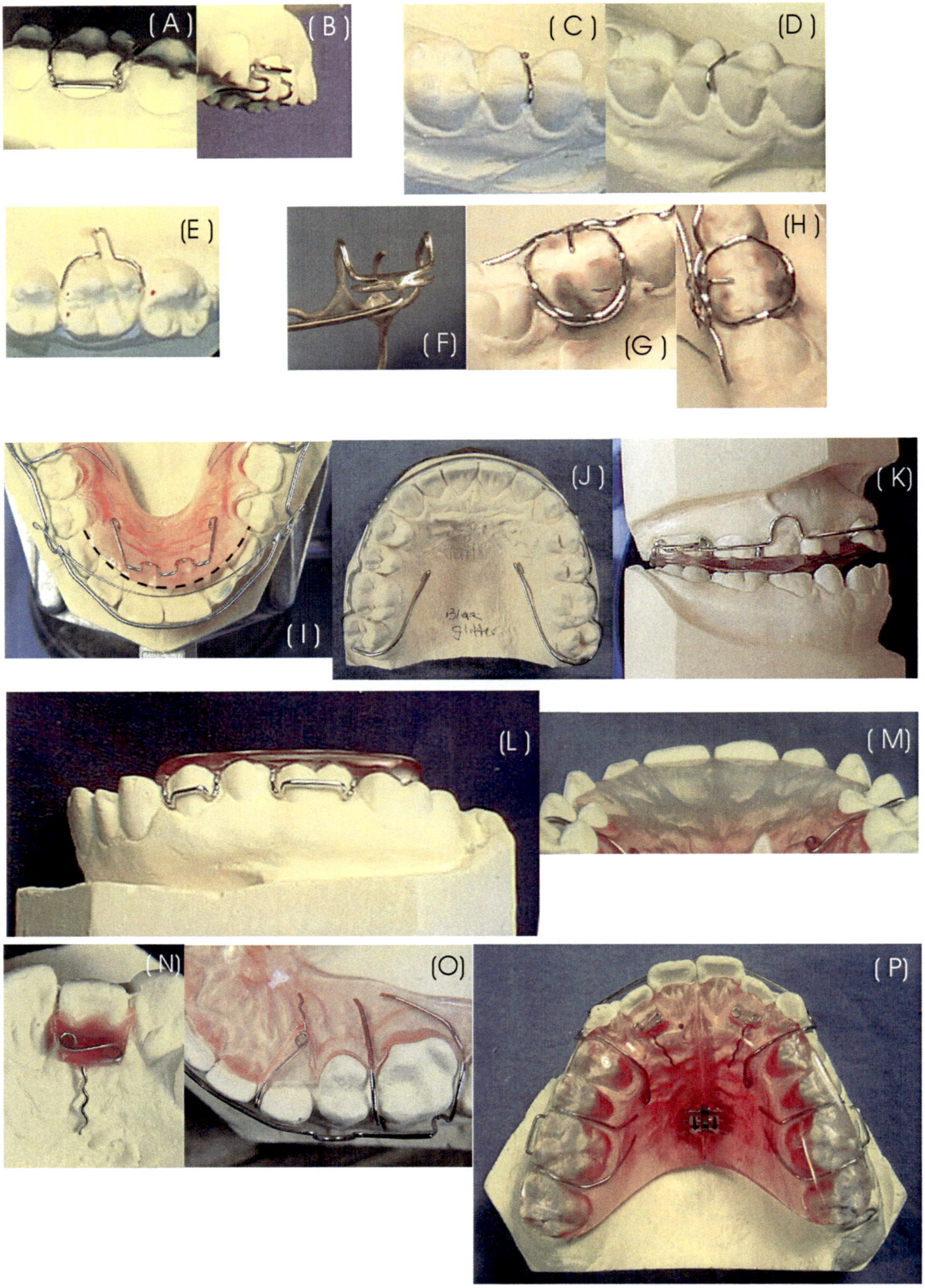

(A&B) Voss Clasp. **(C&D)** Finger Clasp. **(E)** Sage Clasp. **(F, G, H)** Crozat Clasp.
(I) Automatic Hawley, note dotted line represents where acrylic is trimmed away from lingual of teeth to allow movement. **(J)** Circumferential Hawley. (K) Posterior Bite Pads (PBP) in occlusion. **(L)** Pbp's lateral view. **(M)** Anterior Bite Plane. **(N)** Double Helix Clasp blocked out for acrylic work. **(O)** Distalizing Sweep Spring. **(P)** Schwarz appliance with 2 springs and PBP.

6 Components of removable appliances

"Force has no place where there is need of skill."
Herodotus
485-425 B.C.

Imagination is more important than knowledge...
Albert Einstein

The Hawley retainer forms the base from which many appliances are adapted. Virtually any combination of clasps, arches, springs, screws, etc. can be assembled to perform specific functions. We will now look at some of the different elements that can be combined to meet our design requirements.

Clasps

Clasps provide the retention that holds an appliance in the mouth against the dislodging forces of the active elements and oral function. There is a great variety of different types of clasps that can be used to fulfill different requirements. Each type performs its own specific function or is the component of choice in a specific situation.

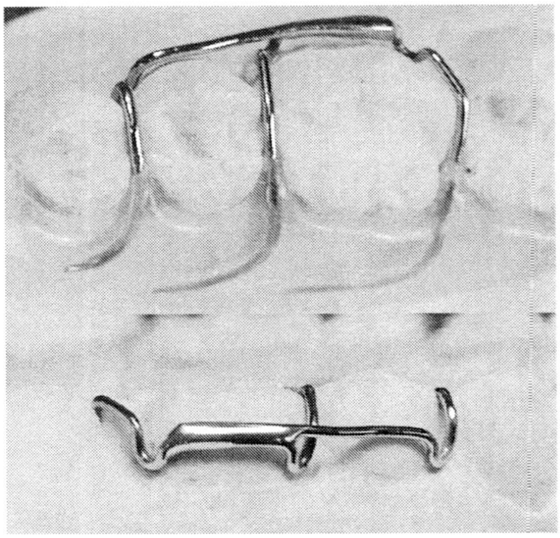

Fig.6.1 Auxillary Adams clasp

Adams clasp variations

Auxiliary Adams clasp

The auxiliary Adams clasp is used to provide additional retention to an appliance by inserting a third Adams arrowhead on the tooth adjacent to the one providing the primary retention. The arrowhead engages the undercut on the distal side of the tooth from the primary Adams clasp. The primary Adams is commonly placed on the 1st molar, with the auxiliary on the 2nd bicuspid.

The auxiliary Adams clasp is bent using 0.7 mm hard wire. One leg of the auxiliary Adams clasp is a tag which is inserted into the acrylic body of the appliance. The second leg is bent to lie against and parallel to the bridge of the primary Adams and is then soldered to the primary clasp. A Hawley arch may be soldered to the bridge of an auxiliary Adams.

Delta clasp

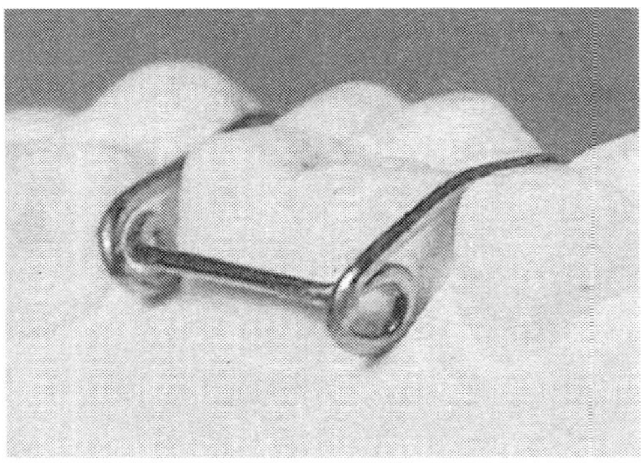

Fig. 6.2 Delta clasp

The delta clasp is a variation designed by Dr. Clark for use on the twin block appliance. It resembles an Adams clasp excepting the retentive elements are single helixes. Starting at the buccal bar they coil gingivally once to pass over themselves and then continue to the occlusal embrasure.

Voss clasp

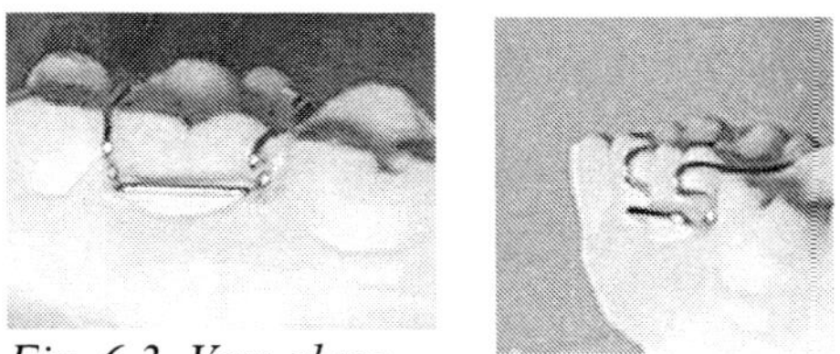

Fig. 6.3 Voss clasp

The Voss clasp is often mistaken for the Adams clasp and used in its place. The Voss clasp has a longer buccal bar, with the eyelets positioned at 90° to it vertically and oriented bucco-lingually. The eyelets angle inwards to contact the tooth on the proximal surfaces to gain retention. From the eyelets the arms make a 180° bend that takes them to the occlusal embrasures.

Single eyelet Adams

Lower molars on younger patient's often have little vertical height on the distal, making them difficult to clasp with a standard Adams clasp. A variation is to place the retentive element on the mesial of the tooth in the normal fashion, but contour the distal of the tooth as a circumferential clasp. Contour the wire to the buccal surface of the tooth just off of the gingival margin.

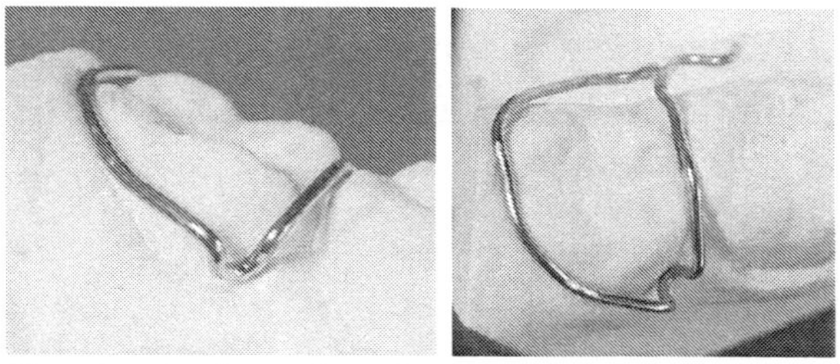

Fig. 6.4 Single eyelet Adams clasp

Other clasp designs

C-clasp

The c-clasp is the familiar Akers or circumferential clasp used extensively in partial dentures. On younger patients these clasps are of limited value because the teeth have limited or no undercuts to engage. To alleviate this a shelf can be created on the buccal of the tooth with composite to provide retention. The shelf is removed at the end of treatment.

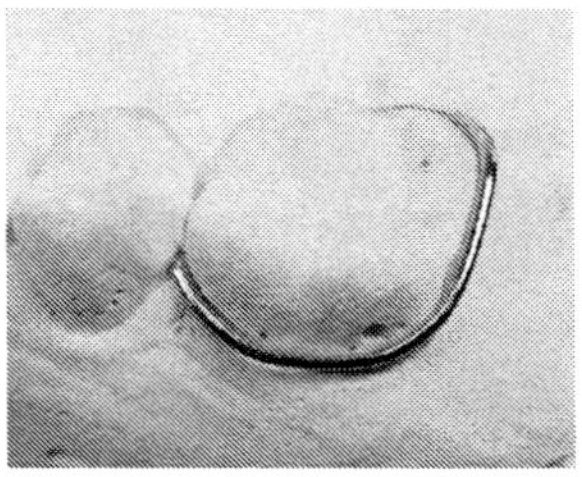

Fig. 6.5 C-clasp

If the appliance has an active element lingualizing the anteriors the c-clasp should be brought from the distal of the abutment, otherwise the active force will work to open the retentive tip of the clasp rendering it of little value.

The c-clasp can also be a short, almost a spur clasp, soldered onto the Wilson loop of a Hawley arch to engage either the cuspid or 1st bicuspid.

Ball clasp

The ball clasp is one of the most commonly used clasps. It consists of a length of wire with a ball of solder on one end.

This ball is bent to engage undercuts on the mesio-buccal or disto-buccal of the tooth, or more commonly to engage under the contact point in the interproximal embrasure. Ball clasps can be made by placing a drop of solder on the end of a wire or may be bought prefabricated. They are classified by the size of the wire not the size of the ball. Common sizes are; 0.7 mm, 0.8 mm, 0.9 mm. 0.7 mm is used for light clasping or on children, 0.8 mm is the best size for all around use, and 0.9 mm can be

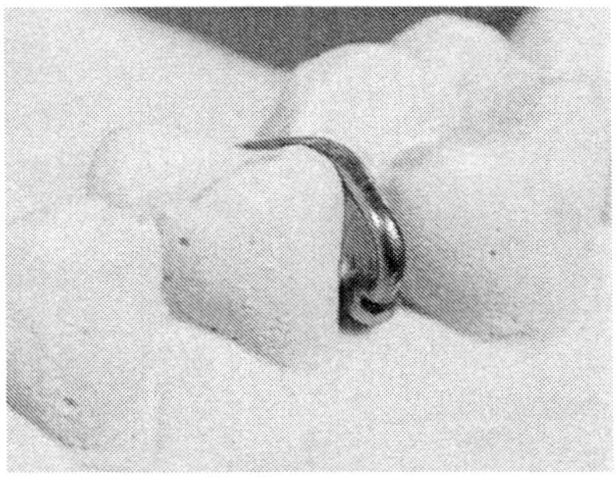

Fig. 6.6 Ball clasp

used for adults when a long clasp is required.

Start bending the ball clasp by scraping the interdental papilla slightly to received the ball. Bend the wire just above the ball so that the arm curves buccally before contacting the embrasure at the occlusal surface. This gives the clasp more flexibility, more retention and makes it easier to adjust. The retentive arm of the ball clasp is contoured tightly through the occlusal embrasure, and a retentive tag bent to follow the palatal surface. Use a fairly large, well defined tag on the ball clasp such as a curly-q. This helps to make a single arm clasp more stable.

The ball clasp can also be bent to resemble a c-clasp, j-clasp or even an Adams when the situation warrants.

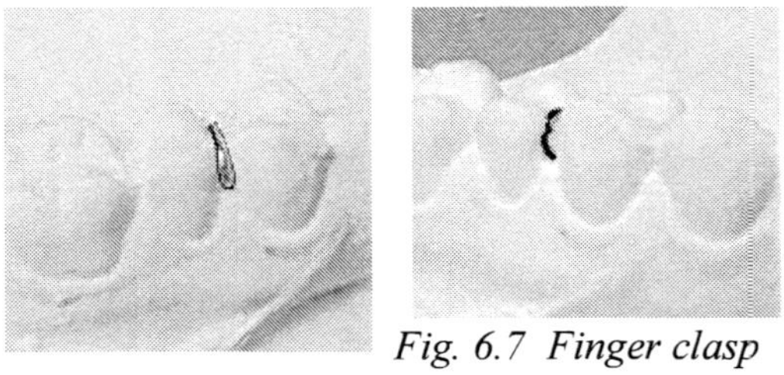

Fig. 6.7 Finger clasp

Finger clasp

The finger clasp resembles a ball clasp with the ball removed. It can be made with wire ranging from 0.5-0.8 mm.

Single arrowhead, anchor clasp, triangular clasp

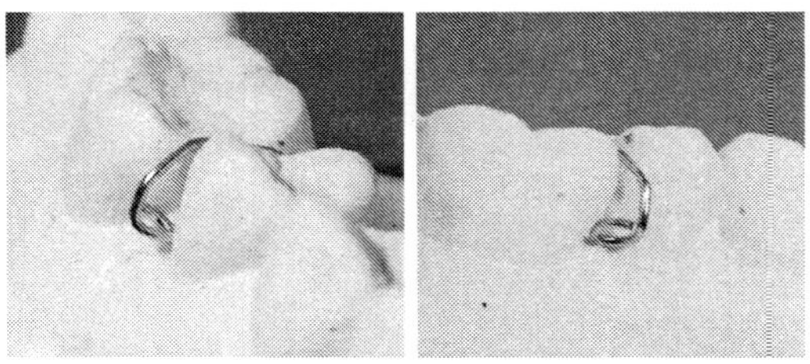

Fig. 6.8 Triangle clasp

These clasps bear a resemblance to each other, being all single arm clasps. They are treated similarly to the ball clasp. The triangular or eyelet clasp is bent from 0.7 wire, the single arrowhead or anchor clasp can be purchased pre-made.

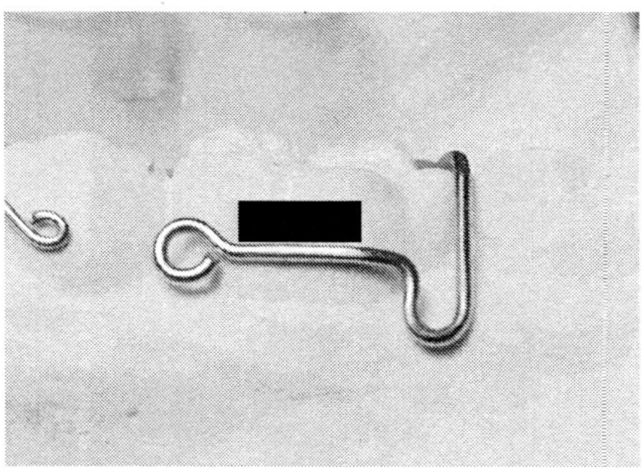

Fig. 6.9 Buccal tube clasp. The black box indicates the position of the molar bracket

Buccal tube clasp

The buccal tube clasp is used to gain retention on a case in which the patient is already wearing full arch brackets and requires a removable appliance. Most other clasps would interfere with the brackets and arch wire (with the exception of the ball clasp) in such a case. The clasp is placed on the most posterior molar bracketed.

The clasp approaches from the distal of the tooth crossing over the occlusal and forming a small loop or helix before passing gingival to the buccal tube. The clasp terminates in an eyelet loop into which the clinician will insert a probe, upon insertion, in order to bend the retentive arm of the clasp buccally. This allows easier insertion of the appliance. The flexibility to accomplish this is provided by the loop at the distal of the clasp.

If the tooth being clasped is not part of a straight wire appliance — but is being distalized by headgear — the clasp should approach from the mesial. This allows the clasped tooth to move freely to the distal.

Townsend clasp

The Townsend clasp is used to provide retention to the anterior segment of an appliance. The clasp can be fabricated from 0.5 or 0.6 mm wire.

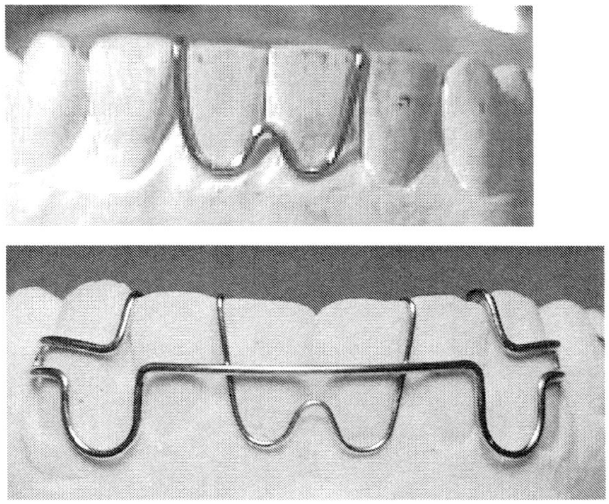

Fig. 6.10 Townsend clasp and a Townsend clasp with a Ricketts A rch

The Townsend clasp passes interproximally between the central and lateral, running closely along the distal of the central and then along the gingival margin of the central. The clasp rises to a v-shape in the interproximal of the two centrals to avoid the interdental papilla and then passes along the gingival margin and distal surface of the other central. The Townsend clasp may be used on either a mandibular or maxillary appliance.

Duyzings

The Duyzings consist of two wires which engage the mesial and distal undercuts of a single molar. The two wires are mirror images, one passing over the mesial occlusal embrasure, and one the distal. The wires come from the embrasure curving toward the center of the tooth but not meeting. They then curve back to engage the undercut at the line angle of the side of the tooth from which they originated. Use 0.7 mm wire.

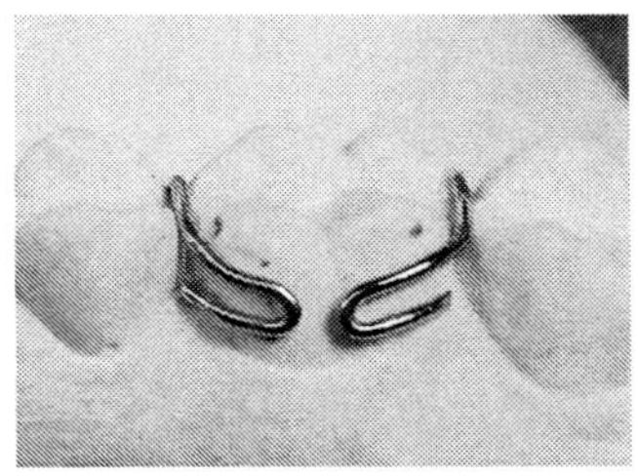

Fig. 6.11 Duyzings clasp

Sage (lingual)

The sage clasp engages the undercuts on the proximal surfaces of the lingual of a molar. The single wire starts at the mesial proximal undercut, and contours along the lingual to the center of the tooth. It then bends out into the palate to form the tag, before bending back to the tooth, and contouring to the lingual surface into the distal proximal undercut. Made with 0.5 mm wire.

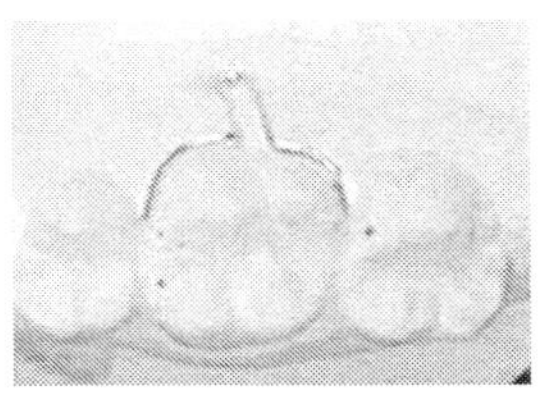

Fig. 6.12 Sage clasp

Crozat

The crozat clasp is used exclusively on the crozat appliance. The crozat appliance is a removable, all wire appliance. It is one of the oldest orthodontic designs still in use.

The crozat clasp is also known as the "*double crib clasp*". It is placed on the first molars and gains its retention by 0.7 mm wire which pass under the contact areas.

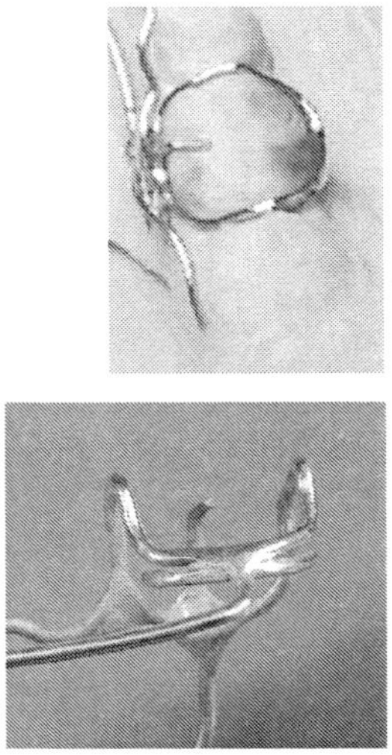

Fig. 6.13 Crozat clasp, occlusal and buccal view

The clasp has three parts which are joined by solder. They are an 0.7 mm wire which is formed into a ring and completely surrounds the molar. It is contoured to a close fit around the molars lingual gingival margin, and has its free ends on the buccal of the tooth at the level of the height of contour. At this point it is soldered to the second wire. The second wire provides the retention. It passes from the undercut formed gingival to the mesial contact, across the buccal of the tooth to the distal contact. Slight preparations are made in these contact regions.

The last part of the clasp is the occlusal rest. It is also made with 0.7 mm wire and passes through the lingual groove to rest on the occlusal surface. It is soldered to the ring portion of the clasp on the lingual.

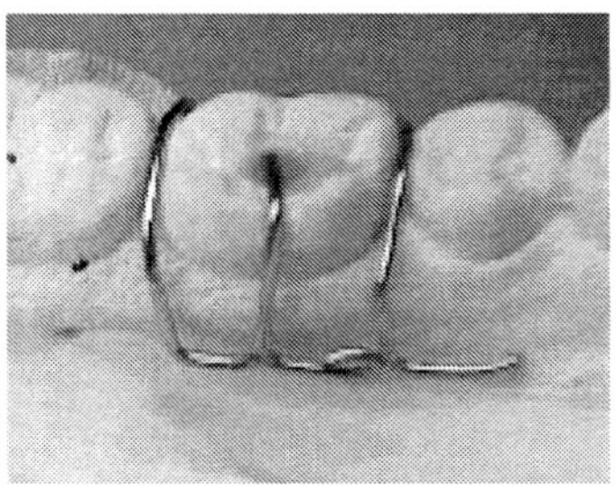

Fig. 6.14 Occlusal rest

Occlusal rest

Rests can be important supplements to orthodontic clasps, particularly on lower appliances. The small acrylic body of a lower removable appliance does not give sufficient vertical support to the appliance. A simple rest can be made by bending 0.7 mm wire though the lingual groove, down to a retentive tag on the lingual.

Arches

Soldered Hawley arch

The soldered Hawley arch is a modification of the standard Hawley arch. The difference is that the distal arm of the Wilson loop does not cross the occlusion at the distal of the cuspid, it instead makes a 90° bend towards the posterior passing along the buccal surfaces of the premolars to the bridge of the

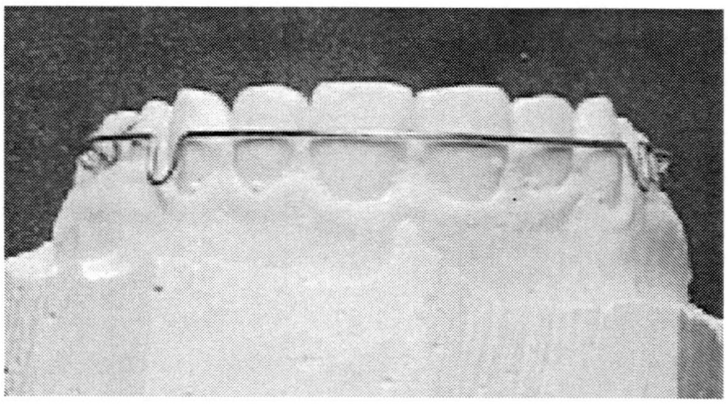

Fig. 6.15 Soldered Hawley arch, labial view

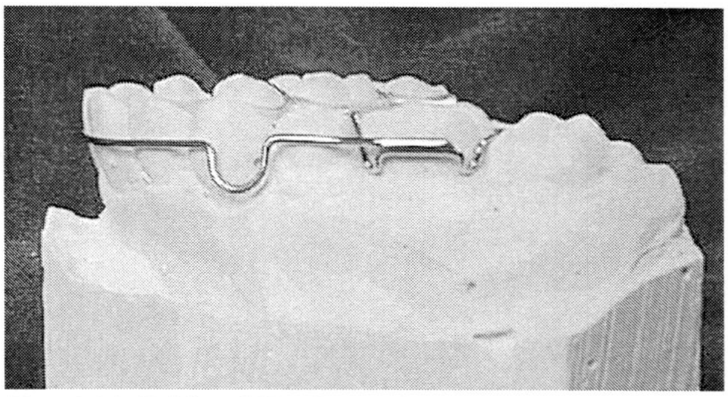

Fig. 6.16 Soldered Hawley arch, saggital view

Adams clasp. The wire is bent into close, parallel contact with the bridge of the Adams clasp and then soldered to it.

The labial portion of the arch is the same as a standard Hawley in that it contacts the incisors in the same manner on their labial surfaces. The Wilson loop, however, is placed slightly more to the posterior, with the loop beginning at the center of the cuspid and ending at the center of the 1st premolar.

This gives the appliance more control over the retaining of the cuspid, particularly with regards to rotational relapse.

The soldering of the arch may be done in a number of ways, the two most common being either on or off of the model.

To solder the arch off of the model, you can first do the acrylic work for the appliance, the soldering may be done before or after polishing. Spot weld the arch to the bridge of the Adams clasp, once the arch has been spot welded the appliance can be removed from the model without distortion of the arch.

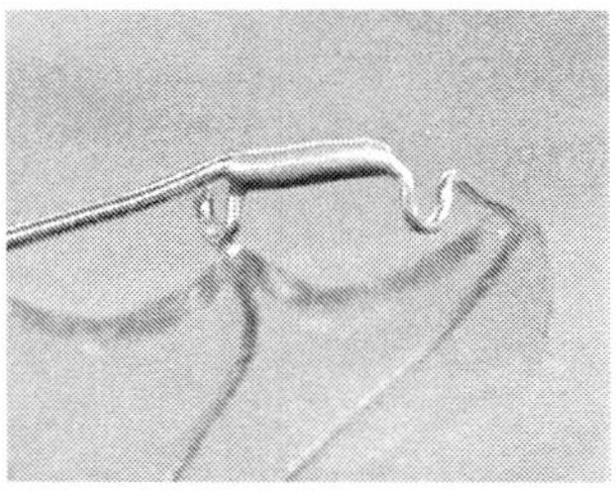

Fig. 6.17 Solder joint

The appliance is then secured in a third hand positioning device (soldering tweezers embedded into a plasticine base works well) with the area to be soldered above the acrylic body of the appliance. Remember that heat rises, if you position the acrylic above the area to be soldered the acrylic will burn.

Soldering is then easily accomplished. This method gives a good even solder joint without damaging the model.

Soldering can be done before the acrylic work is completed by spot welding the wires, removing them from the model and then soldering them. When this method is used, the wires relax slightly on application of the heat for soldering towards their original form. After soldering they do not quite fit the model properly.

Soldering the arch on the model may be done before or after the acrylic work. The arch is waxed into its position on the model. If acrylic has been done, it is best to place a thermal barrier over the acrylic near the region to be soldered (wet paper towel at a minimum, commercially available thermal barriers are more effective) as well as, the wax holding the arch. If you do not protect this wax the arch may shift in the middle of soldering. The joint is then soldered.

Soldering on the model will damage the working model.

Automatic Hawley (Auto-Hawley)

The automatic Hawley is a Hawley arch with a self-adjusting spring wire attached. This spring wire is used to move the anterior teeth lingually. It can retract the teeth into an even arch, working on the most labial elements first. This allows the appliance to correct rotations while retracting.

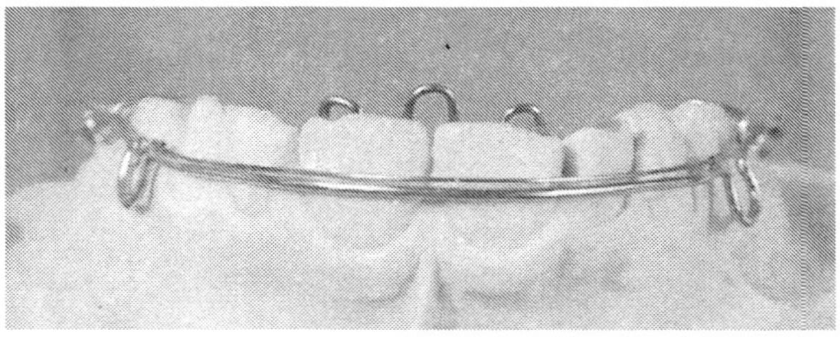

Fig. 6.18 Two wire Auto hawley arch

There are two types of auto Hawleys; one and two wire.

The two wire design uses the standard Hawley design as the base for the spring wire. To this is added a pair of .020" tubes 2 mm long, which are soldered to the arch. The distals of these tubes are flush with the 90° angle at the mesial of the Wilson loop. The tubes are oriented so that the long axis of the tubes point inside the arc of the arch wire. This is what gives activation to the spring wire. The tubes are spot welded to the arch. A carrying wire (0.5 mm wire) makes it easier to position the tubes correctly.

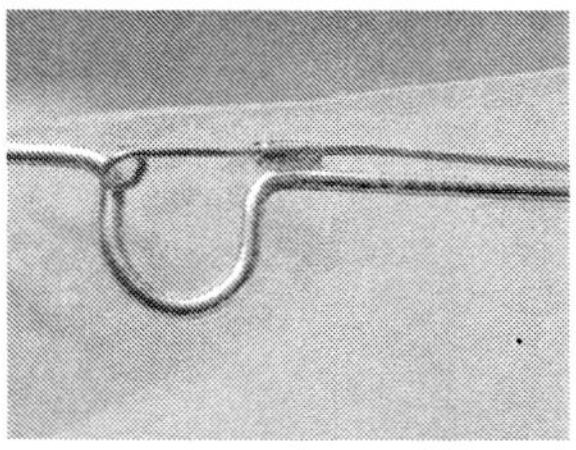

Fig. 6.19 Tube placed at mesial of Wilson loop

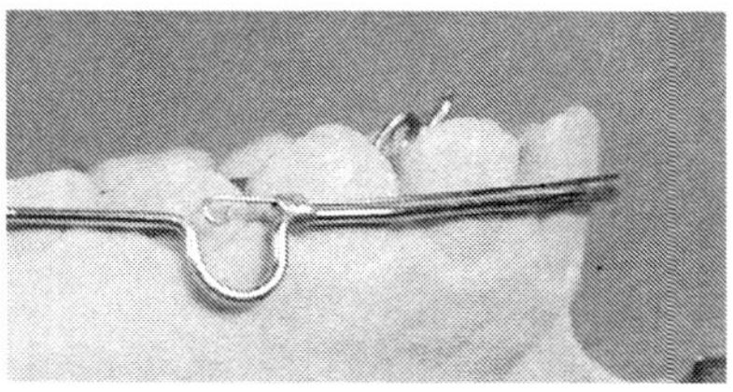

Fig. 6.20 Spring bent to helix inside Wilson loop

After carefully soldering the tubes to the arch check that they are clear. If there is flux in the tube it may be cleared by heating it gently, and when the flux softens push a 0.5 mm wire through the tube. Let the flux solidify around the wire, then twist the wire to break it free and withdraw it. The tube is now clear.

If the tube is filled with solder, it must be trimmed off and started over.

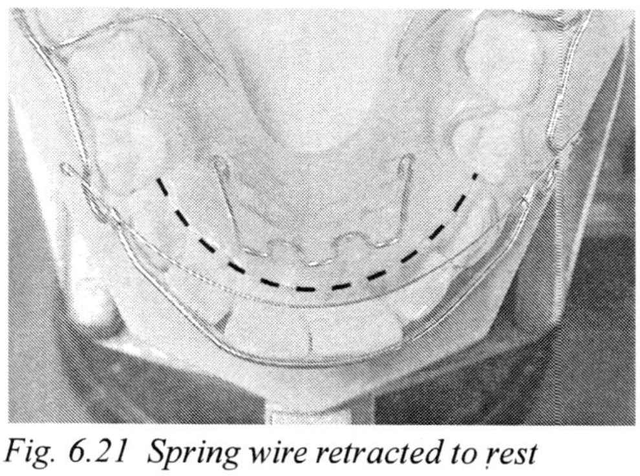

Fig. 6.21 Spring wire retracted to rest position, dotted line indicates trimmed lingual acrylic.

The spring is an .012 or .014 round spring wire. Form a helix in one end of the wire, then pass the straight end through the two tubes. Cut the wire to a length which allows it to follow the form of the Hawley arch. Bend a helix in the second end. The helixes should rest in the center of the Wilson loops when the arch is on the model. When the appliance is off of the model the spring should freely slide through the tubes to a position inside (lingual to) the Hawley arch.

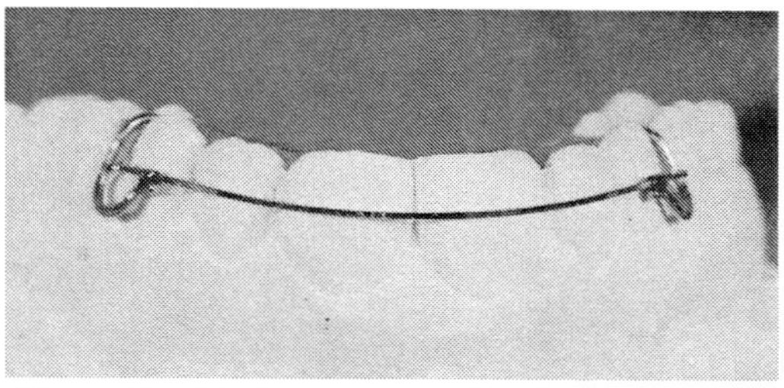

Fig. 6.22 Single wire auto Hawley arch

The single wire design attaches the tubes directly to the Wilson loops and leaves out the labial wire of the Hawley arch. This has the advantage that there is no labial arch left sitting off of the teeth when they begin to retract.

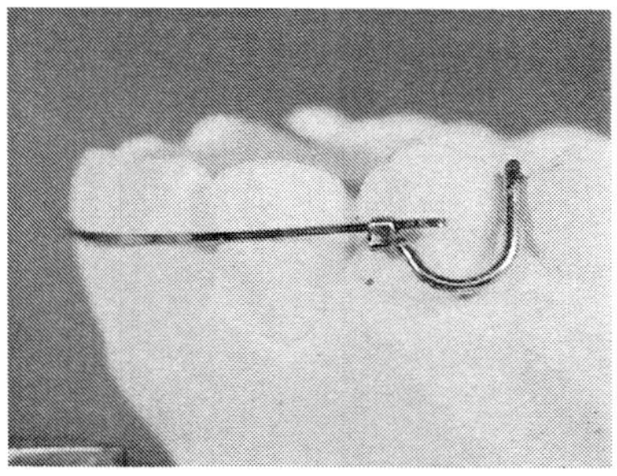

Fig. 6.23 Helix of rectangular wire bent parallel to occlusal plane

The arch wire should be kept as close to the gingival as is practical to prevent the teeth from tipping excessively. Teeth that have a distinct labial incline can present a problem because the spring wire will try to slide up the inclined plane presented by labial surface without retracting the teeth. This can be alleviated by using a rectangular spring wire (.010x.020). This wire is flexible in the occlusal plane but stiff in the vertical plane.

An important aspect of the auto Hawley is the acrylic design. To move the teeth lingually we must remove the acrylic to the lingual of the teeth (see Fig 6.21 - dotted line). This should be done in an even arc from cuspid to cuspid — do not scallop the acrylic behind each tooth. The acrylic should be contoured to match the desired final arc that the teeth will form. This forces the teeth to align. When their lingual surfaces contact the acrylic, the most lingual portion will touch first and act as a control stop. If the tooth is rotated its movement will be a rotation around this control stop as it straightens. The dentist can easily adjust this acrylic to achieve the desired affect.

Circumferential arch

The circumferential arch is similar to the soldered Hawley arch in that it continues along the buccal of the posterior teeth after the Wilson loop. Unlike the Hawley arch it does not require additional clasping for retention, although clasps may be added. The retentive elements of the circumferential are part

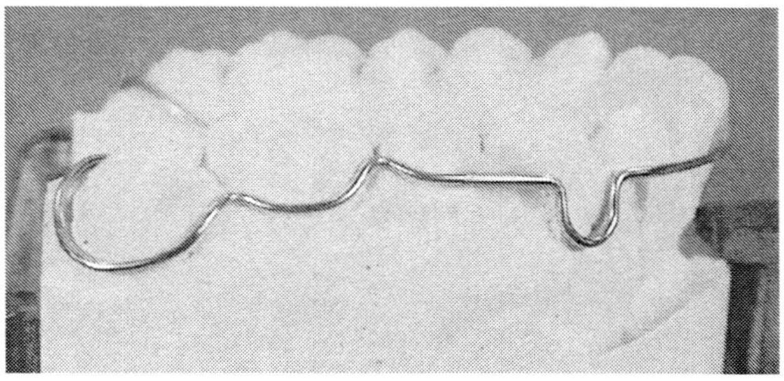

Fig 6.24 Circumferential arch

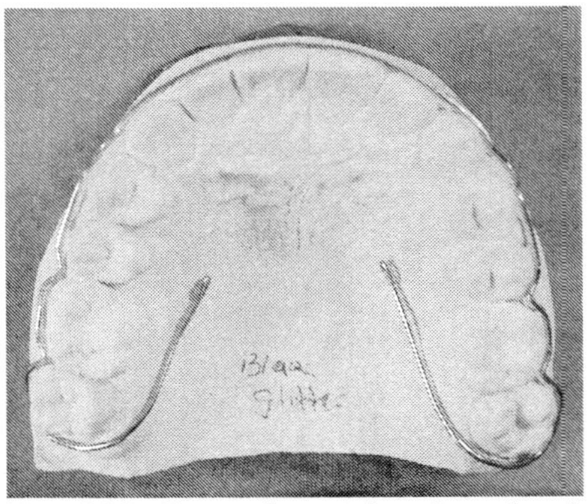

Fig. 6.25 Circumferential arch occlusal view

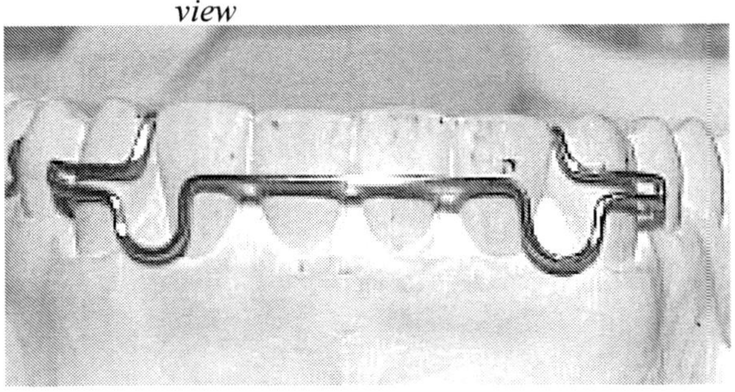

Fig 6.26 Ricketts arch, labial view

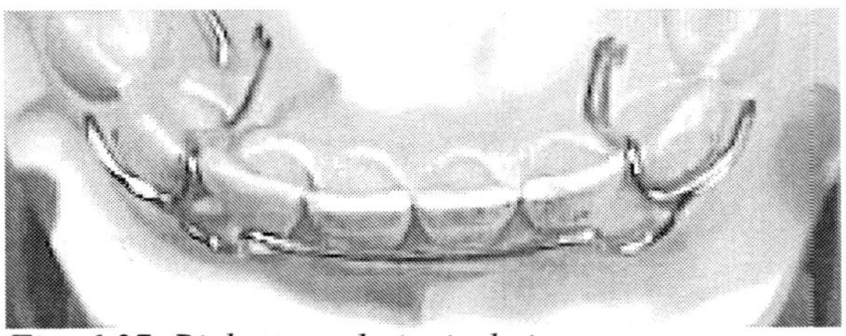

Fig. 6.27 Ricketts arch, incisal view

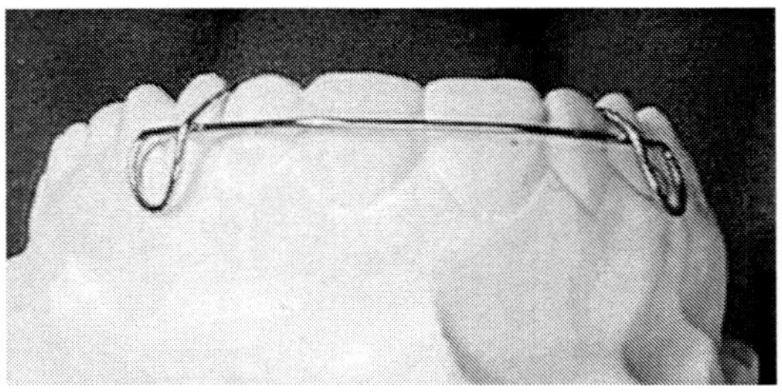

Fig 6.28 Reverse Wilson loop

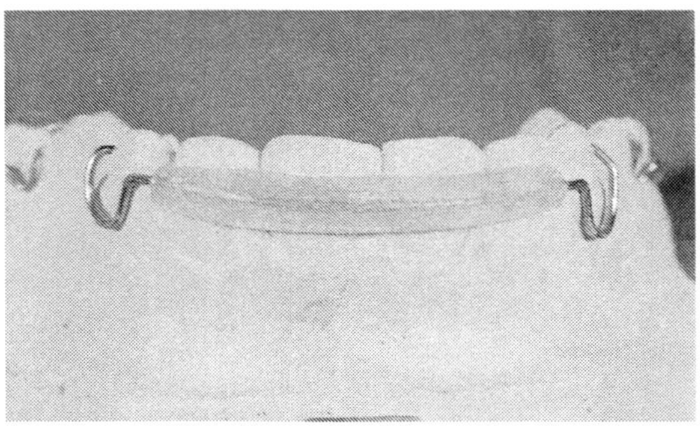

Fig. 6.29 Acrylic arch

of the arch itself.

The arch is bent the same as the soldered until the distal of the 2nd bicuspid, at this point the wire is angled into the interdental embrasure to contact the mesioproximal of the 1st molar. The wire then is contoured to the 1st molar just above the gingival margin. If the second molar is present it is treated in the same manner as the first. The wire is bent into the palate at the distal of the most posterior tooth on each side of the arch. A retentive tag is formed to provide retention to the acrylic.

Ricketts Arch

The Ricketts arch is similar to the 3x3 Hawley arch.

The differences lie in the position of the Wilson loop, which is placed on the lateral, and a recurving arm on the cuspid. The cuspid arm can be used to gain extra retention for the appliance or as a spring to control the cuspids. The occlusal portion of the spring arm should be at the level of the labial arch wire and the gingival portion of the spring arm slightly gingival to the arch wire.

The tags of the Ricketts arch pass through the embrasure interproximal to the laterals and cuspids.

Reverse Wilson loop

The reverse Wilson loop is similar to the 3x3 Hawley arch, but with the Wilson loop coming from the distal to mesial. This arch is used when control of the cuspid is needed, particularly if the cuspid has been rotated.

Acrylic arch

The acrylic arch is similar to the labial arch of a spring retainer. It is a Hawley arch — either 3x3 or soldered — which is bent to lay slightly off the buccal surface of the teeth. During sprinkling of the acrylic the arch is covered from 2-2 or mesial of 3 to mesial of 3. This provides a tightly conforming surface on the labial of the anteriors that discourages movement, particularly rotation, of the teeth. The acrylic is bevelled occlusally and gingivally to provide a smooth, non-irritating surface to the lip.

A labially malpositioned tooth can be cut from the model and repositioned before the arch is bent. When finished the arch will act as a spring to pull this tooth in the position it was placed on the model. When used in this manner the arch should be bent with 0.5 mm wire if 3x3, and 0.7 mm wire if soldered.

Spring arch (Roberts retractor)

This arch is similar to the Hawley arch with the addition of a helix bent into the Wilson loops. This is used to retract the anteriors. As with any retracting arch, the arch should be bent to an idealized arch form to represent the final contour of the labial surfaces of the teeth.

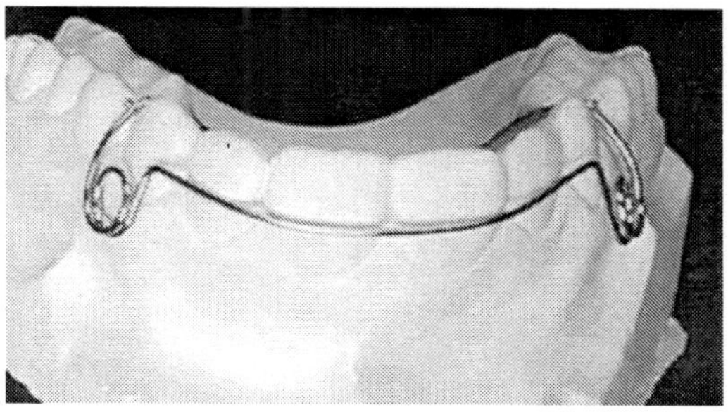

Fig. 6.30 Roberts retracting arch

High labial arch

The high labial arch is an arch wire which is bent into the labial vestibule rather than across the labial of the teeth. The high labial is used when teeth are to be lingualized, it is not used as a retaining arch.

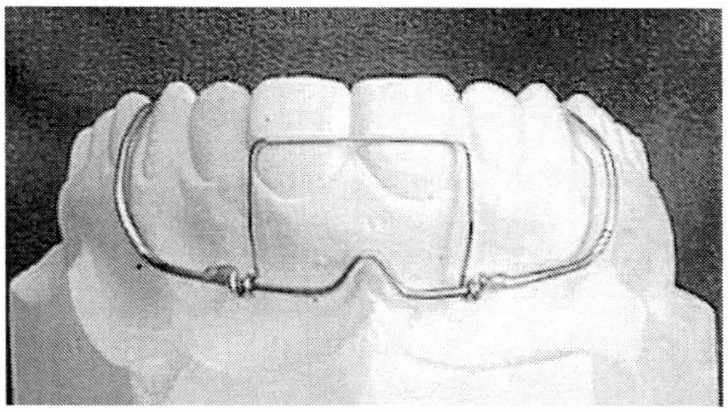

Fig. 6.31 High labial arch with apron spring

Springs called apron springs are soldered onto the wire which come over the labial of the teeth to be moved from the gingival and act to retract the teeth. An apron spring can act on one tooth or a number of teeth (see *apron spring* for bending instructions).

When bending a high labial arch, relief must be provided in the arch wire for the labial frenum. Start bending by forming a 30° angle that will fit over the labial frenum, then contour the wire to the tissue (with 1 mm relief) to the area cervical to the cuspids. The wire is then curved occlusally and bent to pass through the cuspid/1st bicuspid embrasure.

Contoured

This is a Hawley arch that is contoured to fit precisely about the labial surfaces of the teeth. It may be of a 3x3 design or a circumferential. This arch gives maximum control of the teeth with a wire arch.

Posterior bite pads and anterior bite planes

Any region of the acrylic plate which is designed to occlude with the opposing teeth is a *bite plane*. A bite plane can be in the posterior or anterior. A posterior bite plane is know as *posterior bite pads (PBP)* and are used in pairs on both sides of the arch. A PBP can be used on the maxilla or mandible. An anterior bite plane can be placed only on the maxillary arch.

Bite planes are used to change the occlusion of the patient during treatment. They provide an artificial occlusal surface that "opens the bite" or increases the vertical dimension of occlusion.

In active appliances bite planes can be used to:

- allow teeth in crossbite to cross the occlusion,
- allow posterior teeth to erupt (anterior bite plane),
- assist in a mild repositioning of the mandible (anterior bite plane),
- add to retention by seating the appliance during function (PBP).

TMJ therapies often use splints with full arch bite planes to relieve pain during treatment. TMJ splints will be discussed in the section on *splints and niteguards*.

Posterior bite pads (PBP)

Posterior bite pads are an acrylic covering of the occlusal surfaces of the posterior teeth in either arch. They can be used to: open the bite to free an anterior which is in crossbite, eliminate posterior cuspal interference during arch expansion, and help to make an active appliance more effective by seating the appliance firmly every time the bite pads contact the opposing.

They extend from the mesial of the first bicuspid to the most posterior tooth in the arch. All teeth in the arch must be covered to prevent unwanted eruption of any uncovered tooth. They occlude with all teeth on the opposing arch, at least one cusp of each opposing tooth must be in contact with the bite pad. It is possible to cover only a portion of the most posterior tooth — at least the mesial cusps — provided all opposing teeth have a surface to occlude against.

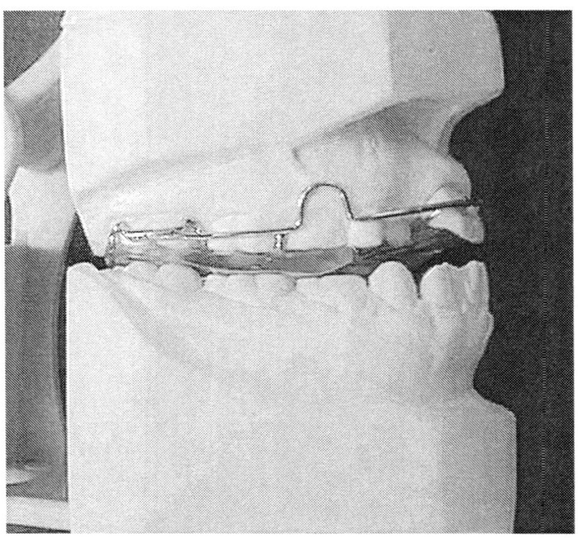

Fig. 6.32 Posterior bite pads in occlusion

Opposing models are essential for the fabrication of posterior bite pads. Ideally a bite should be supplied which is taken at the proper vertical opening, the thicker the bite pads are to be, the more important is this point. A wide opening performed on the articulator is never as accurate as a bite.

The occlusal surface of the bite pads can be smooth or finished with slight depressions for the centric cusps (indexing). A smooth bite pad allows the surface to slide over the opposing posteriors, essential when the arch is being expanded. Indexing allows the bite pads to provide positive positioning of the opposing teeth, stabilizing the position of the mandible on the appliance. A combination of these is used when you wish one quadrant to be moved and the other to act as anchorage, as in a saggital or unilateral expansion appliance.

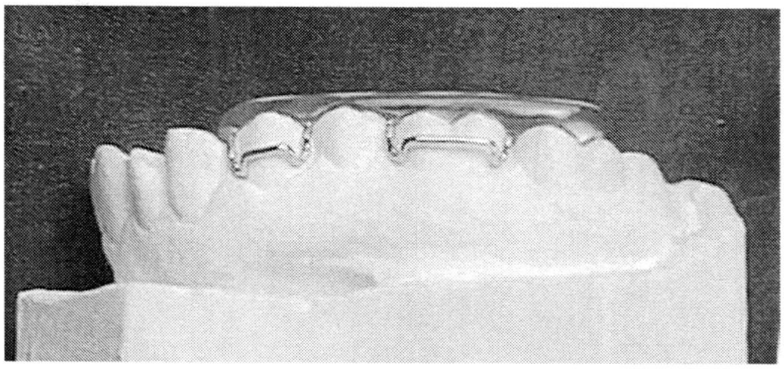

Fig. 6.33 Posterior bite pads, note smooth occlusal surface finished at buccal occlusal line angle

The buccal margin of posterior bite pads may be finished in either of two ways. The acrylic can be ended at the buccal-occlusal line angle of the posterior teeth, or it can be carried 2 mm gingivally over the buccal surface. When the bite pad is extended to the buccal surface it should be scalloped to match the buccal contours of the teeth, rather than being left straight. This is more esthetic, as well as more comfortable for the patient.

Anterior bite plane

The anterior bite plane is a flat plane of acrylic to the lingual of the maxillary anteriors which contacts the incisal edges of the mandibular incisors. The anterior bite plane can be placed only on the maxillary. It is used to provide an open bite in the posterior, for teeth in crossbite to pass over one another, or to allow posterior eruption to decrease anterior overbite.

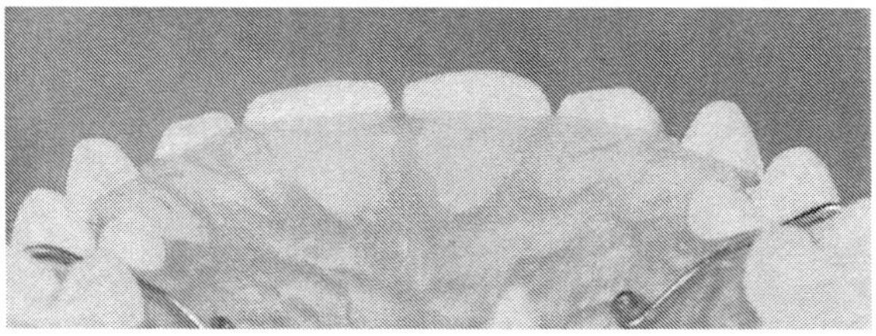

Fig 6.34 Anterior bite plane

The bite plane extends from the lingual of the 1.3 to the lingual of the 2.3. It should be flat and smooth contacting all teeth, approximately parallel to the occlusal plane. The bite plane must not slant down (palatally) toward the lingual. This could cause the mandible to be forced to the posterior. It must have sufficient lingual width that the lower anteriors are not able to bite lingual to the bite plane.

The anterior bite plane can be used in conjunction with full bracketing to *"release the occlusion"*, eliminating occlusal interferences to movement. This is a simple appliance consisting of an acrylic plate, two ball clasps, and an anterior bite plate.

The anterior bite plane can also be made with an acrylic "cap" over the incisals of the maxillary anteriors. This acts to stabilize the teeth and the appliance.

Anterior inclined bite plane (Sved bite plate)

This bite plane is similar to the simple anterior bite plane excepting that it has a distinct angle sloping from lingual to labial. This causes the mandibular to be drawn anteriorly when the mandibular incisors contact the inclined plane. This can result in a slight anterior repositioning of the mandible. Again the inclined bite plane must have enough labio-lingual width that the patient cannot rest the mandible behind it.

The inclined bite plane can also have a flaring effect on the lower incisors, tilting them to the labial.

Active components for tooth movement

Tooth movement

Some of the components that were discussed in the previous section can be activated to provide tooth movement, particularly the arches. The movements produced by these components tend to be relatively straight forward; an arch will invariably lingualize the teeth. Springs, elastics and other such components are not so simple. The forces generated and directed by these must be considered in order for us to make proper use of them.

We have previously looked at the basics of the biological reaction to tooth movement, now we can look at what the forces are that move the tooth and how they interact.

We tend to think of a tooth being stable as if it were set into concrete. This is not the case. A tooth's position is dictated by the combination of external forces that act upon it. If these forces are not in a static balance, the tooth will not maintain its position.

Static balance can be thought of as the effects of all forces on the tooth cancelling each

Anchorage

"Throw out the anchor!!" The image of stalwart sailors, heaving out a massive anchor to hold their ship from smashing on the rocks, always springs to my mind when I talk about anchorage.

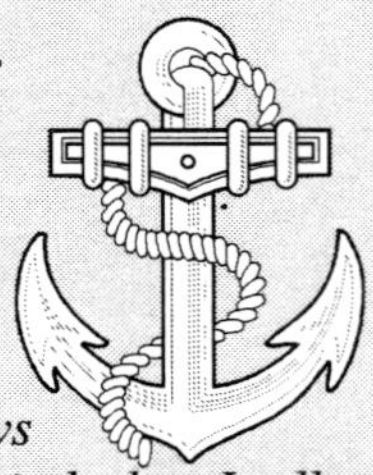

Anchorage can be thought of as a holding force. When we push (or pull) on a tooth with an orthodontic force, we need to have a stable anchorage point to push from. The force of the push must come from somewhere, it cannot exist in a vacuum of nonattachment. If there is no point to push from the force simply dissipates. So we anchor the force. We tie the wire into a bracket on other teeth, or we use an acrylic plate and hold it in with clasps. Now we have somewhere to push from, generally other teeth in the mouth.

But just as with the ship, our

anchorage must be strong enough to hold us.
When we exert a force on a tooth, an equal force is always placed on the appliance in the opposite direction. This means that the force that can move the tooth that we want moved can also move our anchor teeth. If we use two teeth with equal root surface area, the one we want moved and the one for anchorage, they will both move the same amount.
The solution in this case is simple, increase the root surface of the anchor — use more teeth. So to move one tooth, anchor with four teeth. But remember that it is the root surface area that is important. If you want to move a lower first molar (large root surface area) and you anchor it against the four lower incisors (small root surface area) which will move? Most likely both, and that is not what you want. Actually all the teeth involved in an orthodontic treatment will move to some degree, the trick is to have the anchor teeth move as little as possible.
Another type of anchorage is called reciprocal anchorage, *this is when we want both sides to move — such as a midpalatine expansion appliance.*
Sometimes we need to place a force on all of the teeth in the mouth, or the teeth just aren't enough anchorage for what we need. Then we need to look outside of the mouth for our anchorage. Extraoral anchorage uses the skull as our anchor point. Facebows bring our attachment point outside the mouth, and headgear provides anchorage against the skull.

other. A simple example is the lingualizing pressure exerted by the buccinator muscle of the cheek being balanced by the buccalizing pressure of the tongue.

Orthodontic movement is accomplished when we disrupt this balance, by either introducing a force or reducing a force. Activating a spring can be an example of adding a force, and some functional appliances can be used to eliminate forces.

Force on the tooth

Let's look at a spring placed on the lingual of an upper central, parallel to the occlusal plane. The lingual of the tooth has a forward and downward slant in relation to the spring — let's say 45° — which makes it act as an inclined plane. When we activate the spring, the force which is parallel to the occlusal plane is deflected. It pushes partly in the direction of its action, forward (labially), and partly up (gingivally) the slope of the tooth. At a 45° angle these two actions will be equal. The tooth would move labially and be intruded if the spring were set in concrete.

Now let's remember the law of action and reaction; Newton's Third Law says for every action there is an equal but opposite reaction. Therefore, for every force on the tooth there is an equal and opposite force on the appliance. The force pushing forward on the tooth, pushes back on the appliance and the force acting gingivally on the tooth pushes the appliance occlusally. The appliance will be moved away from the tooth and the spring can slide down the lingual of the tooth losing its effectiveness.

These forces are the reasons for the anchorage of the appliance. Anchorage of the appliance avoids displacement, and prevents movement of teeth that should stay still.

It is important that we place a spring so that its forces are as close to 90° to the long axis as possible. This directs the forces generated by the spring into the tooth in the most efficient manner. Less force is lost through misdirection.

Lastly, to complicate matters further, the direction of force a spring exerts on any single tooth is at 90° to the point at which the spring contacts the tooth. We can never bend a spring to contact the entire surface of a tooth when it is activated; only one point of the wire is really in contact at any time. This is useful when we wish to rotate a tooth, but something to be aware of when we don't.

Springs

A spring is a resilient wire that can be deformed to place a force on a tooth or group of teeth, with the objective of repositioning them then. Springs move teeth with a tipping action, the higher the spring toward the incisal, the greater the tipping. They can be placed to the lingual or facial of the teeth being moved and used on either fixed or removable appliances. Virtually any wire can be bent with a helix or loop or even left straight to form a spring, as long as it exerts a force on a tooth and the tooth has somewhere to move.

The wire temper that is used for springs can vary by practitioner. "Spring hard" temper wire is a harder temper that is designed to be used for springs (good name, right). Some technicians and doctors prefer to use the softer "hard" wire and rely on work hardening to increase the temper. The argument for hard wire is that it can be adjusted more with less fear of breakage. Springs can be constructed using wires from .3 mm (.012") to .7 mm (.028") depending on the purpose and length of the spring. The longer a spring is the more flexible it is and the more gently it releases its force.

The use of springs on removable appliances will be discussed here. Springs on fixed appliances are covered in the section on those appliances.

Lingual springs

Lingual springs are placed to the lingual of the teeth being moved. On removable appliances these springs are anchored in the acrylic plate. Lingual springs can move the teeth either labially or mesial/distally.

A spring needs an arch

When used to move a tooth labially, a spring should always be used in conjunction with a labial arch. If this is not done, there is the possibility that the spring may push the tooth past its intended corrected position — patients have been known to adjust their springs themselves. The labial arch acts as a stop to ensure that the tooth does not move farther than is acceptable. It can also act as a rotation point when correcting a rotated tooth. In this situation, the arch is bent to the labial of the tooth so that it rests where the labial surface of the tooth will be in its corrected position. If the arch is not bent off of the tooth, the tooth will not move.

Basic z-spring

One of the simplest and most commonly used springs is the z-spring. The z-spring derives its name from its form. The active portion of the spring closely resembles a "z", the top being the active arm contacting the tooth, and the bottom leading to the retentive tag of the spring. The active arm or free arm of the spring is the longest arm, with each successive arm becoming slightly shorter. This gives the spring a somewhat triangular appearance when viewed from the occlusal. The z-spring may consist of two or three arms.

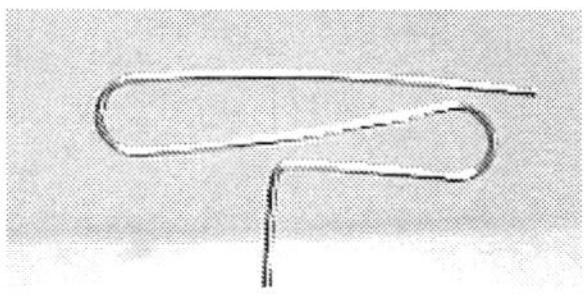

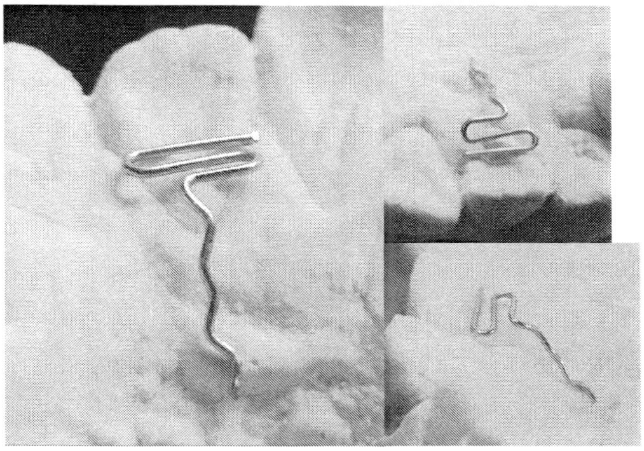

Fig. 6.36 Z-spring from various angles. Note the springs orientation to the tooth, particularly the long axis

The action of the force of a z-spring is approximately perpendicular to the long axis of the arms, depending upon how it is activated.

The spring is placed on an anterior tooth just occlusal to the cingulum, where there is a wide flat surface of the tooth for the spring to work against. This gives the dentist more control of the movement of the tooth. The spring should not be raised any higher than absolutely necessary. The closer the spring is to the incisal of the tooth the more the spring will act in a tipping manner.

On the horizontal plane the active position of the spring should meet the tooth at 90° to the long axis of the tooth. In other words, the lingual end of the active portion of the spring should be placed slightly more occlusally than the active arm that is contacting the tooth. This ensures that the forces generated by the spring will be acting on the tooth rather than just displacing the appliance and dissipating themselves. The tag of the spring is bent down and contoured to the palate.

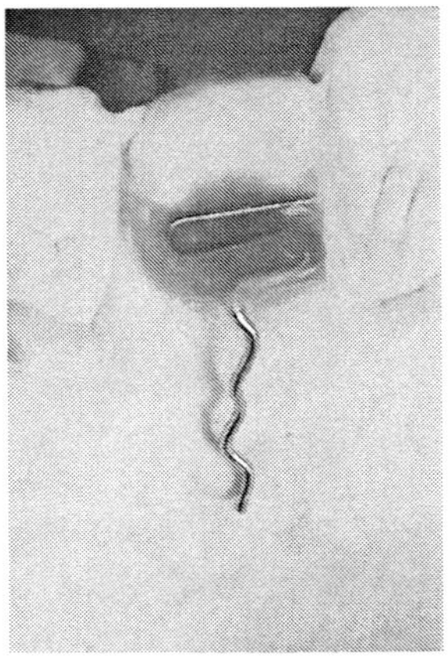

Fig 6.37 Area gingival to spring is blocked out with wax

The area gingival to the active arm of the spring is blocked out with wax. This is done so that when the acrylic is sprinkled on the appliance, the spring will not be encased in acrylic. After the acrylic has cured, the wax is cleaned out freeing the spring for movement. Ensure that there is no acrylic in front of the spring to interfere with its movement.

Double helix spring

The double helix spring is similar to and performs the same function as the z-spring. The difference between the two is the inclusion of two circular helixes at the ends of the arms of the double helix spring (hence the name). The helixes increase the length of wire in the spring, giving it a longer and more gentle range of action.

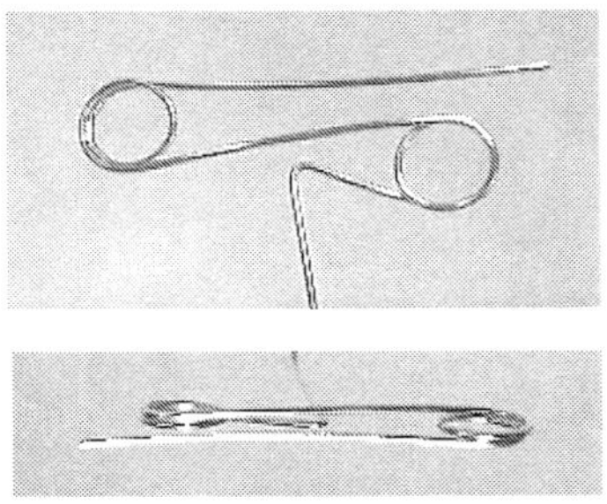

Fig. 6.38 Double helix spring, incisal and labial views. Note the free arm in labial view is towards gingiva

The helixes of the spring are formed so that they turn in opposite directions. The first helix winds towards the occlusal and the second helix winds towards the gingival, giving the spring an overall flat profile. The free arm of the spring is always placed to the gingival against the tooth.

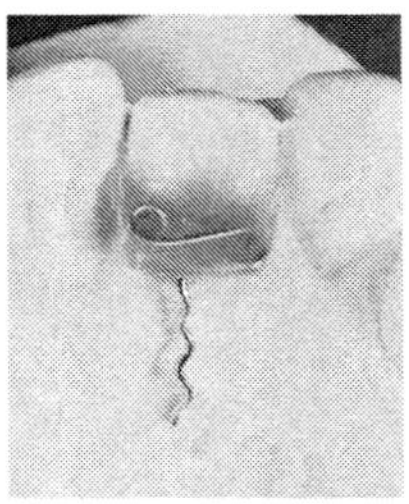

Fig. 6.39 Double helix spring blocked out for acrylic

Sweep spring (kick-back)

This spring is used to move a tooth mesially or distally along the arch. There must be a separate spring for each tooth being moved and the springs must be activated to move the teeth one at a time.

The sweep spring contacts the proximal of the tooth on the opposite side to the desired movement; the arm may continue over to the buccal surface of the tooth. The spring follows along the palate 5-8 mm, then forms a helix. The helix must be placed at least in the center of the tooth being moved to achieve effective activation. The helix is bent to unwind as the tooth moves, and is positioned parallel to the palatal tissue.

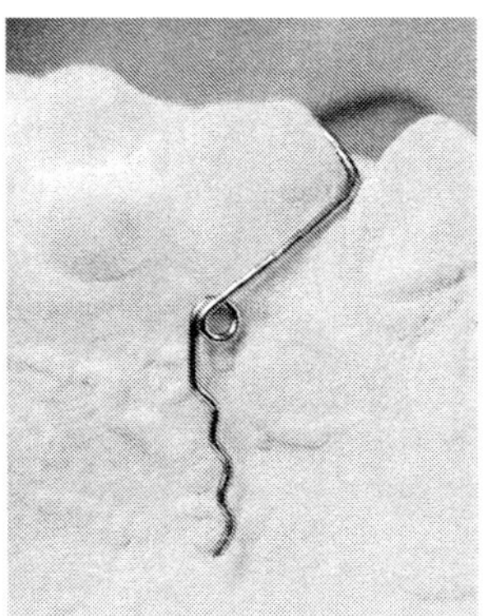

Fig. 6.40 Spring to move cuspid distally

The acrylic lingual to the tooth being moved must

be trimmed as not to interfere with the tooth movement. Trimming it straight will help it serve as a guide for the tooth. A guard may be made for the spring from a long tag or a separate piece of wire. The guard is to ensure that the spring is not deflected into the patient's tissue. It is placed gingival to the active arm, containing the spring between it and the acrylic to the occlusal.

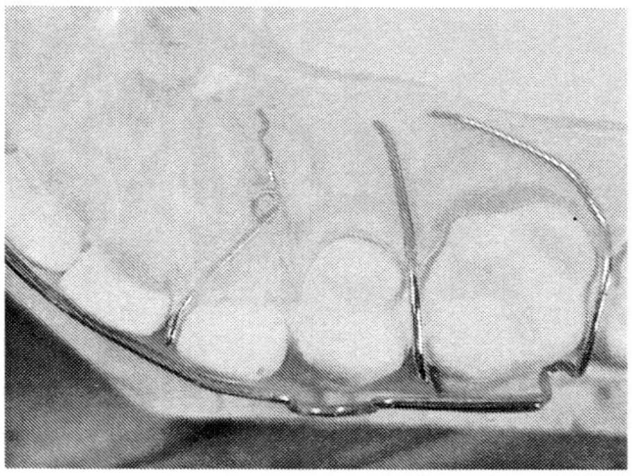

Fig 6.41 Spring to move bicuspid distally. Note how the acrylic is trimmed to allow for movment.

Lap spring (cross over)

Lap springs are used to even out the arch form of the incisors. They move the incisors labially towards a labial arch bent to an ideal arch form. They move the laterals more than the centrals when activated, but can be adjusted or modified to correct any of the incisors. The springs are used in pairs, each half has a free arm starting at the distal of the one lateral and passing along the linguals of the incisors to the distal of the opposite lateral. The spring then loops back toward the midline; this arm extends to the distal or middle of the centrals where it bends palatally and enters the acrylic. Alternately the first arm can continue to the distal of the central where it forms a helix before entering the acrylic.

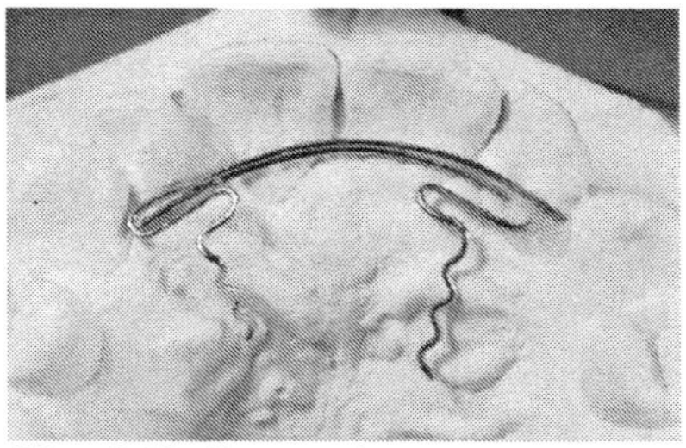

Fig. 6.42 Lap springs

Labial springs

Labial springs permit movements to the lingual as well as, to the mesial/distal. These springs exert their forces from the labial side of the tooth. Most are attached to a labial arch wire by soldering. When soldering these fine wire springs it is doubly important that the wires do not become overheated and lose their temper.

Labial finger spring

The labial finger spring can move a tooth lingually or mesial/distally. They can be used on any teeth from central to bicuspid. The spring is soldered to the arch in front of or to the opposite side to which the tooth is being moved.

The wire is brought gingivally from the arch to just below the gingival margin, then formed into a helix. The helix should open in the direction that the tooth is being moved. A simple finger spring will omit the helix.

From the helix the wire is brought occlusally on the lingual of the first

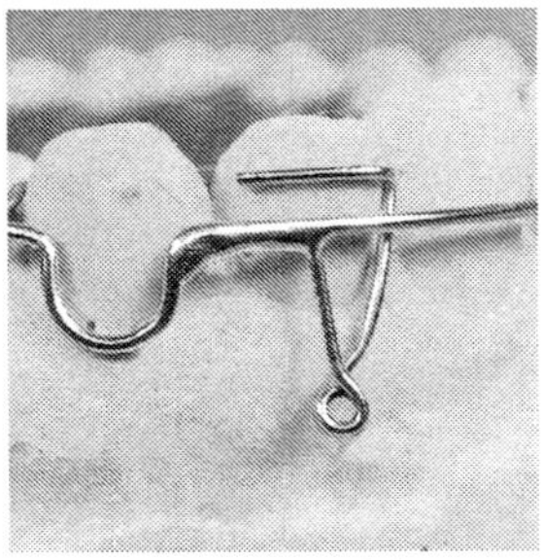

Fig. 6.43 Labial finger spring

arm (inside the arch) to the proximal side of the tooth opposite to the way the tooth is being moved. The wire should run up this proximal surface, and then curve around, fitting to the tooth, and contour across the labial surface of the tooth. This proximal and labial contact is what allows the spring to act on both lingually and mesial/distally.

Direct pressure

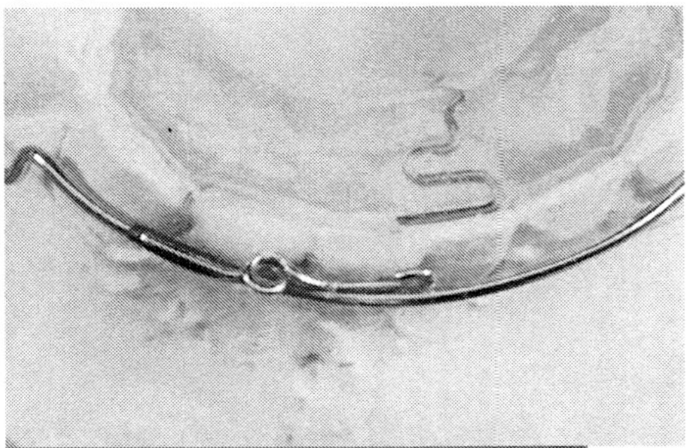

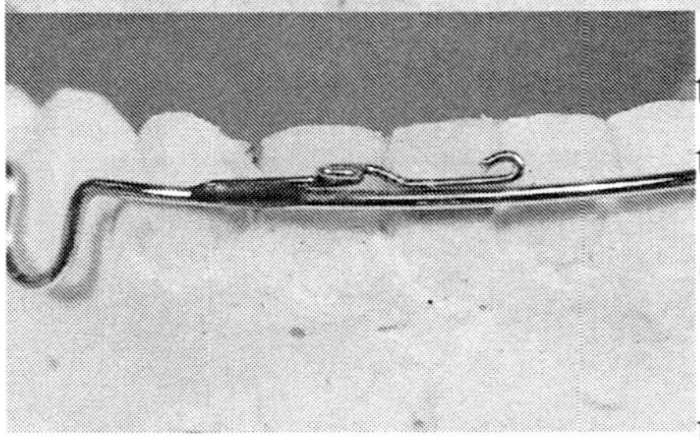

Fig. 6.44 Direct pressure springs.

The direct pressure spring is a simple lingualizing spring of 0.5 mm. It can be just a straight wire soldered parallel to the labial arch in front of the tooth to be moved, or a helix may be added to the spring. If a helix is used it should be placed in the interproximal embrasure so as not to interfere with the teeth.

Cuspid retractor spring

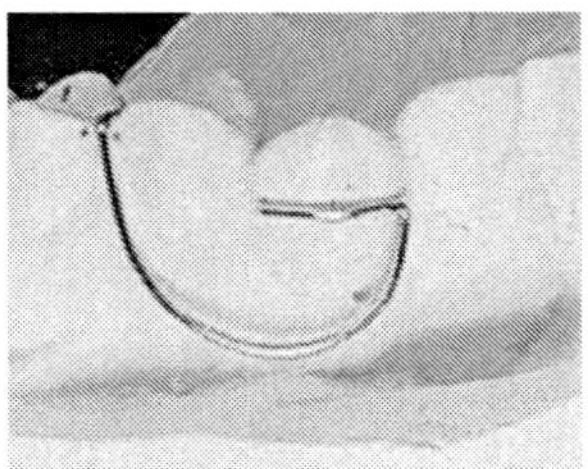

Fig. 6.45 Cuspid retractor spring

The cuspid retractor spring acts on the mesio-labial of the cuspid, even though it is anchored to the acrylic palate in most cases. The spring originates on the lingual surface and passes through either the cuspid/1st bicuspid or 1st bicuspid/2nd bicuspid embrasure. It then curves gingivally over the tissue in a wide arc, finally bending occlusally to rest on the mesiao-labial of the cuspid. The spring can also include a helix over the gingival tissue. Due to the unsupported length of the spring it is bent with 0.7 mm wire for extra rigidity. This spring can also be soldered to the bar of an Adams clasp on the first or second bicuspid.

High labial spring and apron spring

The high labial or apron spring is used with the high labial arch. This is a spring not commonly seen anymore. 0.5 mm wire is first soldered to the arch wire under the tooth to be moved. The wire is then wrapped around the arch in a tight coil using the solder as an anchor before it is brought occlusally to the tooth. It passes across the labial of the tooth and then gingivally back to the arch. The spring is again wrapped around the arch on the other side of the tooth and then the tag is soldered.

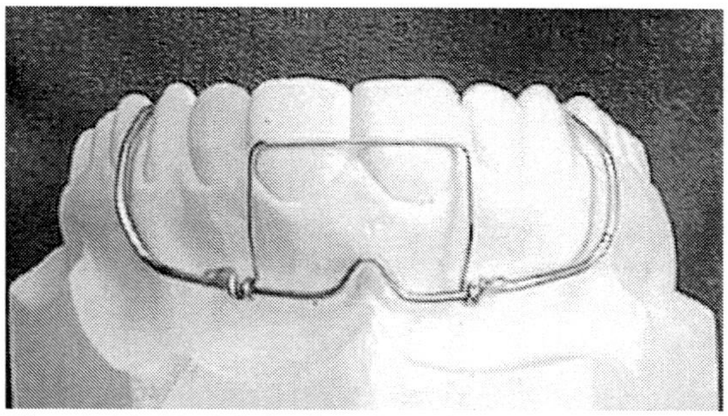

Fig. 6.46 High labial arch with apron spring

Expansion Screws

In 1902, Pierre Robin used a split plate appliance containing an expansion screw of his own design and gained 4 mm to align a central incisor. Expansion screws have since become invaluable in numerous applications.

The most common use of the expansion screw has been to create space, with it being most frequently positioned in the mid-palatal area.

Frequently, a discrepancy between the size of the teeth in the arch and the size of the arch is the reason for the crowding that the treatment is to correct. To make the teeth fit, therefore, a change must be made in either how much tooth material is in the arch, or how big the arch is. The amount of tooth material can be changed by the dentist by stripping (grinding off small amounts of the teeth interproximally) or by extraction. Arch length can be changed by widening or lengthening the arch.

Expansion screws are the most common tool used to change the arch width or length of the patient in order to relieve crowding.

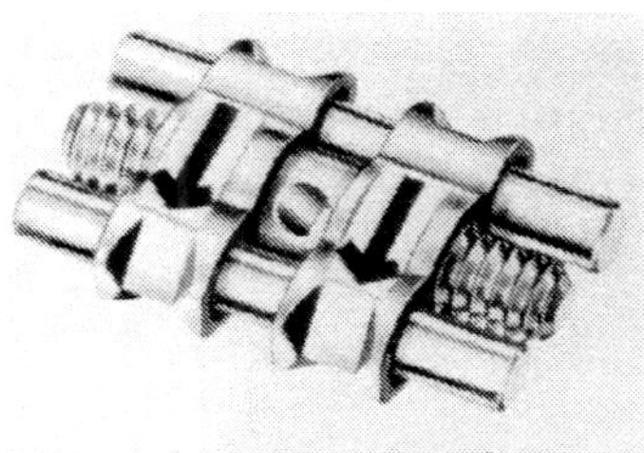

Courtesy of SNF-Forsestadent®

Fig. 6.46 Basic expansion screw

The general description of an expansion screw is, a two piece body (or housing) joined by one or two guide pins and a threaded post (screw). The threaded post has a small turnbuckle-like section in the middle which has two holes passing through its center at right angles to each other. The screw is opened by inserting a small wire key into the holes and turning the screw a ¼ turn. This moves the body housings .2-.25 mm apart, expanding the screw and the appliance of which it is a part. An arrow — usually placed on the housing — indicates the direction to turn the key in order to open the screw.

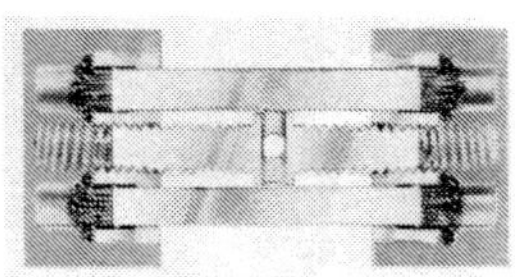

Fig. 6.47 Expansion screw opened. Courtesy of SNF-Forsestadent®

The expansion screw is embedded in an acrylic plate — containing clasps, arches, etc. — which is split to match the two halves of the screw.

NOTE: Wires on the appliance must be designed so that their tags do not cross the cut for the expansion screw.

On some designs the guide pins are a single U-shaped piece which can be

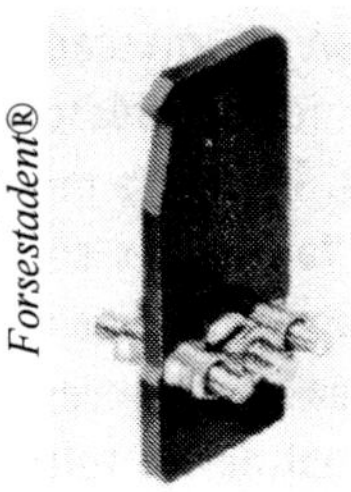

Courtesy of SNF-Forsestadent®

Fig. 6.48 Expansion screw with plastic tab

straight or curved. The curved design allows the screw to be placed closer to the anterior resulting in an appliance with less bulk.

Expansion screws also have a tab, usually plastic, which covers the turnbuckle assembly to prevent it from filling with acrylic during processing. This tab also assists in the placement of the screw on the model.

Positioning a mid-palatal expansion screw

Positioning an expansion screw on the midline to widen the arch is known as transverse expansion. To do this an expansion screw must be positioned in three dimensions: anterio-posteriorly, saggitally, and horizontally.

Anterio-posterior positioning

The screw is placed centered about a line which bisects the 2nd bicuspid/1st molar embrasure. This position can be moved slightly to the posterior in an extremely narrow arch.

Saggital positioning

The screw is centered exactly over the mid-palatine raphe. The opening between the two halves of the screw should be aligned with the midline of the patient, and the guide pins are at 90° to the midline.

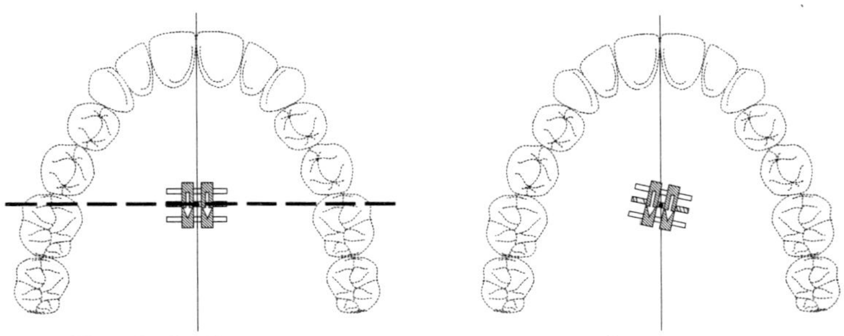

Fig. 6.49 Correct *Incorrect*

Horizontal positioning

The guide pins of the screw must be oriented parallel to the occlusal plane. This must be done exactly. If the screw is tilted in the horizontal plane, one side of the appliance will lift off of the tissue when the screw is opened.

The body of the screw should be oriented to follow the palatal surface from a lateral perspective. This helps to keep the acrylic plate from becoming ex-

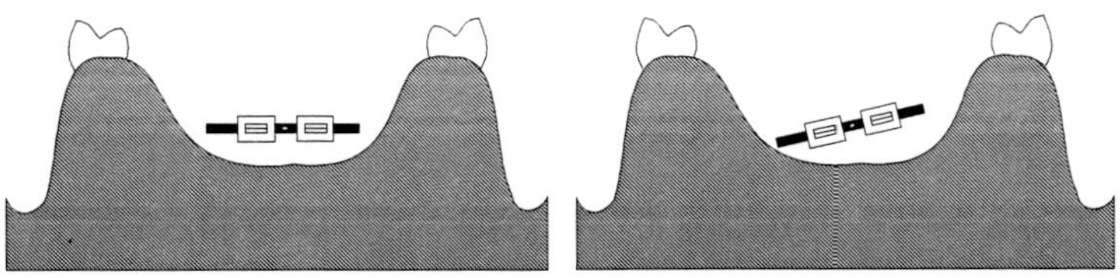

Fig. 6.50 Correct *Incorrect*

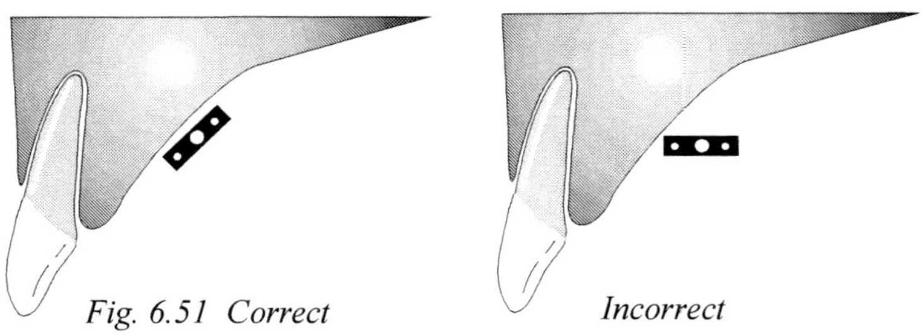

Fig. 6.51 Correct *Incorrect*

cessively thick.

Uses of expansion screws

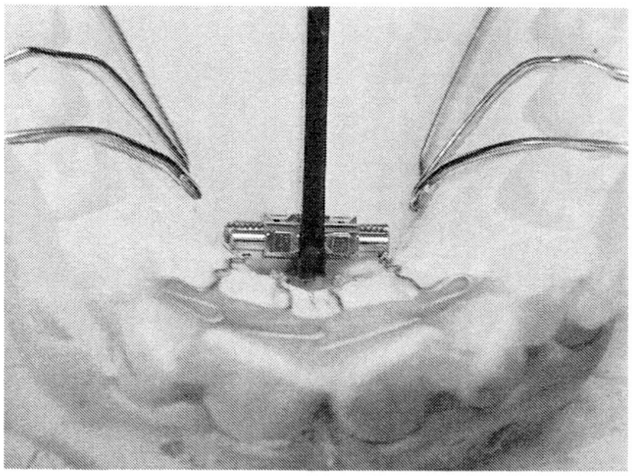

Fig. 6.52 Expansion screw on model, anterior view.

The basic expansion screw design can be put to a number of different uses. It is most commonly used to widen the palate when used from a mid palatal position.

They can also be used to move single teeth or groups of teeth facially by turning the screw 90° so that the guide pins point toward the tooth/teeth.

Saggital movement of one or both posterior segments can be accomplished with the standard expansion screw. Care must be taken in the positioning of the screws. They must follow the line of the alveolar ridge for the teeth to move posteriorly into acceptable positions. Horizontally the screw should align with the lingual gingival margin of the posterior quadrant.

Placing an expansion screw

Expansion screws can be positioned on the model using several methods. The one thing that should remain constant is that a mid-palatal screw should always be placed with the arrow facing to the posterior. The method that I prefer is to cut the plastic tab with my wire cutters, leaving about 1½ mm of plastic under the screw. The screw is then held in position on the model and a drop of wax placed on the distal of the tab where it contacts the model. The exact position of the screw can now be adjusted before the screw is fixed into place with a drop on the mesial.

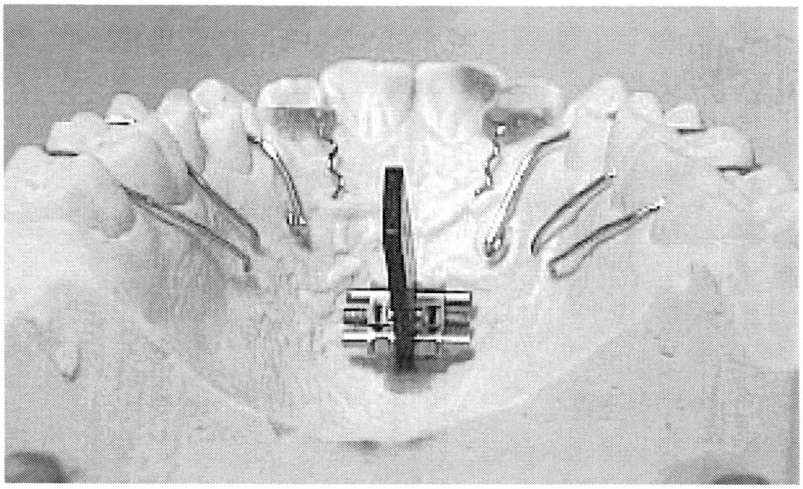

Fig. 6.53 Expansion screw fixed to model with wax

Another way to position a screw is to cut a groove into the palate of the model to accept the plastic tab, and then seal around the tab with wax.

A third method is called "freehand". This involves sprinkling a small amount of acrylic onto the palate at the beginning of processing, and then placing the screw in this pad of acrylic. I do not recommend this method as it is difficult to position the screw accurately.

When a screw is used for mid-palatal expansion, the screw should be positioned so that the arrow points to the posterior. It does not really make any difference on a removable appliance which way the arrow points, however, on one appliance, the RPE, it does. The RPE is fixed in the mouth which means that the screw must be activated inside the patient's mouth. This is difficult to do if the arrow does not point to the posterior. Therefore, we place all screws pointing this way to ensure that there can be no mixups.

Acrylic processing has some differences when expansion screws are included in an appliance. The first difference is that the screw becomes the first part of the appliance to be sprinkled. It is easy to get air trapped under a screw that will then form a bubble in the acrylic. One way to accomplish this is to premix a small amount of acrylic and run it under the screw in liquid form, or shake the powder under the screw, add monomer and then poke a small instrument or wire under the screw to release any air.

When the acrylic work is finished you must cut the acrylic palate in order that the screw can be activated. The cut should be smooth, straight and narrow. The cut must be designed to allow the screw to be opened without the sides of the cut binding.

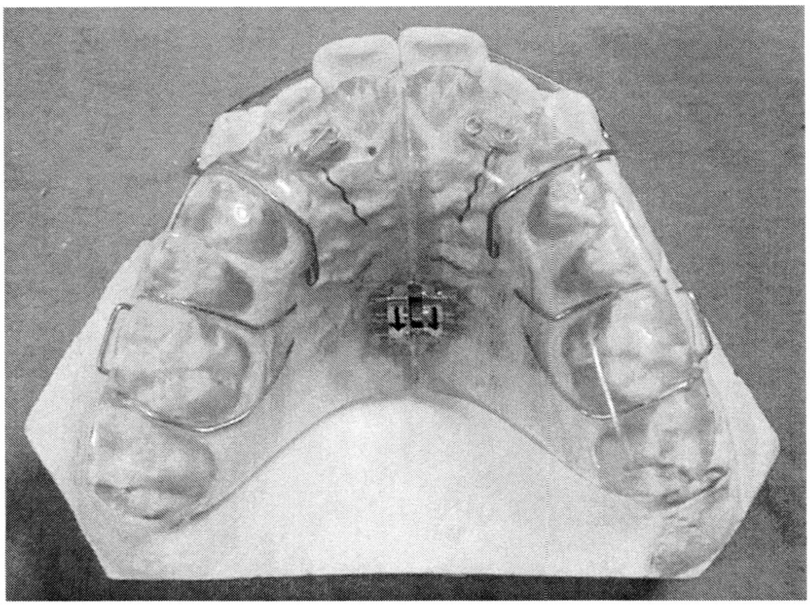

Fig. 6.54 Finished appliance with acrylic palate cut

The cut may be made with a disk or a saw.

The best type of disk to use is a steel "circular saw blade". These come in sizes from 1/4-7/8". When used in a bench lathe at slow speed these disks will make a clean and smooth cut. A separating disk will also work well, although it will tend to heat the acrylic and cause it to melt. This clogs the disk and does not give a clean cut. You must also be careful not to cut or nick any wires when using a separating disk.

When using a disk you will often find that you cannot cut all the way through the area just anterior to the screw. This can be done by pushing a thin fissure bur (700 or 701) through the tab at the mesial of the screw and then drawing it forward to meet your cut.

A hand saw can be used to make this cut, and many people prefer it. You can place the appliance on the desk and use the saw normally or brace the saw against the desk with your abdomen — blade facing up — and draw the appliance back and forth along the blade. Many people find this method gives them a straighter cut. On an appliance with a labial arch, you must detach the blade from the saw and pass the free end between the arch and the acrylic before reattaching it. Then cut toward the screw.

Types of expansion screws

Standard expansion screw (Glen Ross)

Standard expansion screws can be put to a great variety of uses. Even though there are many specialized designs available, a great many of their uses can also be meet with the standard type screw. Screws of the standard design can be obtained in sizes that will fit any design from 3 mm width to 13 mm.

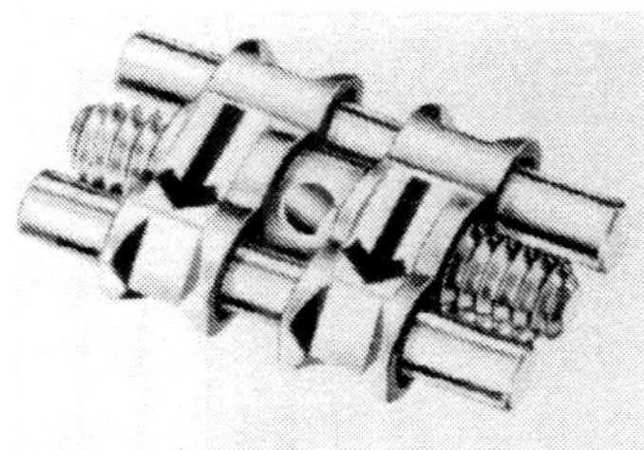

Courtesy of SNF-Forsestadent®

Fig. 6.55 Standard expansion screw

Fan screw

The fan screw is used to provide differential expansion between the anterior and posterior. The fan screw comes in one or two piece configuration. The two piece (screw and hinge) configuration has the advantage of being able to expand both the anterior and posterior segments. Specialized screws are available that allow anterior and posterior expansion of the lower arch.

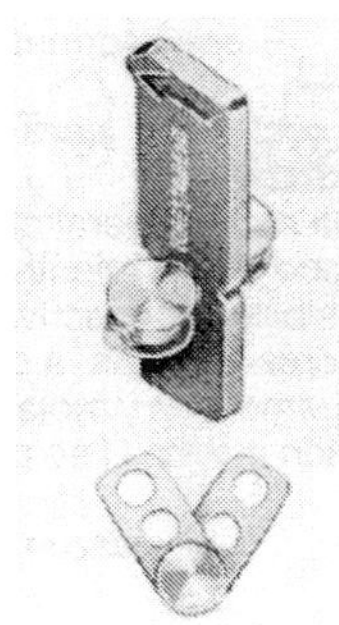

Courtesy of SNF-Forsestadent®

Fig. 6.56 Two part fan screw

3-way screw

The three way screw allows transverse expansion of the posteriors and labialization of the anteriors in a single screw. 3-way screws come in a flat configuration, as well as an anatomical configuration that reduces the appliance's thickness in the palate. These screws may be used on both upper and lower appliances, however, they are quite bulky in a lower appliance.

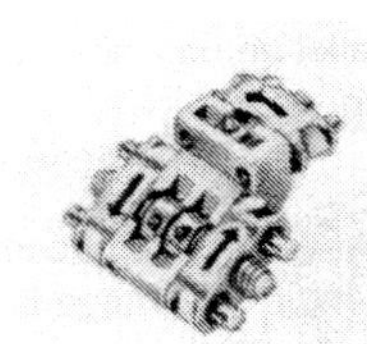

Courtesy of SNF-Forsestadent®

Fig. 6.57 3-way screw

Hyrax screw

The Hyrax screw is unusual in that it is used in a fixed banded appliance. The hyrax is soldered to bands on the 4's and 6's, although it may be used on other posterior teeth or just the 6's.

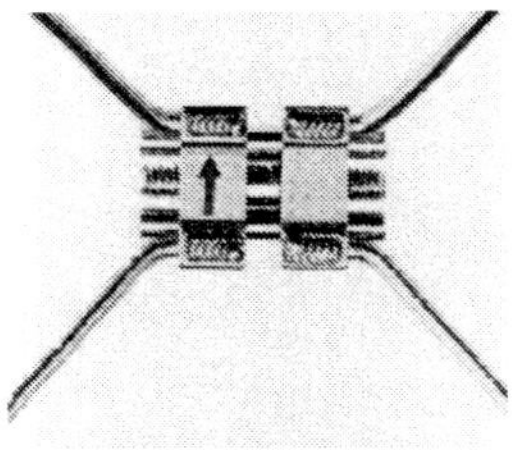

Courtesy of SNF-Forsestadent®

Fig. 6.58 Hyrax screw

The hyrax is one way to make an appliance nicknamed the "skullsplitter" formally called the RPE (Rapid Palatal Expander). The Hyrax is a large, heavily built screw with four heavy wire arms attached to the body of the screw by either solder or in some cases laser welding.

This appliance works by breaking the mid-palatine suture to expand the maxilla. This requires rapid, stable expansion of the appliance, hence the heavy design of the screw. The heavy wire arms must be bent using heavy pliers to avoid damage to your pliers.

They should be bent to allow the body of the screw to rest as high in the palate as possible for the patient's comfort. The posterior arms should contour to the distal of the 6's, with the anterior arms coming to the mesial of the 4's. Excess wire from two arms can be removed and contoured to pass along the lingual of the teeth from 4-6. This is usually easier than bending this continuously from one of the arms. The arms are then soldered solidly to the bands.

The RPE appliance will be discussed later in the appliance section.

Micro screw or piston screw

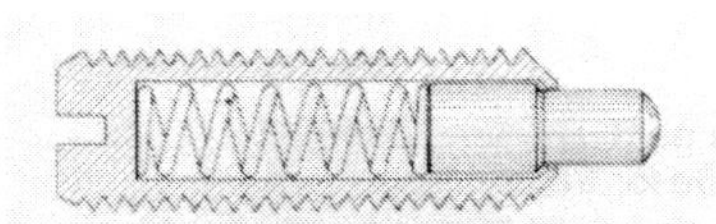

Fig. 6.59 Piston screw cutaway. Threaded housing of screw is screwed into appliance, piston is depressed against tooth and provides motive force. Courtesy of SNF-Forsestadent®

The piston screw is used for the movement of single teeth. It has a spring loaded piston inside of a threaded body. The threaded body fits into a threaded, knurled sleeve which is positioned lingual to the tooth to be moved. As the screw is threaded into the sleeve the piston compresses inside the screw. The piston then exerts force on the tooth until it reaches its rest position. The screw is then screwed in another turn to reactivate the piston. Be-

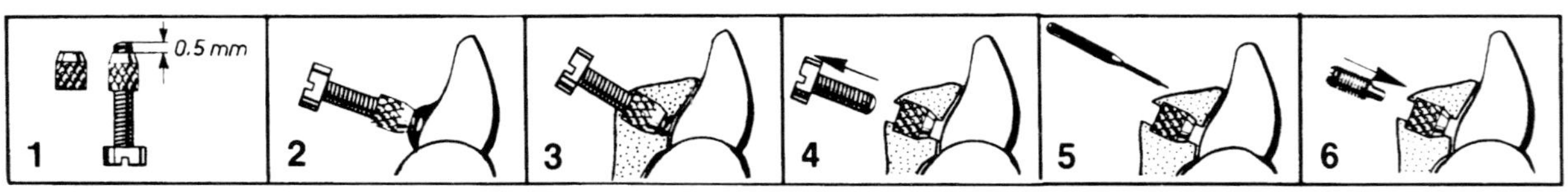

Fig. 6.60 Placement of pistion screw. 1&2) Serrated housing nut is threaded onto positioning screw and luted to model. 3&4) Acrylic is processed around housing nut, and positioning screw is removed.5&6) acrylic is finished and piston screw is treaded into housing nut. Courtesy of SNF-Forsestadent®

cause this screw exerts pinpoint pressure, it is much more accurate than a spring, particularly when used to rotate a tooth. Piston screws come in lengths of 4, 6 and 8 mm.

To insert a piston screw in an appliance, a positioning screw is threaded into the threaded sleeve and then positioned on the model with wax. The screw is adjusted to exert its force perpendicular to the long axis of the tooth. After the acrylic has been processed the positioning screw is removed and the appliance trimmed and polished. At the end of the process the piston screw is inserted into the threaded sleeve.

Molar uprighting

This screw is used to move mandibular terminal molars buccally, particularly when they are tipped lingually. The spring is a hinged lever arm with one end anchored in the acrylic plate and the other resting on a small swivel pad on the lingual of the molar. A screw in the mesial end of the appliance is turned to push this end lingually, thereby pushing the distal end buccally and the molar with it.

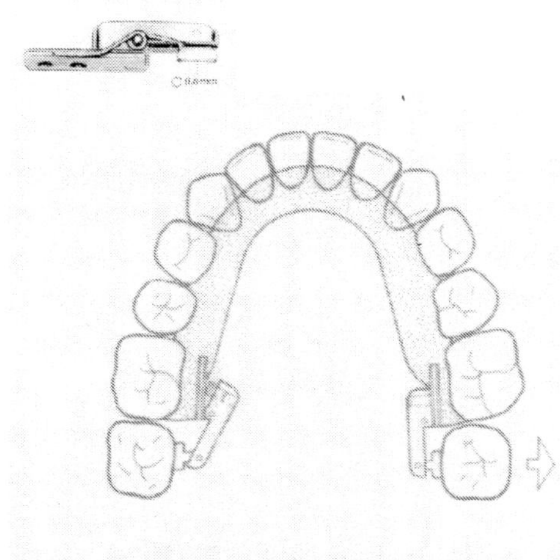

Courtesy of SNF-Forsestadent®

Fig. 6.61 Molar uprighting screw and diagram illustrating it's effect

Closing screws

Closing screws are used as a traction device to close a space. A closing screw can be made by opening a standard expansion screw using a type which has the guide pins and threaded post enclosed by the housing, and waxing out the turnbuckle; or special purpose screws may be purchased. A closing screw works exactly opposite to an expansion screw, pulling the two sections together as the screw is activated.

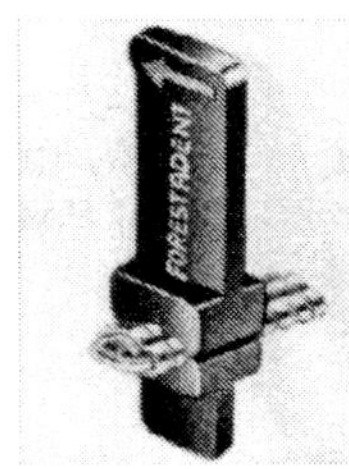

Courtesy of SNF-Forsestadent®

Fig. 6.62 Closing screw. Note thick plastic tab around screw. This provides space for the screw to close. Acrylic must have similarly wide separation.

Elastics, coil springs, hooks and lugs

Some of the other components that are used in the orthodontic laboratory are elastics, coil springs, hooks and lugs.

Elastics

Elastics are familiar to all of us from seeing them on people's braces. They are used to hold the wires into the brackets as well as, to provide motive forces.

Elastics to provide forces are supplied by manufacturers in a variety of sizes and forces. They are made of high quality latex. They come in bags of 100 which the patient changes themselves as often as directed by the dentist. The sizes range from 1/8" (3.1 mm) to 3/4" (19 mm). Elastics provide a consistent, gentle force level when stretched to approximately half of their limit.

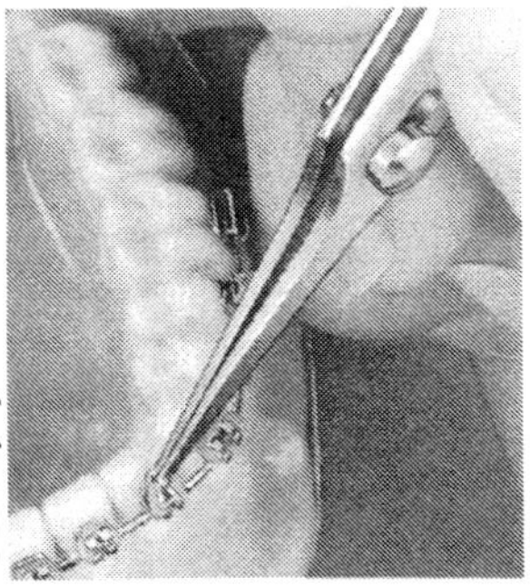

Courtesy of SNF-Forsestadent®

Fig 6.63 Placing donuts onto brackets to secure arch wire

The small, round, often coloured elastics that are used to hold the arch wires into the brackets are called *"donuts"*. They can also be called elastic ligatures. Ligatures used in orthodontics were originally made of dead soft wire that the orthodontist would twist individually around each bracket. The donuts are easier to use and more comfortable for the patients because there are no sharp ends to lacerate the inside of the cheek. In these days of infection awareness the lack of sharp ends also makes them safer for the dentist.

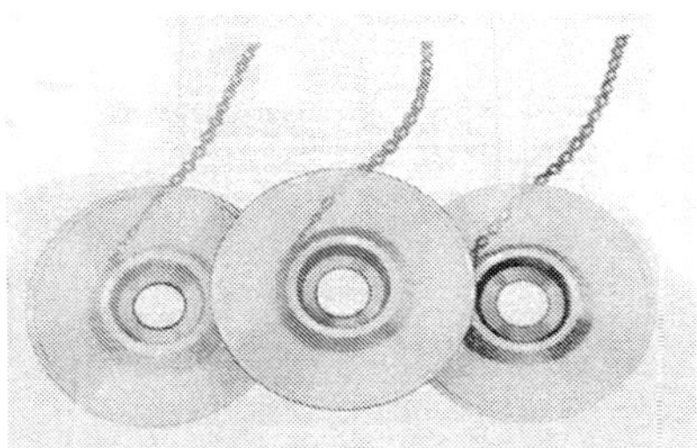

Courtesy of SNF-Forsestadent®

Fig. 6.64 Rolls of chain elastic

Another familiar elastic is the *"chain elastic"*, it is a flat ribbon of elastic that resembles an endless series of 8's linked together. The chain elastic is used hooked over brackets to close small spaces between the teeth near the end of treatment, or for hooking onto a hook/lug on a band or removable appliance.

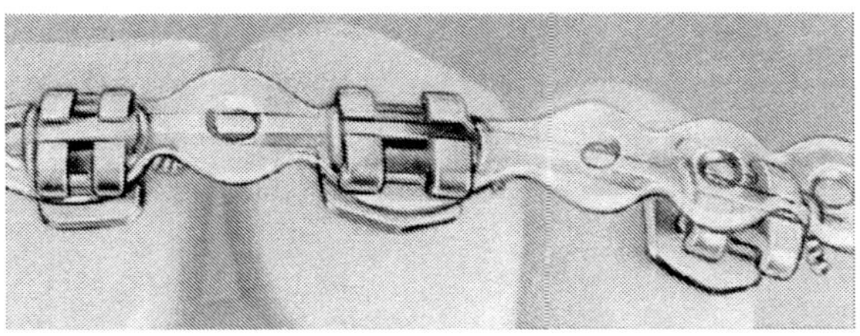

Courtesy of SNF-Forsestadent®

Fig. 6.65 Chain elastic placed on brackets to close spaces

Coil springs

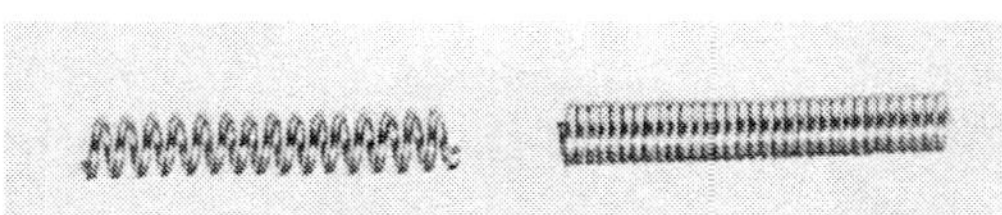

Fig. 6.66 Open and closed coil springs

Coil springs are wound, fine wire springs, that look like the closing springs on a door. They can be purchased or fabricated in the laboratory, and are measured by their inside diameter and the thickness of the wire used in the coil.

Coil springs come as open coil or closed coil.

Open coil springs have spaces between the coils which allow the spring to be compressed. This spring is used to provide a pushing force. They are usually used to open spaces between teeth.

Closed coil springs have no spaces between the coils. These springs are stretched to provide a pulling (retraction) force. They are usually used to close spaces between teeth.

Hooks and lugs

Hooks and lugs are used to provide points on the arch wire, appliance or teeth for the attachment of springs and elastics. They can be premanufactured with mesh pads for direct bonding to the teeth or placed on an arch wire. They can also be fabricated in the laboratory from wire and placed in the acrylic; then soldered to the arch or welded to a band.

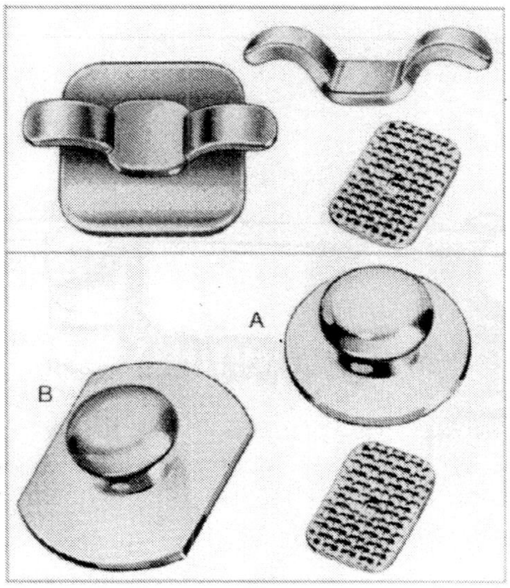

Courtesy of SNF-Forsestadent®

Fig.6.67 Cleats and buttons on mesh pads for bonding to teeth, and without pads for soldering to bands.

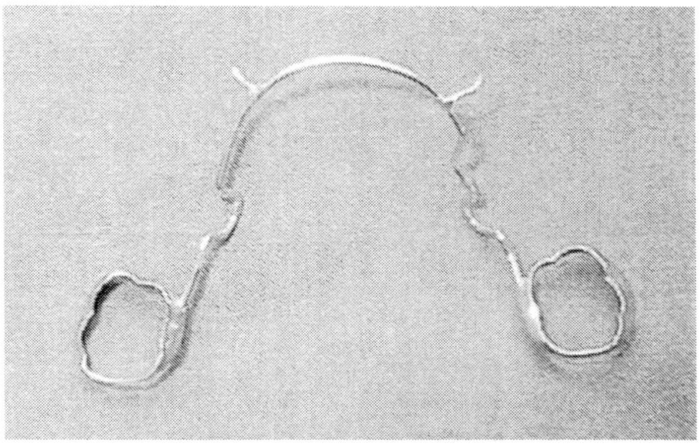

Fig. 6.68 Lingual arch with hooks or spurs to keep anterior teeth from drifting distally into edentulous space.

"Life is what happens while we're busy making other plans"
John Lennon

Experience is not what happens to a man; it is what a man does with what happens to him.
Aldous Huxley (1894 - 1963), "Texts and Pretexts", 1932

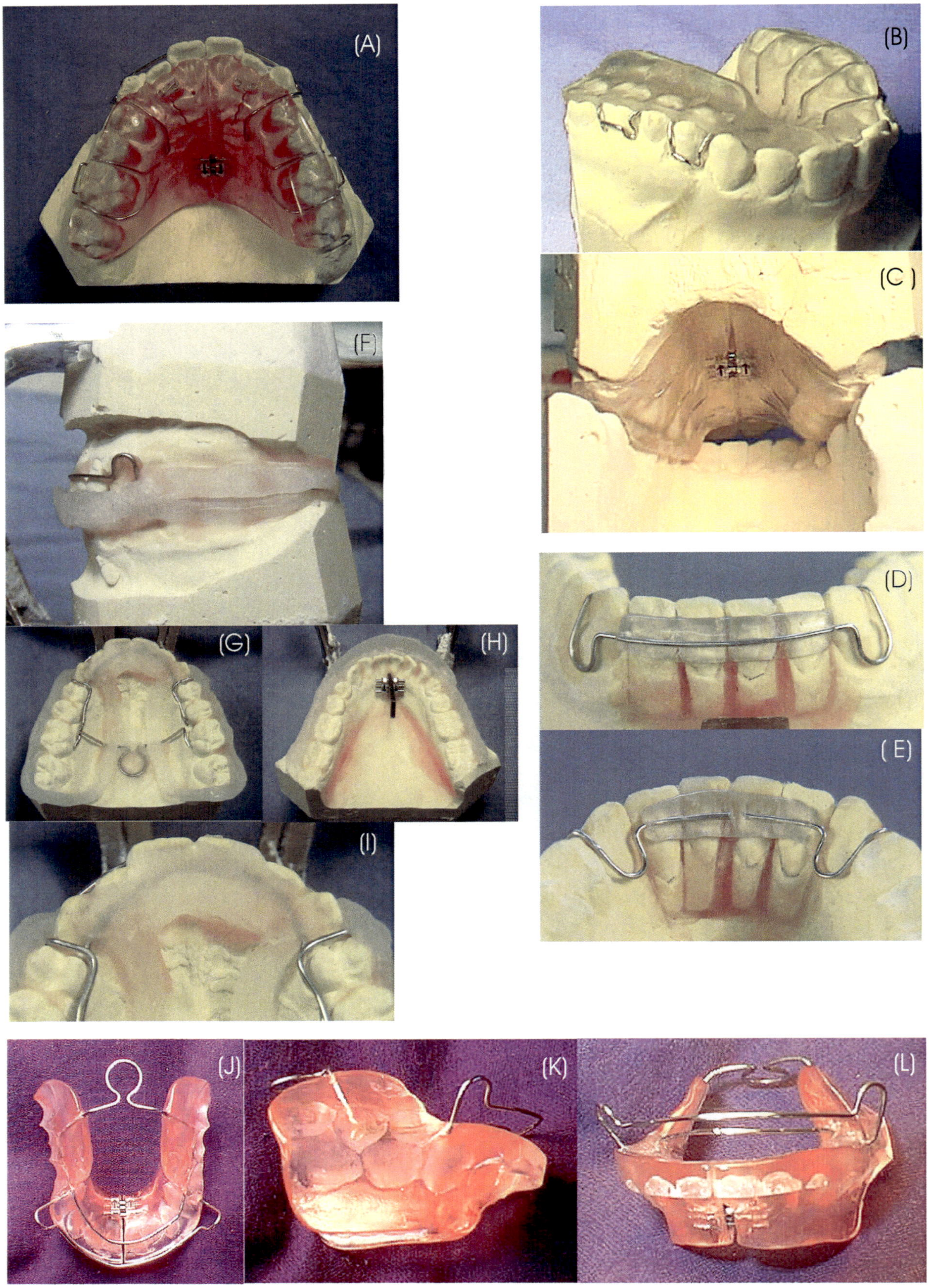

(A) Schwarz appliance. **(B&C)** Nord Appliance. **(D&E)** Spring Retainer, labial and lingual views. **(F)** Posterior waxups for bionator occlude when at correct vertical. **(G&H)** Maxillary and mandibular bionator waxups. **(I)** Smooth wax over lingual arch of bionator to form incisal cap. **(J, K, L)** Occlusal, lateral and anterior views of finished bionator.

7 Removable appliance designs

"My son, observe the postage stamp! Its usefulness depends upon its ability to stick to one thing until it gets there."
Henry Wheeler Shaw

"People forget how fast you did a job - but they remember how well you did it."
Howard Newton

Appliance designs are usually just standard components assembled to perform specific functions. Certain commonly used designs have been informally standardized, while others are described with great exactitude. Names are given to these standard designs to aid in identification and communication between dentists and laboratories, although in many cases people will modify each of these designs slightly (both fixed and removable) to fit their own needs. It has been my experience that each dentist will chose a few designs — from the multitude that exist — that work well for them and then use mainly those designs in their practice. It is a good idea when working with a new dentist or on a design which you have not fabricated for a dentist before to check that their definition of the design matches yours.

Expansion appliances

In 1938, Dr. A. M. Schwarz published a book on using active plates in orthodontic treatment. In the book were numerous designs for appliances, most referred to as *"split plates"* because of their use of the expansion screw. Many of the appliances described in the book have been modified and improved, and are still being used today.

Crossbites

Expansion appliances are used to treat crossbites and to widen the arch in order to increase arch length to reduce tooth crowding.

Most posterior quadrant crossbites are bilateral, meaning that the maxilla is smaller than the mandible evenly on both sides. Even when only one side is seen to be in crossbite, a bilateral cross bite is still usually the cause. This happens because the upper is only slightly narrower than the lower, causing the upper and lower buccal cusps to meet prematurely on closing. The lower then shifts to one side to allow full intercuspation of the teeth. This is known as a functional shift.

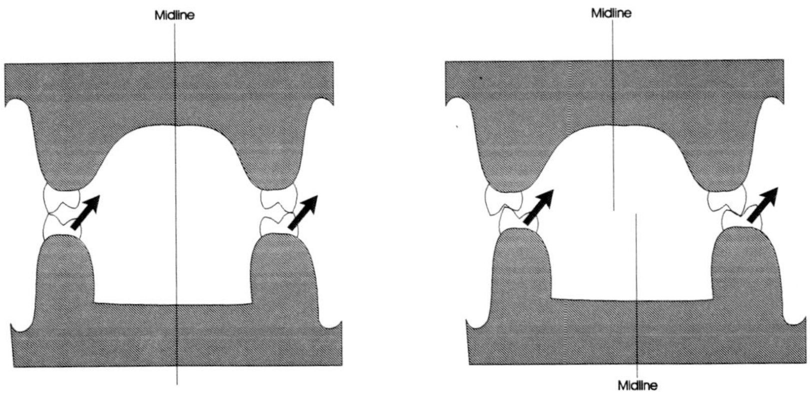

Fig. 7.1 Functional shift

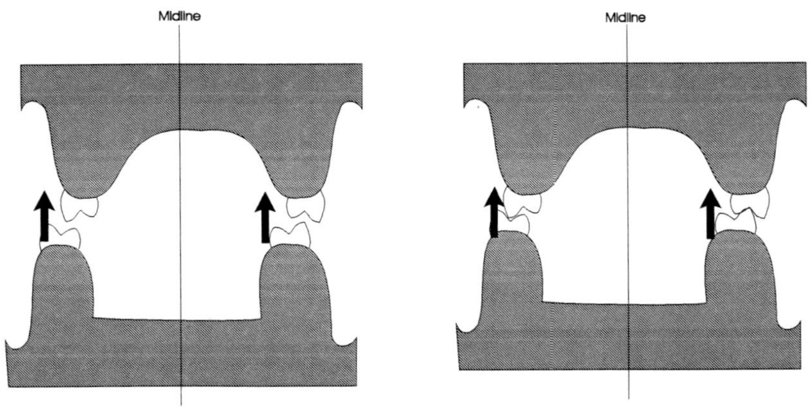

Fig. 7.2 Unilateral crossbite

A true unilateral crossbite exists when one side of the upper is narrower than the other and, therefore, its buccal cusps articulate lingual to the lower buccal cusps.

Schwarz

Dr. Schwarz included several designs in his book that used a mid-palatal expansion screw. It seems that almost any appliance with such a screw is now referred to as a Schwarz appliance. The most basic design of the Schwarz appliance includes:

- two Adams clasps, usually on the 6's
- a Hawley arch, 3x3 or soldered
- a mid-palatal expansion screw.

Some doctors and laboratories will include springs, usually 2-2 crossover springs, as part of the basic design for this appliance. Posterior bite pads may be added to free a crossbite and assist in seating the appliance during function. The usual order of fabrication is:

- Adams clasp
- Hawley arch
- springs — if needed
- position expansion screw
- acrylic.

One side effect of the Schwarz design is that when the screw is opened the Hawley arch retracts. The increase in the width of the appliance causes the arch wire to tighten across the anteriors. This can be used to retract these teeth, if so desired, however the dentist must reduce the acrylic lingual to the anteriors for them to move. If this is not done, the arch tightens across the labial surfaces until it acts as a dislodging force. It becomes a spring working against the unmovable anteriors and forces the anterior of the appliance to unseat.

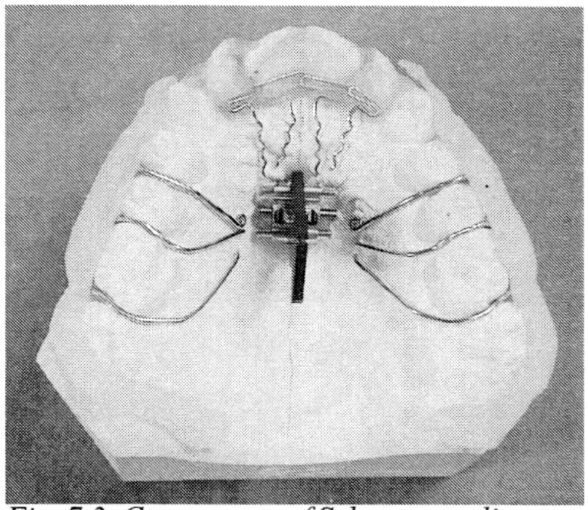

Fig. 7.3 Components of Schwarz appliance, springs may or may not be used.

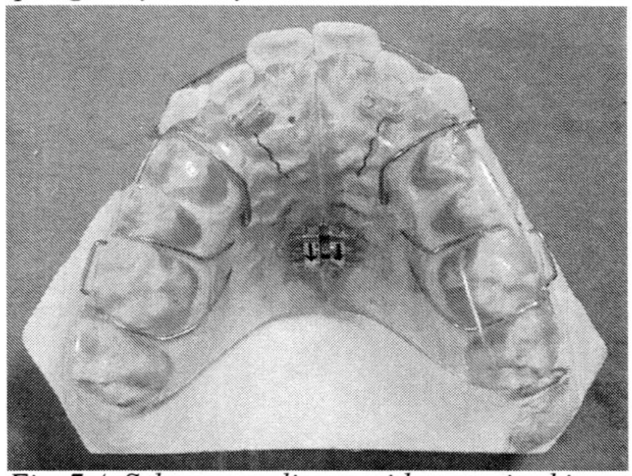

Fig. 7.4 Schwarz appliance with posterior bite pads

If the anteriors are not to be retracted, the dentist must remember to open the Wilson loops slightly once the screw is activated to avoid dislodging the appliance.

Transverse

The transverse is the simplest of the removable expansion appliances. It consists of nothing more than four clasps and an expansion screw. The clasps may be four Adams clasps, two Adams and two ball clasps, or any other combination. Posterior bite pads may be added to free a crossbite and assist in seating the appliance during function.

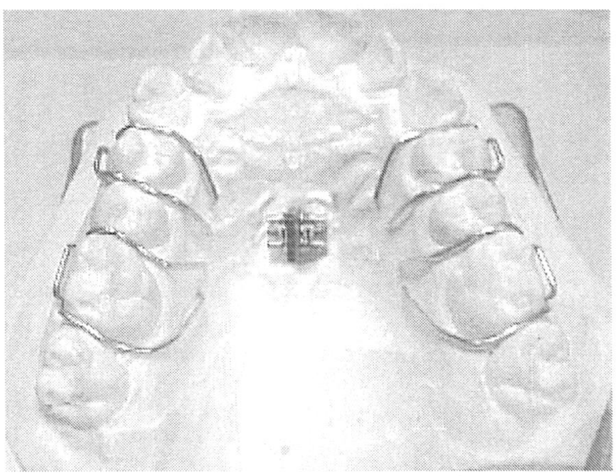

Fig. 7.5 Wire work for transverse appliance

The lack of any springs or active components, other than the screw, means that no Hawley type arch is necessary. This, and the extra clasping, ensures that the appliance stays well seated during treatment making this an effective appliance for simple arch expansion.

The usual order of fabrication is:

1) Adams clasps
2) position expansion screw
3) process acrylic.

Nord

The Nord appliance is used to correct a true unilateral crossbite. It can be designed to resemble a Schwarz or a transverse appliance. The only difference lies in the posterior bite pads. The Nord bite pad is used to provide extra anchorage for movement of the side in crossbite. The Nord bite pads are of a standard design on the side that is being moved; on the other side an extension is added to the lingual of the bite pad. This extension is placed just on the lingual surface of the bite pad and extends down to rest against the lingual surface of the lower posteriors in that quadrant.

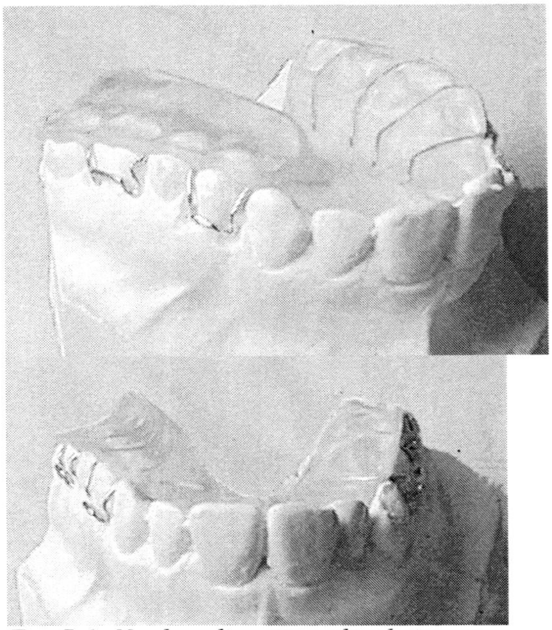

Fig. 7.6 Nord appliance - occlusal views

Therefore, when the screw is opened, it pushes on the side being moved only on the upper posteriors. On the opposite side the force of the expansion screw pushes on both the upper and lower posteriors. To increase the anchorage created, the Nord bite pad is left with occlusal indexing for the mandibular teeth while the side being moved has a smooth occlusal surface on the bite pad.

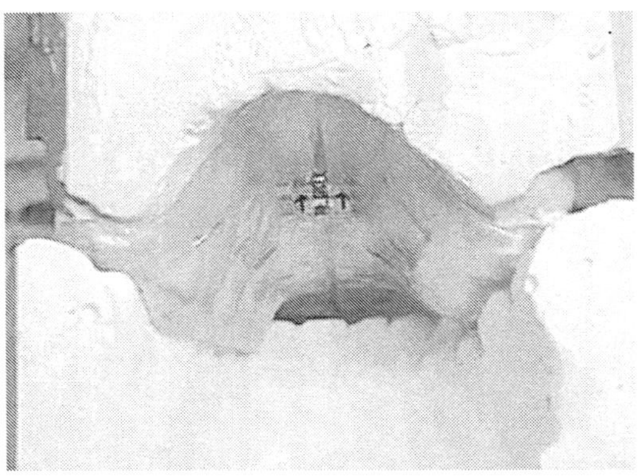

Fig. 7.7 Nord appliance - lingual view

The flange lingual to the lower posteriors should extend to a point just occlusal to the gingival margin. It should not impinge on the tissues.

Common removable designs

Automatic Hawley

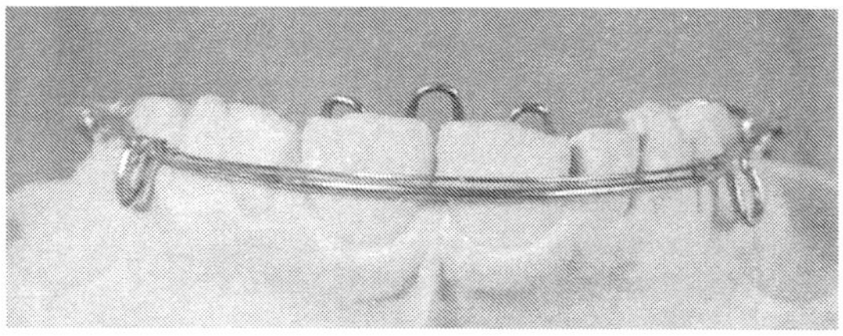

Fig. 7.8 Auto Hawley - labial view

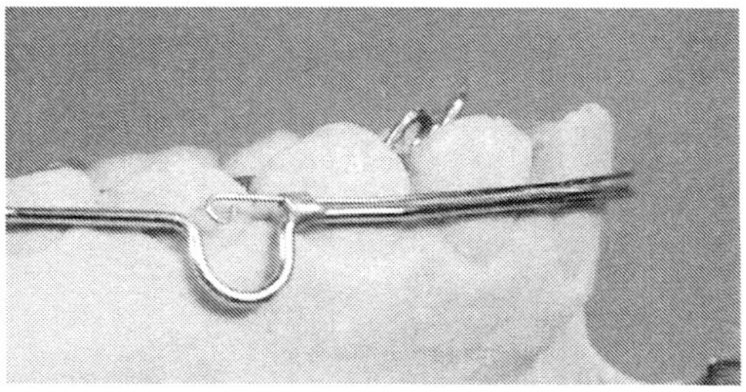

Fig. 7.9 - Auto Hawley - lateral view

The Automatic Hawley (Auto Hawley) is an excellent appliance for the retraction of the anterior teeth. It may be used on the mandible or the maxilla. The Auto Hawley is a self-adjusting spring which is tensioned during fabrication. The spring may be subsequently tighten by tightening the Wilson loops of the arch.

To ensure the lingual movement of the teeth, it is necessary to trim the acrylic lingual to the anteriors. This acrylic is trimmed in a smooth arc, 2 mm from the lingual surfaces, extending from cuspid to cuspid.

When an appliance, such as an Auto Hawley, is prescribed to lingualize the teeth, always check the occlusion with the lower anteriors to ensure that the uppers can be retracted. If the lower anteriors are in function with the linguals of the uppers, the teeth will not retract. It is sometimes difficult to determine this in the mouth, so check the model of such a case before starting.

If the teeth are in contact, one possible solution the dentist may wish to pursue is to increase the patient's vertical dimension of occlusion by encouraging eruption of the posteriors. This works well with deep bite cases that exhibit a collapsed vertical, however, a patient with a long face is not optimal for this strategy. The dentist is the person to decide the course to take in such a case.

Details for fabrication of the Auto Hawley can be found in the *Components* section under *Automatic Hawley.*

Habit Breaker

Several types of habits can be treated with the help of orthodontic appliances. The ones that we will discuss both involve anterior complications. These are tongue thrusting and thumb sucking. These are the most commonly fabricated habit breakers.

Both of these habits tend to produce anterior malocclusions, either excessive overjets or anterior open bites. The two habits can go together in some children. The thumb sucking can encourage an occlusion which inhibits the patient achieving lip seal for swallowing. In order to swallow, we must be able to seal our mouths. The tongue, therefore, comes forward to press on the lin-

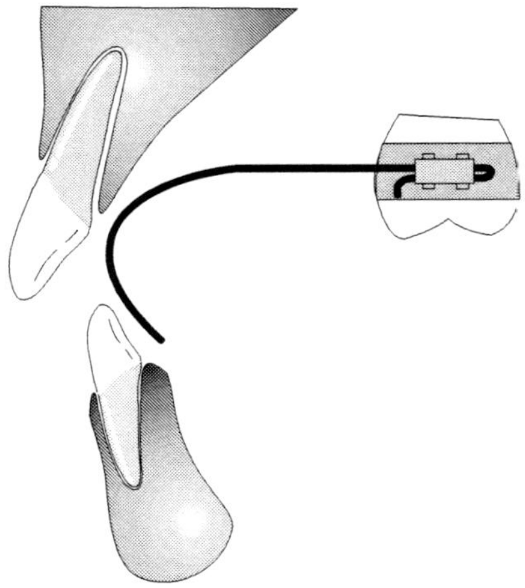

Fig. 7.10 Habit breaker fence for tongue thrust

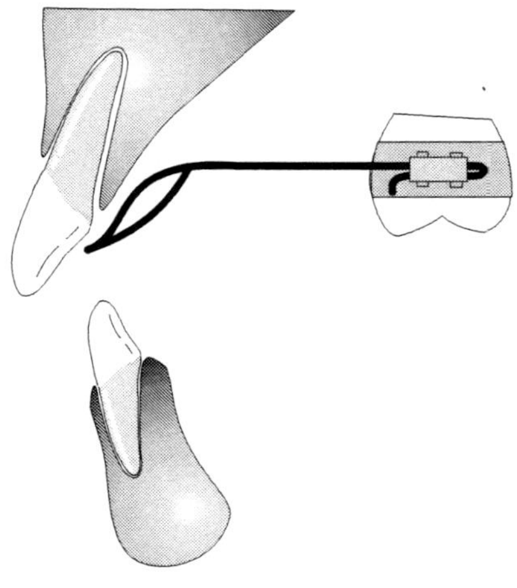

Fig. 7.11 Habit breaker fence for thumb sucking

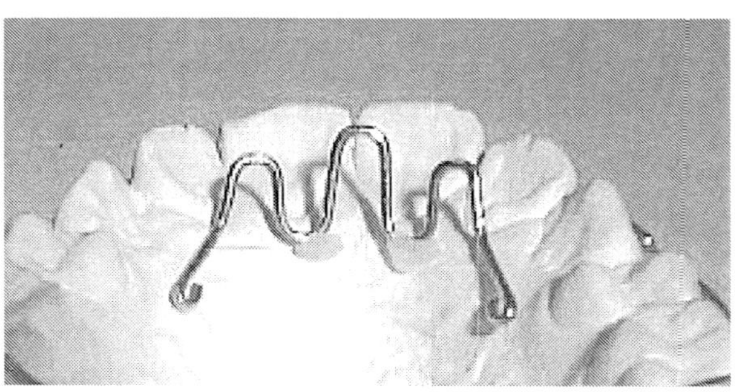

Fig. 7.12 Habit breaker fence for removable appliance

gual of the incisors and seal the gap, causing an aberrant swallowing pattern. Both the thumb and the tongue pushing on the lingual of the upper incisors proclines these teeth increasing overjet. These are some of the possible effects.

Habit breakers can be fixed or removable, and are used on the maxilla. Both designs work by interfering with the habit, usually by placing an obstructive fence to the lingual of the anteriors. For a tongue thrust, this fence keeps the tongue away from the linguals of the anterior teeth. For a thumb habit, the fence makes it impossible for the patient to achieve a suction seal around the thumb. This apparently removes part of the desirability of the habit and acts as a reminder.

There are two ways to make a removable habit breaker. The fence can be acrylic or wire.

An acrylic fence is simply a ridge of acrylic running lingual to the upper anteriors projecting approximately 5 mm down from the acrylic plate. The ridge can be crossed by cuts to remove some material and to ease breathing. This design tends to be heavy and cumbersome, and is not used as frequently as the wire fence.

The wire fence is bent from 0.8 mm wire. In one design the fence is bent to resemble a rounded "m" shape with three points. The center point is placed on the midline and is approximately 2 mm longer than the flanking points. The flanking points (when viewed from the occlusal) are curved slightly so that when placed in the palate, the wire fence curves to match the arc of the lingual of the anteriors.

There should always be an opposing model when a habit breaker fence is being fabricated. The wire fence should be bent so that the point of the fence ends just above the cingulums of the lower anteriors when the models are in centric. This protects the lower anteriors from the tongue thrust as well.

If no opposing model is supplied, you must estimate the position of the fence. Extend the center point 2 mm past the incisal edges of the upper centrals, with the flanking points approximately even with the incisals. Place the fence approximately 4-5 mm lingual to the linguals of the upper anteriors.

To include a wire fence in the acrylic plate there are two methods possible. The acrylic plate can be sprinkled and trimmed, and then the fence added as a repair; or, the fence can be suspended over the model by luting it to a piece of rope wax and luting the rope wax to either side of the model in the bicuspid region. Ensure that the wire is at least 1 mm off of the tissue to ensure that it is encased by acrylic.

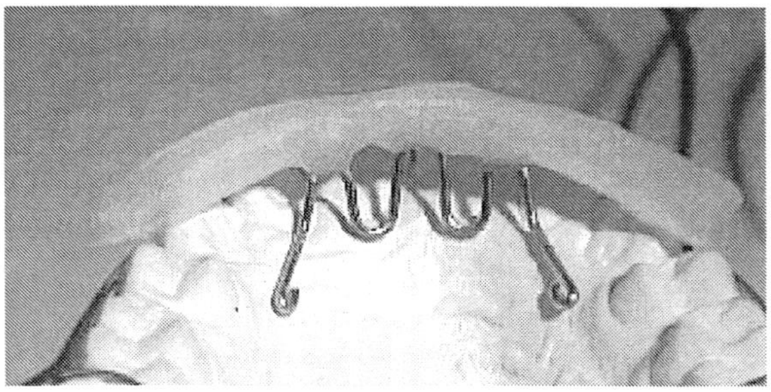

Fig. 7.13 Habit breaker fence positioned with white utility wax

The acrylic around the fence is trimmed and polished smooth and flat.

Spring retainer

The spring retainer is used as a retention appliance, and also as an appliance to correct minor malpositioning of the incisor teeth on the upper and lower.

The spring retainer consists of a Hawley type arch, bent with light wire, that passes along the buccal and lingual of the anteriors. This arch is then covered with acrylic to form a tightly contoured band across the teeth.

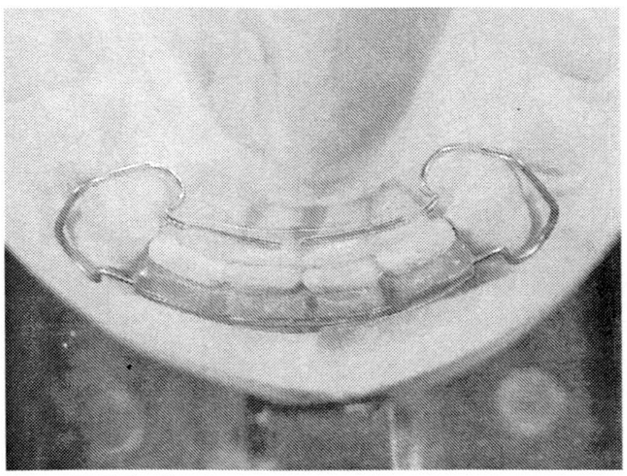

Fig. 7.14 Spring retainer - labial incisal view

To use this appliance as a retainer it is made on the original model without modifying the model. In most cases, however, this appliance is used because a minor adjustment needs to be done. This design works well for adjusting minor rotations and for slight lingual movement. It cannot perform a mesial-distal translation.

To fabricate an appliance to correct a tooth, the model must first be prepared. The tooth to be corrected is cut from the model and waxed back into a corrected position. The wires are now bent over the corrected tooth and the acrylic added. When the appliance is placed in the mouth, the tooth which has been corrected will not match the contour of the acrylic band across the buccal and lingual of the teeth. The wires will therefore flex and stretch, in the Wilson loop region, until the appliance settles over the teeth. The Wilson loops will continue to place forces on the tooth until the tooth moves to match the position that it was adjusted to on the model.

The active portion of the appliance is from cuspid to cuspid. The simplest design of the appliance is known as a 3x3 and consists of the wire — running from cuspid to cuspid — and the acrylic band on the incisors. This design was and still is very popular because it is small and unobtrusive in the mouth as well as, comfortable for the patient. Unfortunately, this design carries a danger of aspiration. It can be swallowed or breathed into the lungs.

A newer design is known as the modified spring retainer. It has an anterior section identical to the 3x3 which is attached to an acrylic body, usually including clasps on the first bicuspids or first molars. This design is not as comfortable, but is more stable in the mouth. Modifications on this are varied. One popular one replaces the acrylic body with a pair of ball clasps soldered to the Wilson loops and passing along the linguals of the teeth to cross the occlusion in the region of the bicuspids and gain retention.

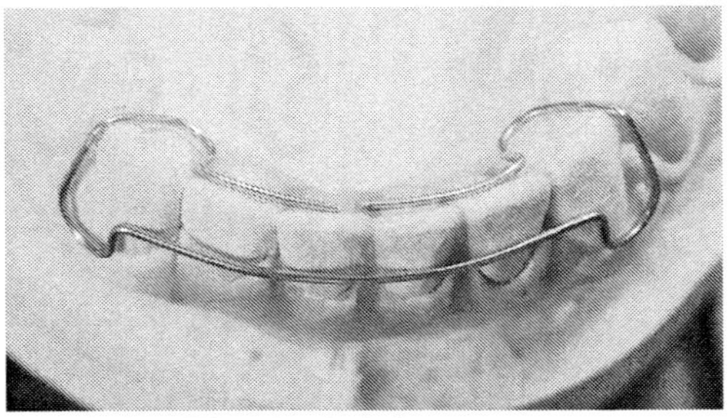

Fig. 7.15 Wire for 3x3 Spring retainer - incisal view

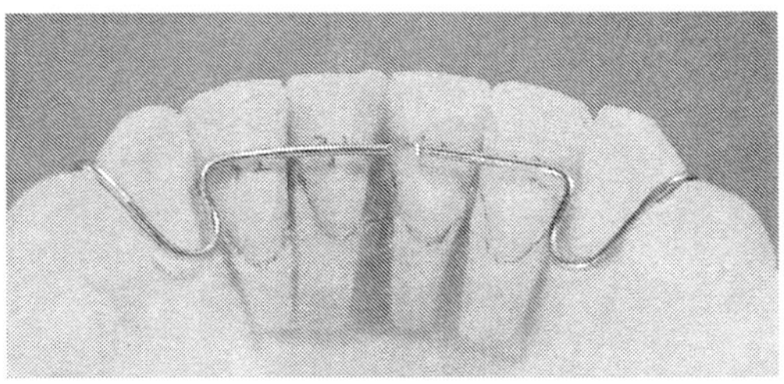

Fig. 7.16 Wire for 3x3 Spring retainer - lingual view

To bend a spring retainer use a light wire, 0.5-0.6 mm, for the arch. Bend a standard Hawley arch on the labial of the anterior with 0.5-1 mm relief from the labial surfaces. Be sure that there is enough excess wire to bend the lingual portion. Bring the wire through the embrasure lingual to the cuspids and form a Wilson loop on the lingual surfaces of the cuspids. At the level of the cingulums, bend the wire to follow the lingual of the anteriors, again with 0.5-1 mm of relief. For a 3x3, simply overlap the wire slightly or cut them where they met. For a modified design, bend the wire to the gingiva approximately 1 mm before the midline and carry it at least 6 mm past the gingival margin.

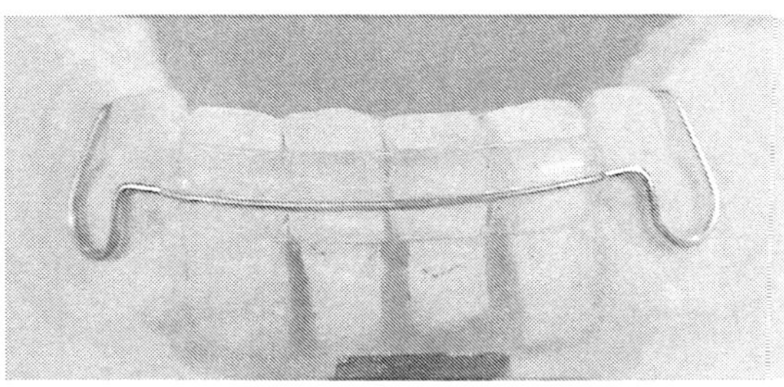

Fig. 7.17 Teeth reset to corrected positions in wax

To assist in making the relief between the wire and the labial and lingual surfaces, place a layer of medical adhesive tape over these surfaces of the teeth. Bend the wire against the tape. When the tape is removed the necessary relief will be present.

To acrylic a spring retainer, first add wax

over the Wilson loops. Cover the entire Wilson loop and 1 mm beyond it. This will ensure that the loop is not damaged by the need to remove acrylic from it. Wax may be used to define the outlines of the acrylic bands, however, in most cases this is not necessary. A knife can be used to trim the occlusal and cervical borders of the band immediately after sprinkling.

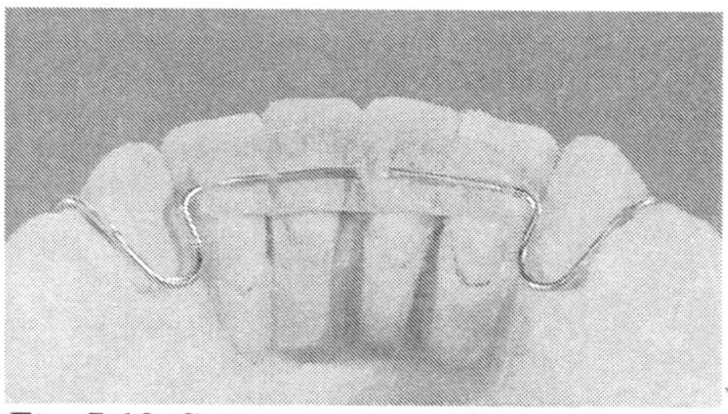

Fig. 7.18 Spring retainer - lingual view

Trim the incisal margins of the labial and lingual bands parallel to the incisal edges of the anterior teeth. The gingival margins can be trimmed straight across just above the interdental papilla or scalloped around the interdental papilla. Do not cover the tissue.

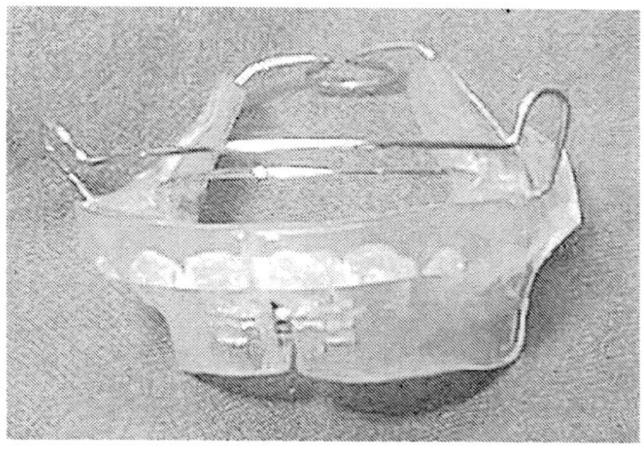

Fig. 7.19 Bionator - labial view

In a modified spring retainer the anterior section must be separated from the acrylic body. Cut a groove across the lingual gingival margins from Wilson loop to Wilson loop with a small (#700) fissure bur.

Functional appliances

Bionator

The bionator is one of the best known and most popular of the functional appliances. The bionator is a sturdy, effective appliance that can be modified to fulfill a number of functions.

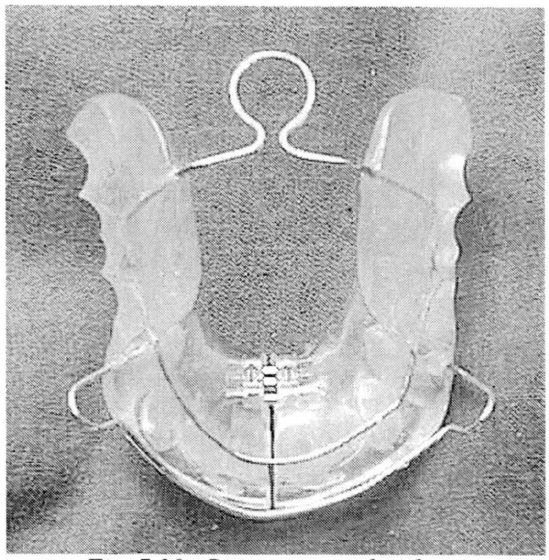

Fig. 7.20 Bionator - occlusal view

The basic design of the bionator is derived from the Anderson activator and the monobloc. The bionator has the advantage that a great deal of the acrylic bulk of these designs was replaced with wires, yielding an appliance that was more comfortable and flexible, yet efficient.

The bionator is most commonly used to correct a Class II occlusion. It accomplishes this by advancing the mandible and increasing the vertical dimension of the patient.

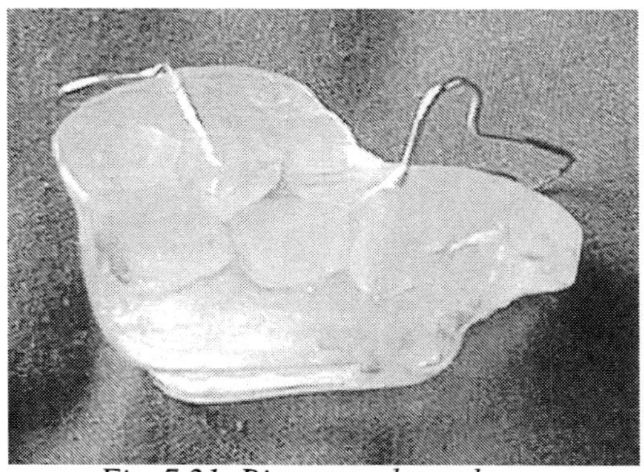

Fig. 7.21 Bionator - lateral

These changes in vertical and protrusion of the mandible are accomplished by the use of a construction bite that is provided by the dentist. A construction bite is a bite which is used in the fabrication of an appliance but is not a bite used by the patient in normal function. A construction bite bears no relation to centric, it is an artificial relationship created by the dentist.

The construction bite for a bionator has several requirements:

- the mandible must be protruded to an end-to-end relationship on the centrals. If this is not possible the patient should protrude as far as they are able. Once they have adapted to this position during treatment a new bite can be taken and a new appliance made. The mandible can be advanced in stages.
- there must be a minimum vertical opening of 1 mm between the centrals, 2 mm is optimum.
- the upper and lower midlines must align unless the dental midline has shifted for dental reasons. A misalignment of the midlines can induce differential forces on the condyles.

The protrusion of the mandible in the construction bite results in the mandible being brought forward into a more normal Class I relationship. For many years, there was an argument over whether the mandible was actually growing longer because of this anterior pull. The short answer for how the change occurs is that the mandible's anterior displacement places a tension on the tissues in the posterior of the glenoid fossa. The condyle is held in a position which is down and forward from its normal rest position, and the tension induced stimulates growth to the posterior wall of the fossa. The end result is that the glenoid fossa is filled in (remodelled) behind the condyle until the condyle's new position resembles its original relationship with the fossa. The mandible itself does not grow, the bones of the joint change shape.

The vertical adjustment of the patient's occlusion takes place due to eruption of the posterior teeth. This is encouraged by opening the posterior bite and then removing all acrylic between the occlusal surfaces. Teeth will erupt until they meet an antagonist. Removing the occlusal acrylic causes the teeth to erupt, opening the patient's vertical and reducing overbite.

The acrylic is removed in carefully sculpted channels that guide the teeth into the eruption path that the dentist desires. Occluso-distally (down and back) on the maxilla and mesio-occlusally (forward and up) or straight occlusally on the mandible.

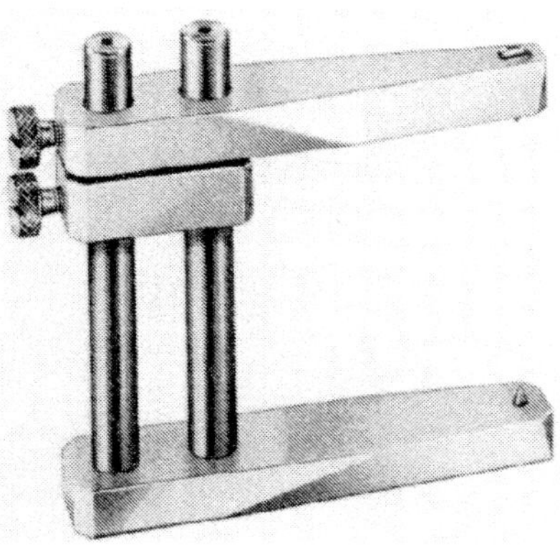

Fig. 7.22 Verticulator

Fabrication of the bionator

To construct a bionator, the models must first be mounted on an device that will provide an accurate vertical dimension. For this you may use a plain line articulator or a verticulator.

A verticulator is a device with a single upright and two arms which hold the models at a set vertical opening. It does not allow any movement of the models other than straight up and down, increasing or decreasing the vertical.

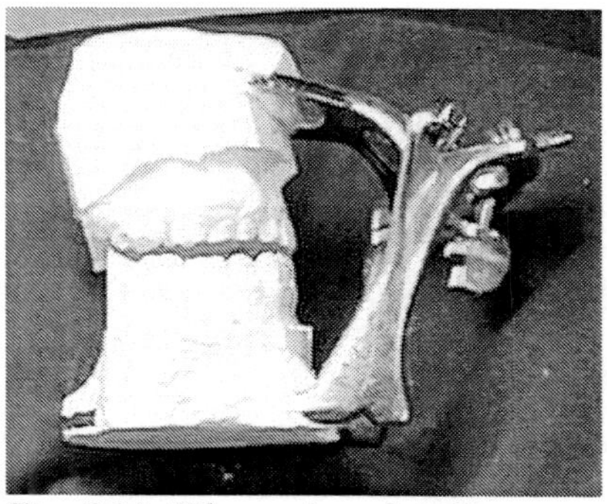

Fig. 7.23 When using plain line

If you are using a plain line articulator you must remember to mount the models backwards, with the anterior of the models facing the back of the articulator. You should do this to provide access to the posterior of the models when they are closed to the construction bite during sprinkling of the acrylic.

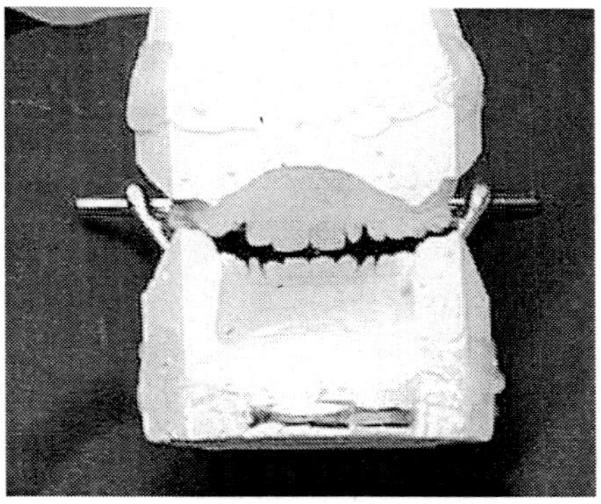

Fig. 7.24 Mounting provides access to lingual surfaces

The construction bite should have the anteriors in an edge to edge or even slightly Class III relationship, with at least 2 mm of vertical opening between the upper and lower incisals. It is important the bite be correct from the operatory because no adjustment can be made to the bite on the articulator. The open and advanced position of the mandible means that the condyles are not operating in a simple hinge axis position. This hinge axis movement is the only one that an articulator can mimic — not duplicate — therefore, any change made to the bite on the articulator will introduce errors into the appliance.

Your articulation must have a stable vertical dimension to fabricate this appliance.

Bionator design

There are several designs that can be used for the bionator depending on the treatment objectives. The basic design consists of these elements:

- the coffin or omega spring
- the lingual arch
- the labial arch
- the lower lingual body
- the lower incisal cap
- the upper palatal wings
- a lower midline expansion screw is a frequently used option.

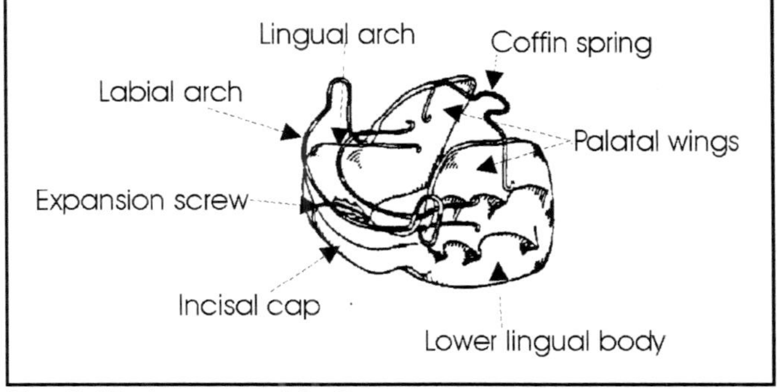

Fig. 7.25 Anatomy of the Bionator

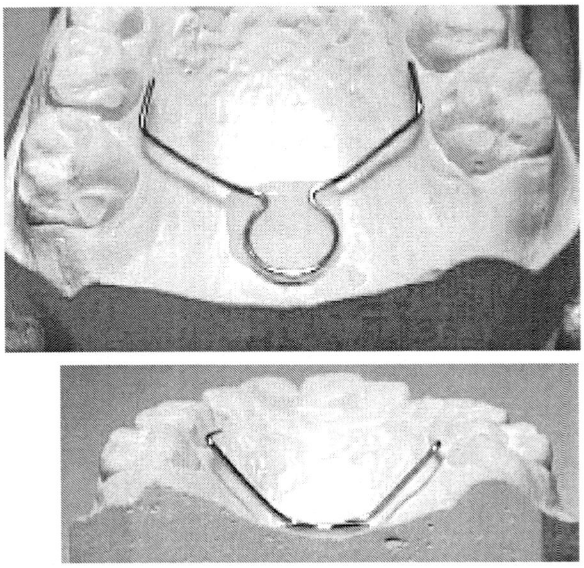

Fig. 7.26 Omega/Coffin Spring

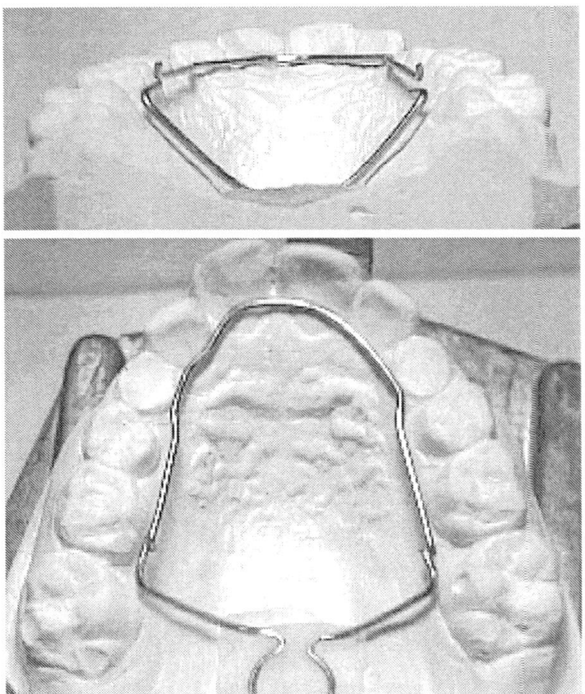

Fig. 7.27 Lingual Arch and Omega Spring

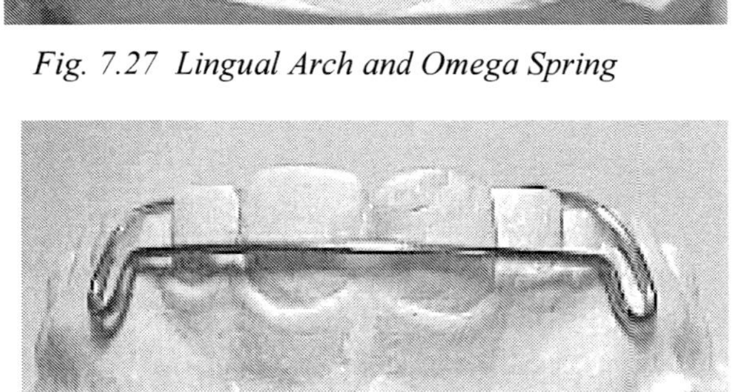

Fig. 7.28 Labial Arch

The wires

The first wire bent is the Omega or Coffin spring. The shape of the wire resembles the Greek letter omega, Ω. Use 1.0 mm hard wire.

The wire is placed between the 6's, 1 mm off of the tissue. The tag ends are bent just to the gingival or lingual of the teeth. All wire tags are kept in or close to the inter-occlusal region because this is where the acrylic will be the thickest.

The lingual wire is made with 0.8 mm hard wire. It runs from the middle third of the 1.3 to the middle third of the 2.3 with the tags continuing into the acrylic to the region of the 5's on either side. The lingual wire should contact the lingual surfaces of the anterior teeth, one of its functions being to help maintain the vertical dimension of the construction bite. On a case with malpositioned anteriors, the lingual wire may be shaped to approximate an ideal arch, provided it still contacts enough of the lingual surfaces of the anteriors to provide vertical support.

If the appliance incorporates an expansion screw on the lower midline, the lingual wire must be cut by the dentist before the expansion screw can be activated. This would occur approximately 4 weeks into treatment. At the same time as the expansion screw is being activated, the two halves of the cut lingual wire can be used as finger springs to begin straightening the anteriors. The clinician must remember to adjust the coffin spring as the expansion screw is opened, or the unequal stresses on the appliance will cause breakage.

The labial arch is made with 0.9 hard wire. It is bent in the form of a Hawley arch with some minor alterations. The labial aspect

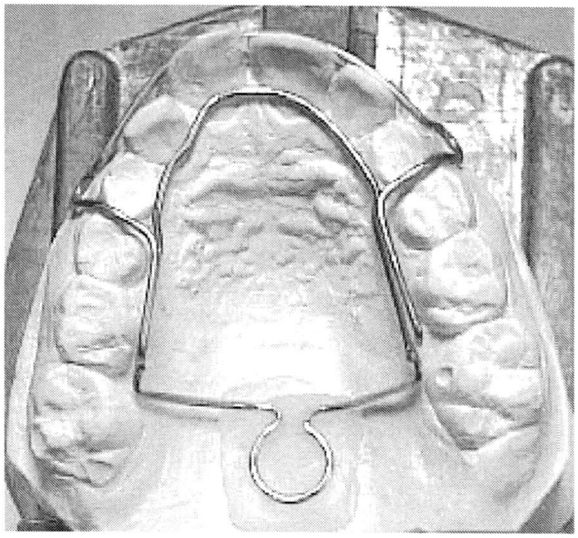

Fig. 7.29 Bionator Wires

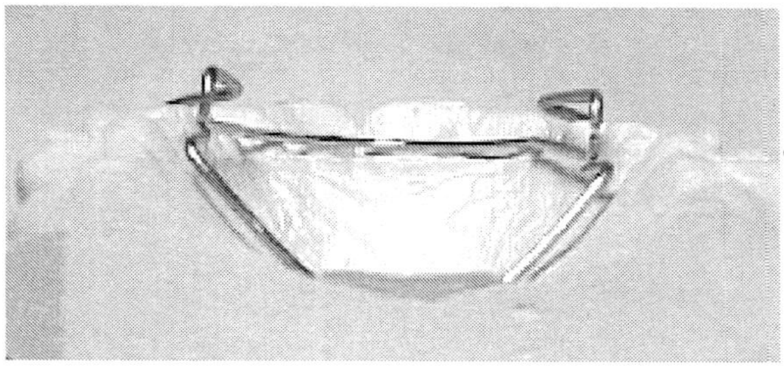

Fig. 7.30 Note tags in interocclusal region

of the wire is kept 1 mm from the labial surfaces of the teeth, and the Wilson loops are made slightly larger for greater flexibility. The labial arch is kept off of the teeth so that a lingualizing force is not transferred to the anteriors from the muscles of mastication.

The patient's mandibular positioning when taking the construction bite stretches these muscles, causing them to exert a constant pressure on the mandible, trying to pull to the posterior. If the labial arch is in contact with the buccal of the anteriors, this force will be transferred to them and will lingualize these teeth. The tags of the labial arch should not pass tightly through the embrasures as it extends to the lingual. This may interfere with the eruption of the teeth.

Wax up

Once the wires have been waxed into position on the models, wax is used to define the areas to be built up in acrylic. Using wax to define your work area helps to keep your models clean and reduce the amount of wasted acrylic. A soft white rope wax is best for this purpose because it contains no dyes that may stain the acrylic. On the maxilla, the wax is placed in a semicircle from the mesial of the first bicuspid to the distal of the last tooth on the arch. The wax passes over the coffin spring. Wax is also placed along the bucco-occlusal line angle of the posteriors.

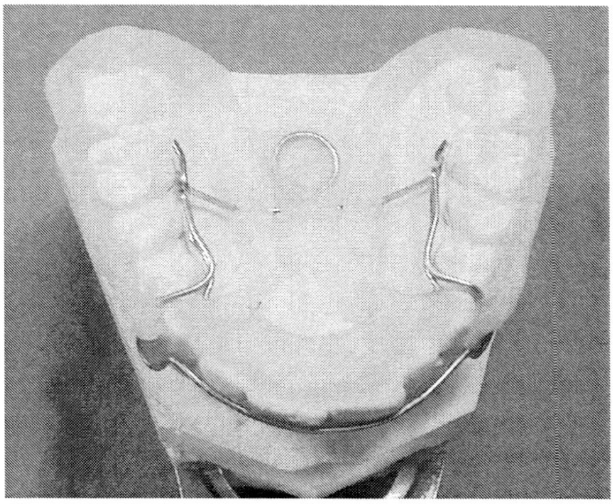

Fig. 7.31 Palatal wings defined with rope wax

On the mandible, wax is placed 2 mm down from the incisal on the buccal of the anteriors. This is to assist in the construction of a incisal cap which will cover the incisal and buccal-incisal third of the lower anteriors. This cap will serve to resist the same muscular forces that act upon the buccal of the upper anteriors. These muscles are trying to pull the mandible to the posterior against the appliance, so the forces act upon the lingual of the lower anteriors, trying to flare them

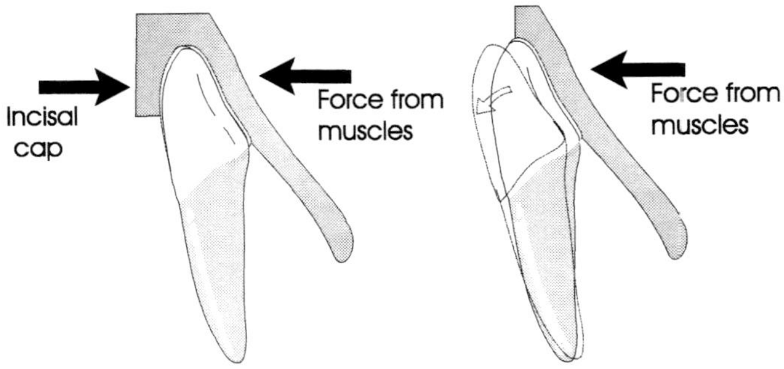

Fig. 7.32 Incisal cap balances muscle forces of lower anteriors

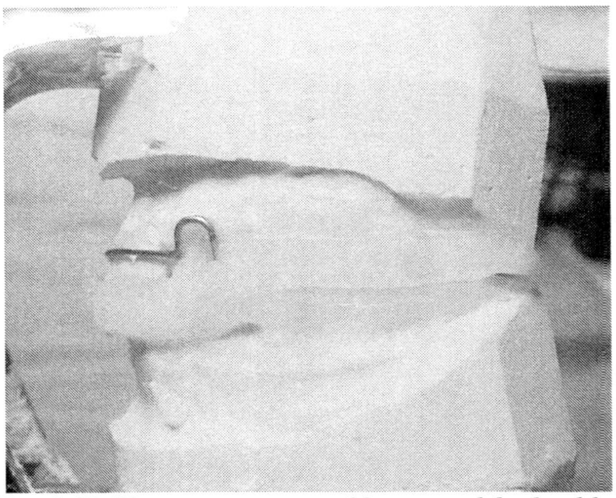

Fig. 7.33 Wax up on upper and lower models should meet when the models are at the proper vertical

buccally. A light wash of wax along the gingival margin on the lower anteriors will relieve pressure in this area avoiding tissue damage.

Wax is placed on the bucco-occlusal line angle of the lower posteriors. This wax and the wax on the upper posteriors can be shaped so that when the models are in the relationship defined by the construction bite, the surfaces of the two wax pads meet. This makes it very easy to know just how much acrylic to add in order to join the two halves of the appliance. You need only fill the posterior regions to the height of the wax pads and they will meet and bond. A thin layer of wax may be added to the lingual sulcus of the lower at this time. It will make the removal of the appliance after polymerization easier.

Wax should also be placed over the lingual wire to avoid its being encased in acrylic when the articulator is closed. This wax can be shaped from cuspid to cuspid on the upper to the height of the incisal edges. This prevents the upper anteriors from being buried in the incisal cap, and automatically forms a smooth occlusal surface on the incisal cap.

Sprinkling the acrylic

When sprinkling the acrylic on a two arch appliance, such as the bionator, Frankel or activator, you must plan the order in which you will proceed.

The large amount of acrylic that must be applied to construct the appliance forces you to work so that the acrylic that is applied first is not allowed to polymerize prior to the appliance being placed into the pressure pot. Should this happen the acrylic would become porous and the bond between the two halves would not be strong.

There are a number of methods that are used to accomplish this. One is to sprinkle the upper and lower halves separately and join them together as a repair. Another is to sprinkle the lower, then trim it and polish the incisal cap and anterior lingual portion. The polished portions are then protected with a thin layer of wax or electrical tape while the upper portion is sprinkled and

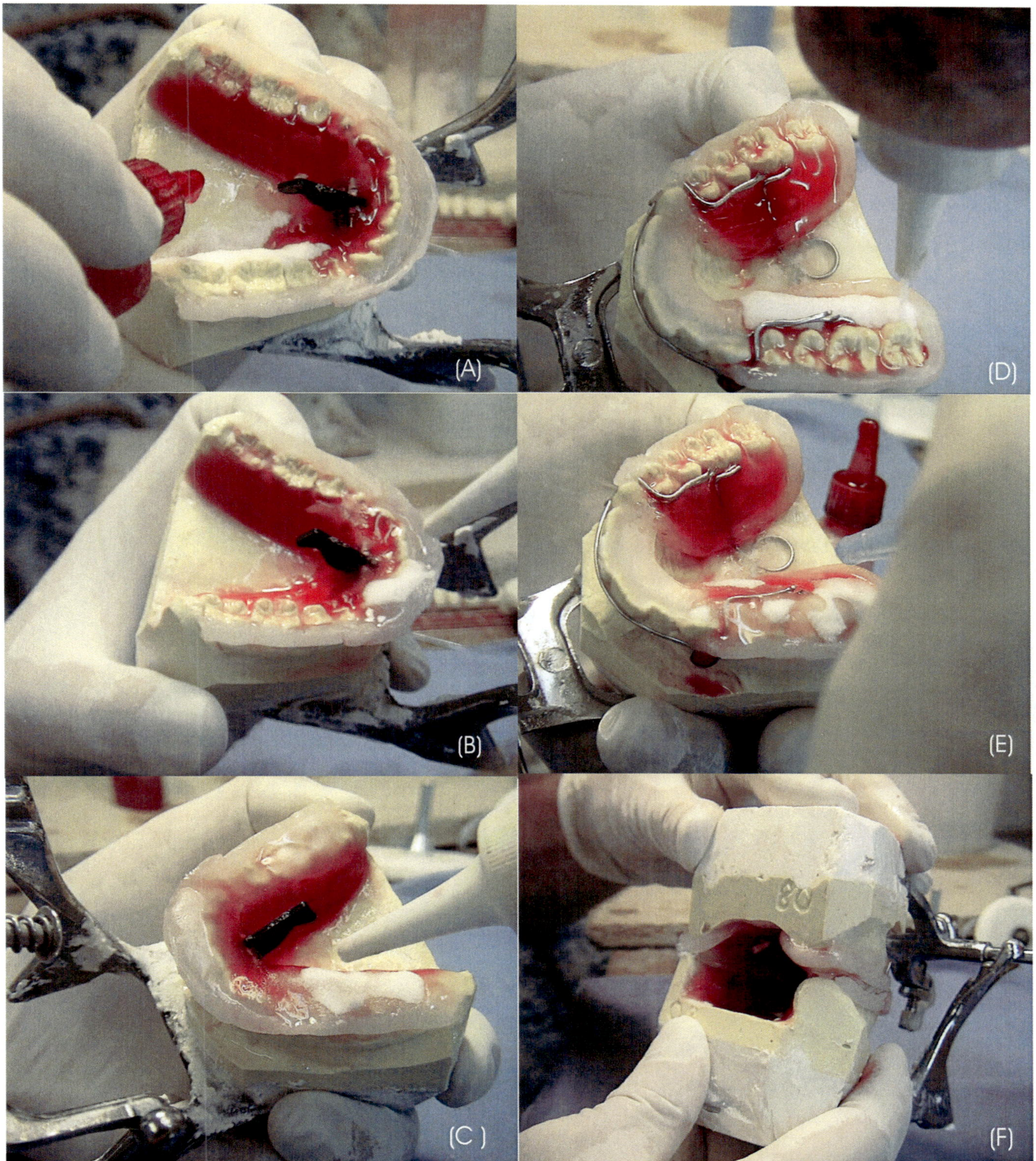

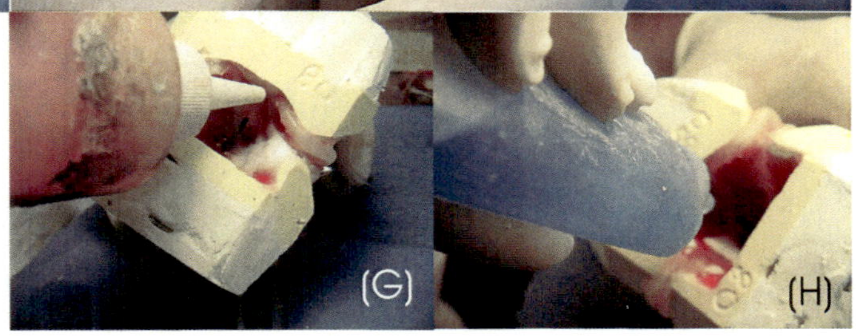

Sprinkling the Bionator
(A) Sprinkle largest area (mandibular body) first, one side, then the other. **(B)** Sprinkle Incisal cap in anterior to height of wax. **(C)** Then a thin layer over the posterior occlusal pads. **(D)** Sprinkle palatal wings of maxilla **(E)** Sprinkle occlusal portion of maxilla wings to the height of the wax. **(F)** Close verticulator into the bite, ensure that it closes to original vertical. **(G)** Add polymer between the two halves. **(H)** Wet polymer with monomer to join maxilla and mandible. I prefer to use clear monomer in this area.

joined to the lower posterior.

These methods both have their strengths and weaknesses, and their use is a matter of personal preference.

The method that will be outlined here is a one step sprinkling that uses the wax forms discussed earlier to assist in controlling the acrylic.

The first part of the appliance to be sprinkled will be the lower body. The lower portion of the appliance is much larger than the upper and, therefore, takes more time. You will then start with this larger area and finish the smaller upper area before the lower area can polymerize.

Start the lower by sprinkling the lingual tissue area of the model, then the incisal cap and then the occlusal area of the posterior to the level of the wax. You can then sprinkle the two sides of the upper portion up to and over the occlusion, and then join the upper and lower together. Once you have closed the models into their construction bite you will add acrylic from the lingual to join and smooth the two parts. This is why you mounted the case backward, to provide access to this lingual area.

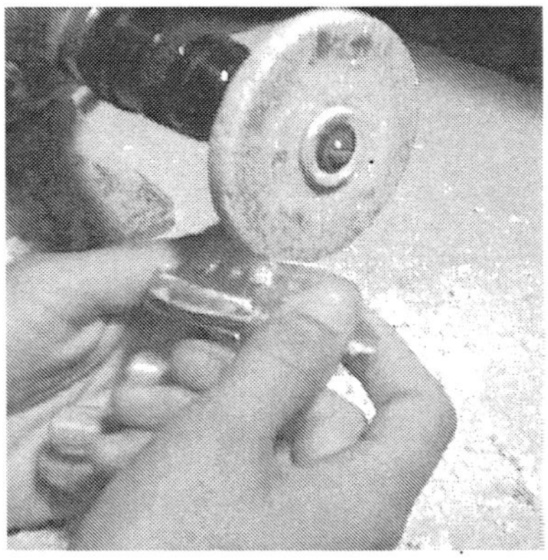

Fig. 7.34 Trimming with large wheel

Trimming the Bionator

The basic trimming of the bionator is the same as any appliance. The only difference in the bionator is that most of the trimming is performed "inside" the appliance, i.e., on the lingual surfaces.

This makes the bionator slightly more difficult to trim and a good deal more difficult to polish than the average appliance.

The trimming can begin with a large fastcut stone. This is used to do the basic shaping for the appliance and gross reduction of excess acrylic. Trim the lingual sulcus region of the lower, the buccal of the inter-occlusal region (slightly) and anywhere else that excess occurs. A large egg bur can then be used to "hollow out" the lingual surfaces of the posterior region. Particular attention should be paid to the inter-occlusal area to give the patient as much tongue space as possible.

The anterior of the lower is smoothed on the lingual and the labial of the incisal cap should be trimmed to a thickness of approximately 1 mm. The superior surface of the incisal cap must be smooth and flat, as well as contacting the incisal of the upper anteriors. If one of the upper incisors is overly short or under-erupted, the tooth may be left out of contact with the incisal cap. The same holds true for deciduous teeth worn down through attrition.

If the case contains an expansion screw, a cut will also be made to free it.

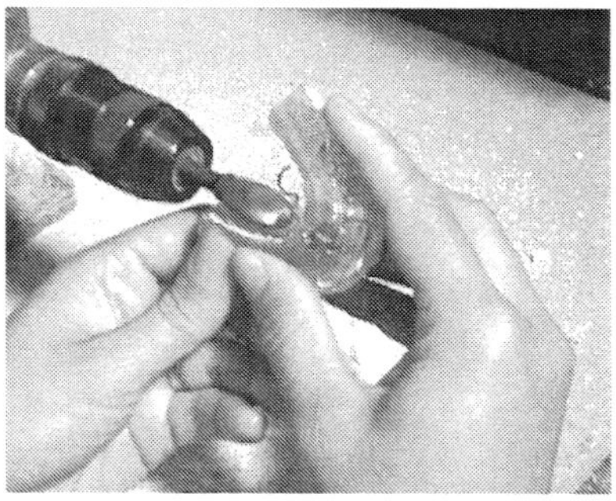
Fig. 7.35 Trimming with a bur

Smaller carbides in a handpiece may now be used to smooth and round all surfaces on the lingual and labial of the appliance. No further trimming is done yet to the buccal surfaces of the inter-occlusal area in the posterior.

After the appliance has been smoothed and shaped to its final form, the trimming of the eruptive paths may be done. The purpose of these paths is to guide the teeth in erupting and increasing the patient's vertical dimension. A soft pencil is used to mark the occluso-lingual line angle on the impression of all of the posterior teeth in the indexing acrylic of the inter-occlusal area.

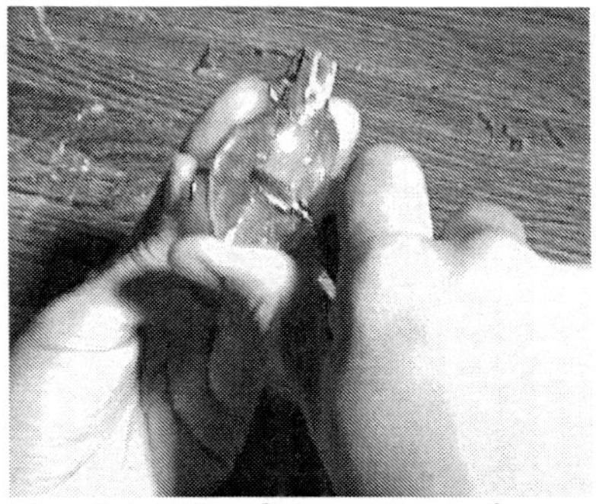
Fig. 7.36 Final trimming with handpiece

The mesio-lingual surfaces of all of the upper posterior are shaded in to mark these areas of the teeth. When all the eruptive paths are completed, the shading on the mesio-lingual of the upper posteriors must still be present on the acrylic. This will ensure that these parts of the teeth are firmly in contact with the acrylic and will serve as a stabilizing factor against the posterior forces exerted by the mandible. Without these contacts the protruded mandible will pull the appliance posteriorly causing the labial bar to contact the labial surfaces of the upper anteriors. The labial bar would then lingualize these teeth.

The teeth tend to move, or appear to move in definite directions as they erupt due to growth. The upper posteriors seem to erupt down and back (posteriorly), and the lower posteriors seem to erupt up and forward (anteriorly). The great majority of vertical growth in the patient's face will be accomplished by the lower vertical change, the upper has much less effect on this.

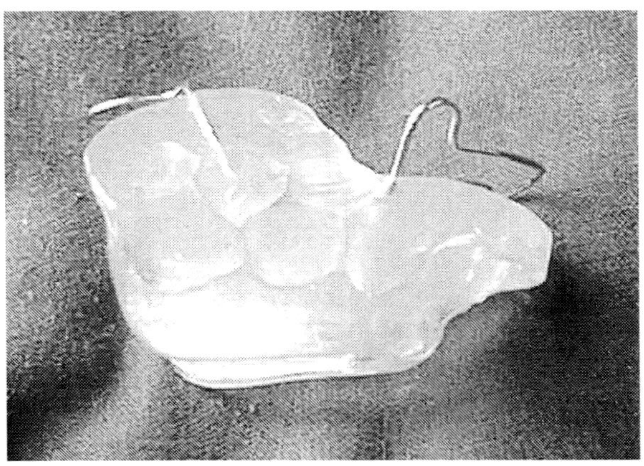
Fig. 7.37 Note trimming of erruption paths

The eruptive paths will obviously be more effective if they are oriented to compliment the natural tendencies of the teeth's growth patterns.

The paths should curve gently to the buccal. This will

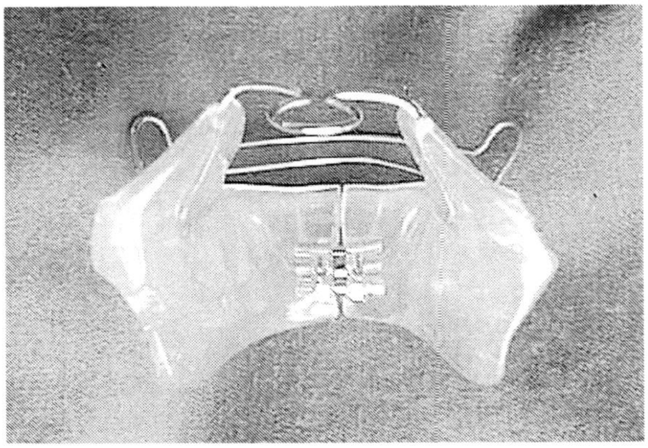

Fig. 7.38 Contour lingual to provide room for tongue

widen the arch slightly as the teeth erupt. This is particularly important on the upper, the upper posterior are now opposing a wider portion of the lower arch due to the protrusion of the mandible.

Polishing

Polishing the bionator is a challenge. Most of the parts of the appliance requiring polishing are on the lingual surfaces, inside the appliance. A large soft buff at slow speed is the best way to start the pumicing. This buff has the flexibility to bend into the lingual curves. Pumice all peripheries with this. When you have polished as much as possible with the buff, felt cones must be used to pumice the rest. This includes the lingual surfaces in the anterior — just lingual to the incisal cap — and the anterior portions of the upper palatal wings.

When the appliance is pumiced smooth, the high shine is applied. The anterior lingual of the lower is again the most difficult area. A small rag buff, 2.5-3 mm on a slow handpiece is what I use in this area.

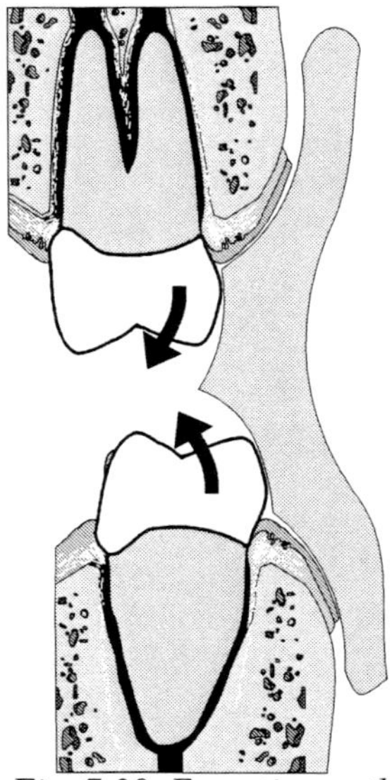

Fig. 7.39 Erruption paths guide molars to the buccal

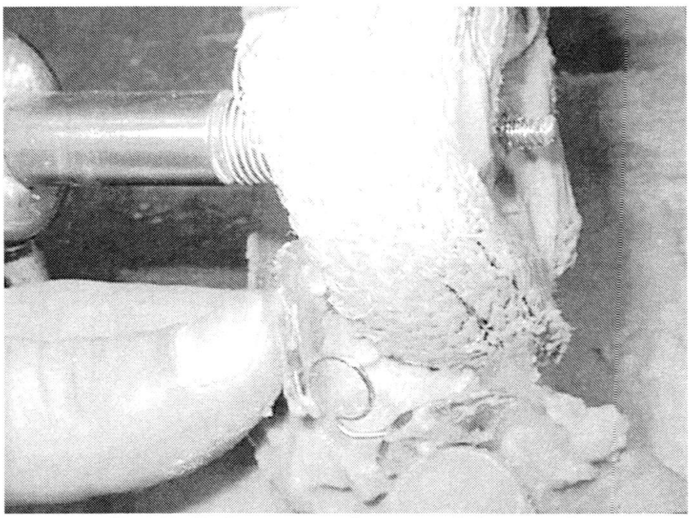

Fig. 7.40 Pumice appliance with large soft buff

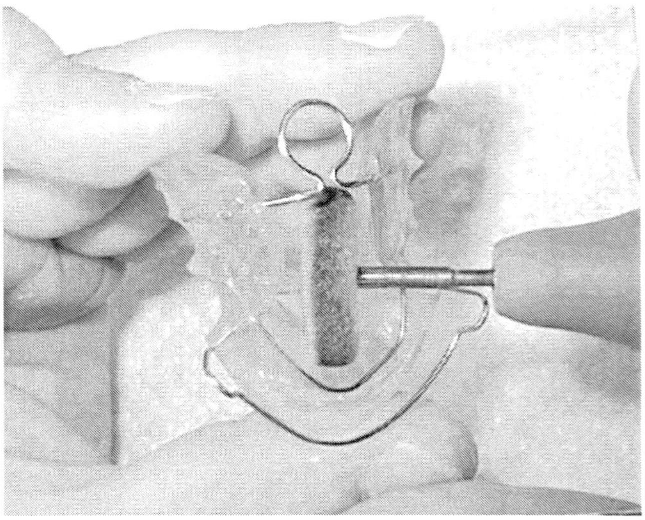

Fig. 7.41 Final polishing may be done with small buffs in handpiece

The Twin Block Appliance

Another functional appliance which has gained popularity in recent years is the Twin Block. This appliance was developed by Dr. William Clark of Fife, Scotland. It is used most commonly for the correction of Class II cases with or without changing the VDO, however the design can be easily modified to address a number of conditions.

The twin block is a relatively small (for a functional), sturdy and comfortable appliance. Most of these qualities come from the fact that unlike the other functional designs, the Twin block comes as two pieces, separate parts for the upper and lower.

The upper has a palate with occlusal pads covering the occlusals of the molars, while the lower has a lingual plate ending at the distal of the 2nd bicuspids with occlusal pads covering the occlusals of the bicuspids. The maxillary and mandibular occlusal pads meet each other at a 70° angle.

These inclined occluding surfaces are the functional portion of the appliance. When they meet, they force the mandible into a protrusive position. This stimulates the changes which result in repositioning of the mandible to a Class I posture.

Dr. Clark designed the Delta clasp to retain the Twin Block. This clasp bears a resemblance to the Adams clasp, except for its retentive elements. Rather than the retentive eyelets of the Adams clasp, the Delta clasps has single helixes placed at the mesio-buccal and disto-buccal line angles of the molars. Many people prefer, however, to use the standard Adams clasp with the Twin Block.

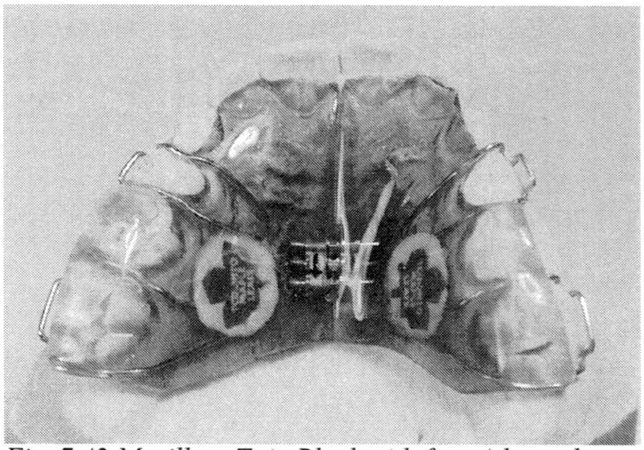

Fig. 7.42 Maxillary Twin Block with four Adams clasps

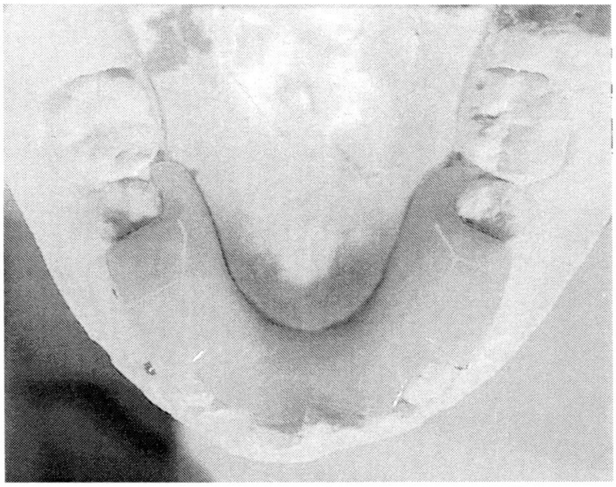

Fig. 7.43 Mandibular Twin Block with four ball clasps

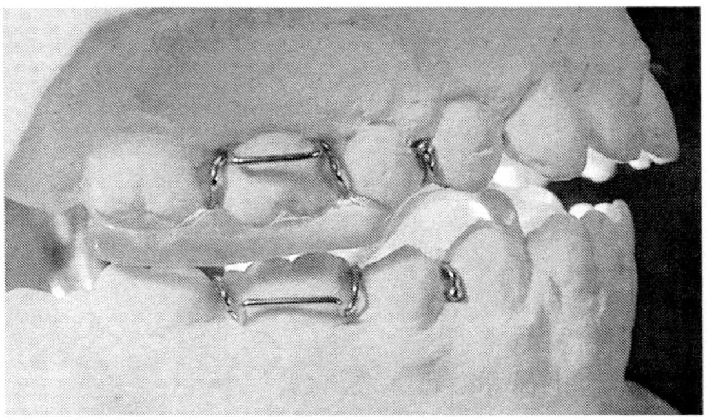

Fig. 7.44 Occlusal pads with inclined ramps in occlusion

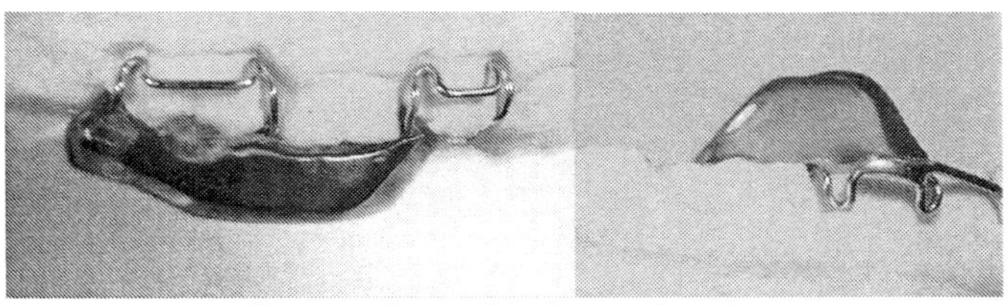

Fig. 7.45 Maxillary and mandibular inclined ramps on occlusal pads

The basic design of the maxillary twin block uses adams or delta clasps on 1st molars and the first premolar, the premolar clasp may be ball clasp placed between the 4/5. The mandibular has clasps on the 2nd premolars, ball clasps may be placed between the mandibular 3/4 for additional retention. A variation of the design is to extend the mandibular acrylic plate to the lingual of the molars and incorporate clasps on the 1st molars and ball clasps 4/5. This modification inproves amndibular stability but interferes with vertical developement.
Expansion screws can be incorporated into the appliances, a maxillary mid-palatine screw can be used to expand the maxillary width. This is useful because the advancement of the mandible places a wider portion of the mandibular arch in opposition to the maxillary posterior than is there pre-treatment. Screws can also be placed to provide sagittal development, or the two may be combined in a 3-way screw.

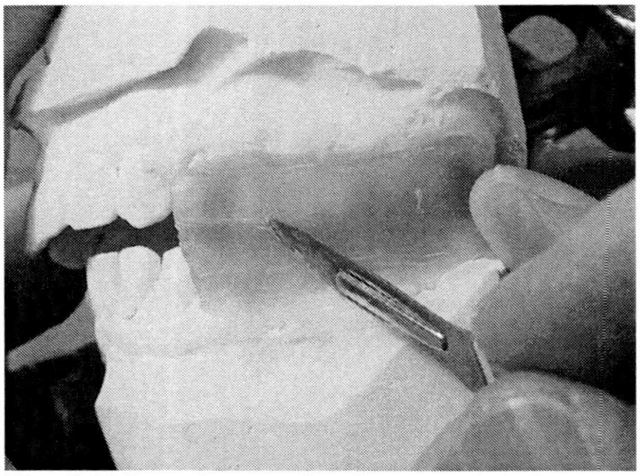

Fig. 7.46 Baseplate wax luted to posterior of maxillary and mandibular models. Cut along occlusal plane with a 70° incline from distal of maxillary 2nd premolar to mesial of mandibular 1st molar.

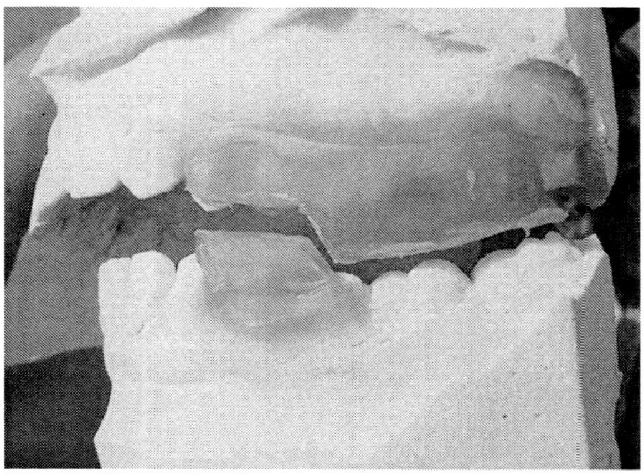

Fig. 7.47 completed wax matrix for inclined ramps

Fabricataion of the Twin Block

Fabrication of the twin block requires a construction bite. In a class II correction the bite should have a mandibular protrusion, as well as a inter-occlusal opening of 1-2 mm on the centrals (3-5 mm in the premolar region). The models are mounted to this bite and the clasps fabricated. I use wax to define the buccal extent of the occlusal pads. A piece of baseplate wax placed along the bucco-occlusal line angle is scored with a line at 70° to the occlusal plane. In most cases this is from the distal of the maxillary 2nd bicuspid to the mesial of the mandibular 1st molar.
Acrylic work for the maxillary and mandibular appliances is most easily accomplished by doing one at a time. Whether the maxillary or mandibular half is sprinkled first doesn't really matter. The sequence that I use is to sprinkle the maxilla so that the acrylic approximately follows the 70° of the wax, then trim the appliance to the stage that it is ready for polishing. The bite is adjusted

to the proper vertical, as supplied by the bite, and the 70° inclines are defined.
The occlusal pads, particularly the inclines are then covered with a separating medium. This may be Vaseline, tape or, as I prefer, a very thin wash of wax (very thin!!). This is to ensure that the newly sprinkled lower does not adhere to or damage this completed area, and yet lets me form the mandibular incline against it. The mandibular appliance is then sprinkled and the bite closed against the maxillary incline to form the mandibular incline.
The mandibular appliance is trimmed as usual, the final step being the selective grinding of the incline planes and occlusal pads to bring the vertical to the proper level.

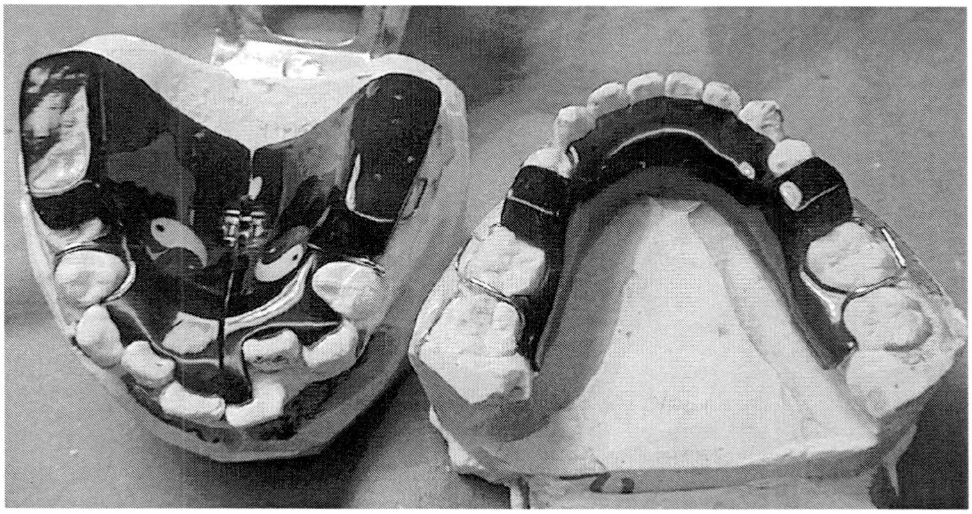

Fig. 7.48 Maxillary and mandibualr Twin Blocks. Mandibular appliance has extensions with Adams claps on the 1st molars.

"Art and science have their meeting point in method."
Edward Bulwer-Lytton

"If you don't know where you are going, you will probably end up somewhere else."
Laurence J. Peter

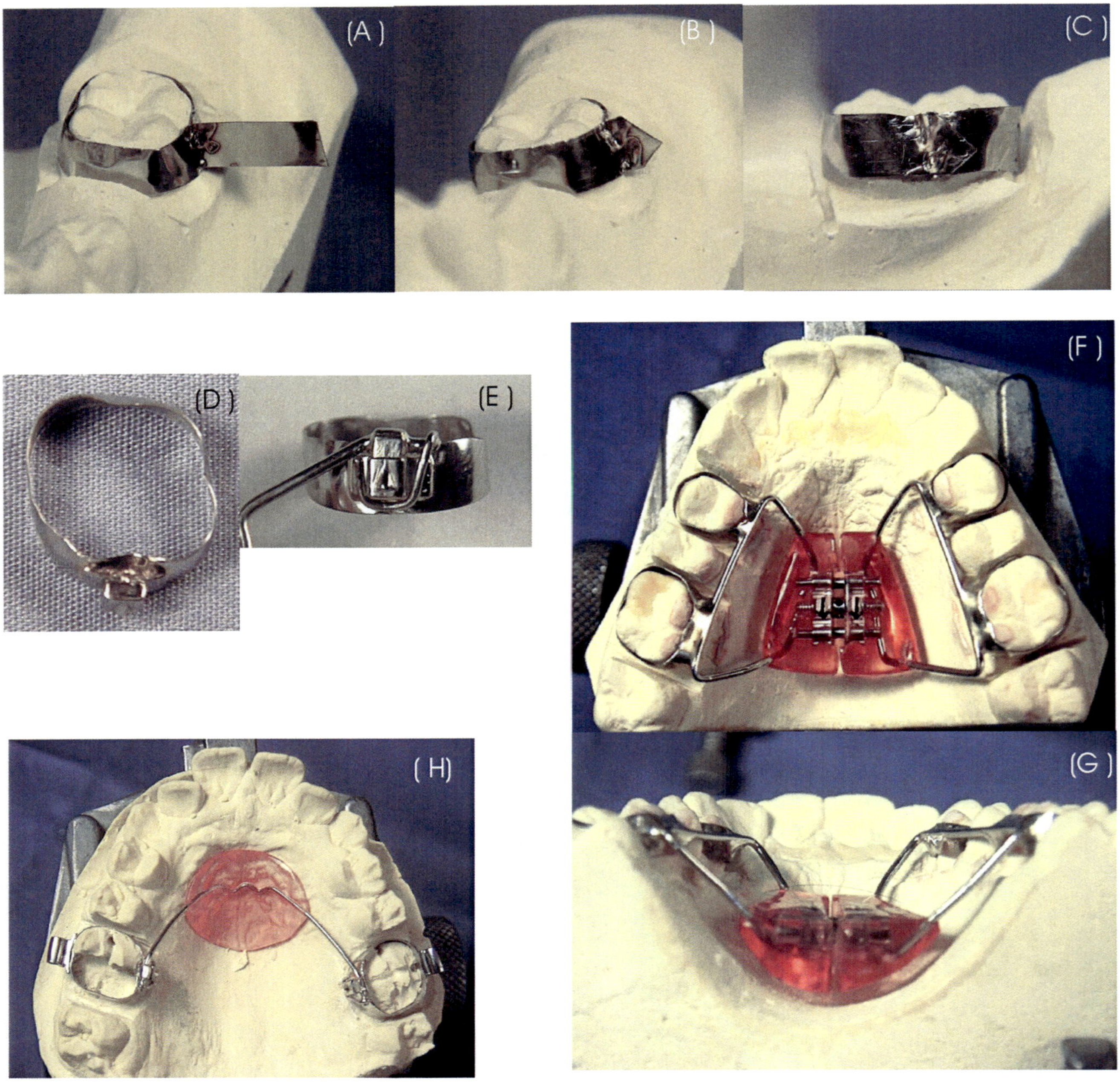

(A) Fabricating custom band.
(B) Form band around tooth and spotweld tag together.
(C) Tighten band by pulling on the tags with pliers, then cut excess tag off in "V" shape. Bend "V" tag over against band.
(D) Band with tube attachment, occlusal view.
(E) Fixed/removable post and tube attachment.
(F&G) Haas RPE, note relief of acrylic from palate in figure G.
(H) Nance Appliance

8 Fixed appliance designs

"I recommend biting off more than you can chew to anyone"
Alanis Morissette
"You Learn"
from jagged little pill, 1996

"Courage is the art of being the only one who knows you're scared to death."
Harold Wilson (1916 - 1995)

Fixed appliances are bonded directly to the teeth. They are placed in the mouth by the dentist and cannot be removed by the patient. Some designs — known as fixed/removable — have attachments which allow portions of the appliance to be removed from the mouth for adjustment, or because their specific function has been completed.

Fixed appliances have several advantages over removables. They can move the teeth in a bodily manner, and with some appliances — straight wire brackets particularly — adjustments can be controlled in 3 dimensions with accuracy. Removable appliances create mainly tipping movements.

Patient cooperation is not an issue in the same manner as with removable appliances. The patient cannot remove them from the mouth. The appliances are in place and functioning 24 hours a day, thereby shortening the treatment time.

There are concerns that must be satisfied with fixed appliances also. The patient must have good oral hygiene, as these appliances encourage the build up of food and plaque. The teeth must be erupted sufficiently to provide enough clinical crown to place the fixed appliance. An appliance with fixed components on the labial must be acceptable to the patient aesthetically.

Fixed appliances are generally attached in the mouth in one of two ways. They can be direct bonded or banded.

Direct bonding involves the preparation of the tooth surface with an etching solution that roughens the enamel surface to provide mechanical retention. The appliance gains its retention from mechanical interlock with either a mesh pad or an etched bonding surface on the attachment. These two surfaces — enamel and attachment — are joined directly with a bonding agent. Direct bonding can also involve an acrylic pad — similar to a posterior bite pad — which is bonded to the buccal and lingual of the posterior teeth and forms an occlusal pad over the occlusal surface.

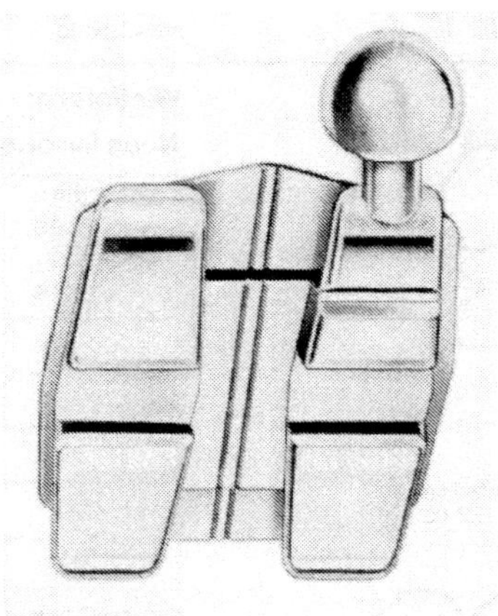

Courtesy of SNF-Forsestadent®

Fig. 8.1 Straight wire bracket

The most familiar direct bonded fixed appliance used today are the straight wire brackets, commonly called "braces". They are small rectangular attachments that are placed on each tooth and joined by a flexible wire.

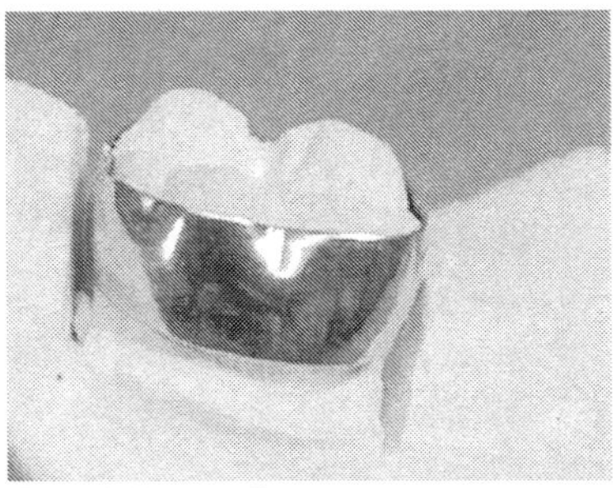

Fig. 8.2 Band

Banded appliances are the fixed appliances most commonly fabricated in the laboratory. Bands are small rings of stainless steel which are cemented around individual teeth. These act as attachment points for the other components of the appliance. The bands may be premanufactured or custom formed from band material. At one time, all fixed appliances were based on bands, however with the advent of simple and reliable systems for attaching direct bond appliances bands are now relegated to the posterior of the mouth in all but a few cases.

Banding

Basic banding techniques - band loop space maintainer

The simplest of the banded fixed appliances is the band loop space maintainer (blsm). This appliance is designed to hold space in the arch for a permanent tooth after the premature loss of a deciduous tooth. It is most commonly used upon the loss of a first or second deciduous molar.

Teeth have two directions that they seem to be determined to move in if nothing is there to stop them. When looking at a model, these are up and forward, occlusally (as in eruption) and mesially. The teeth in the opposing arch provide occlusal contacts that keep the teeth from continuously erupting, and the proximal contacts — where one tooth touches its neighbour — keep them from moving mesially. However, when a deciduous molar is lost early, there is nothing to keep the first permanent molar from moving forward. This is known as mesial migration. If this occurs, there will not be enough space left for the bicuspids to erupt into when their time comes.

Therefore, we use the band loop space maintainer to hold this space for the bicuspid eruption.

The band loop consists of:

- the band which provides the retention
- the loop which holds the space open
- the solder joint which holds the band and loop together.

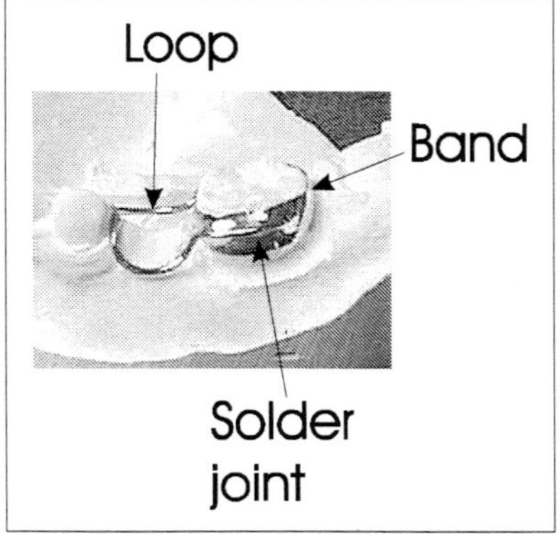

Fig. 8.3 Parts of the band loop space maintainer

The first step in preparing any banded appliance is to place the correct size band on the tooth.

A properly fitted band must fit the tooth snugly and its occlusal margin must be at or slightly below the marginal ridge (within 1 mm). The band may be fitted in the mouth chairside by the dentist, or fitted on the model in the laboratory.

If the band is fitted in the mouth by the dentist, an impression is taken of the arch with the band in place. The impression is removed, the band staying in the mouth seated on the tooth. The band is removed from the mouth and fitted into its position in the impression. The band should be fixed to the impression before the model is poured. If this is not done, the band can be dislodged by vibration during the pouring of the impression. It will then no longer reflect its true position in the mouth when the model is completed.

There are several ways to fix the band to the impression. Molten wax can be poured into the impression of the tooth being banded to hold the band, or impression compound may be used similarly. An alternate method is to place a wire staple over the band with its tines projecting into the impression material. With either method, the model can now be poured without moving the band.

When the band is fitted in the mouth by the dentist before the impression, soldering procedures are affected when fabricating the appliance. Any soldering that is to be done on the band must be completed before the band can be removed from the model. This will always result in some damage to the model. When the band is fixed to the impression with wax or impression compound, these materials must be removed before soldering begins to ensure a clean solder joint. Either of these — damaging the model or removal of combustible material — make it impossible to accurately reseat the band on the model once it is removed.

Model preparation for band seating

When a band is being fitted in the laboratory, the model must be prepared as follows.

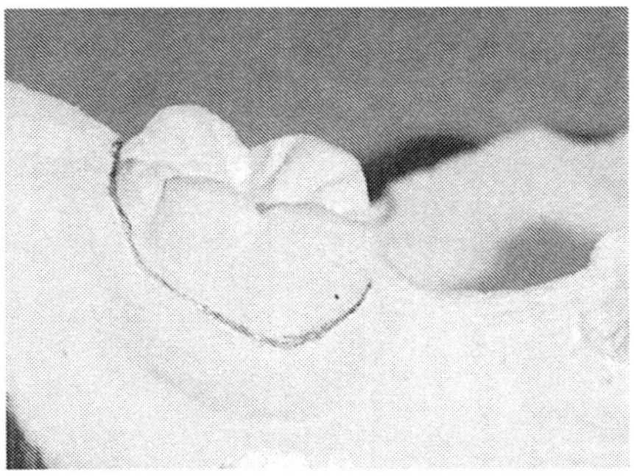
Fig. 8.4 Mark gingival margin

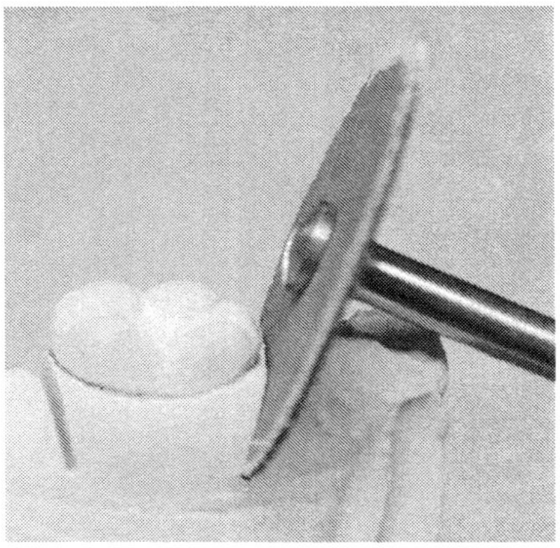
Fig. 8.5 Cut 5 mm on mesial and distal

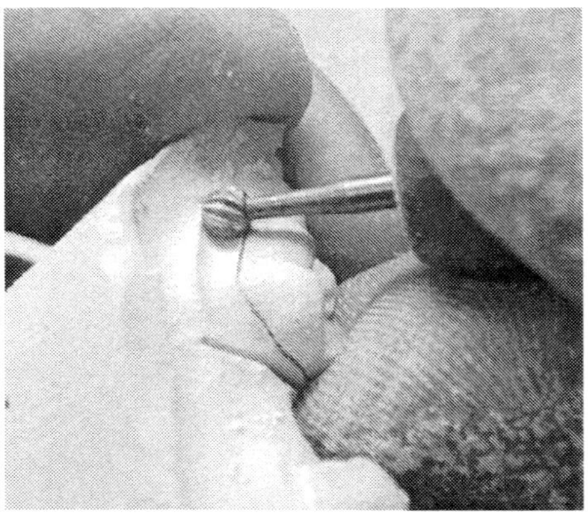
Fig. 8.6 Remove tissue bulk with round bur

Mark gingival margin with sharp pencil all the way around the tooth to be banded. Sharpen the tip of the pencil to a chisel point to allow it to get deep into the gingival crevice. Mark the line as deep into the interproximal areas as possible. This line is a guide to the starting size of the clinical crown of the tooth. When the preparation of the tooth is completed, this line must be intact. Having all of this line present, intact, is your assurance that you have not trimmed any material from the clinical crown of the tooth. Removal of material from the clinic crown will mean that the tooth on which you are working on the model is smaller than the patient's tooth in the mouth. The band which you are preparing will, therefore, not fit in the mouth.

Cut to mesial and distal of tooth to be banded. The cut should be a minimum of 5 mm in depth. This cut is made as close to the gingival margin of the tooth as possible, being careful not to remove any material from the clinical crown of the tooth. You can feel free to cut into the teeth adjacent to the tooth being banded providing that they are not being banded also. The cut may be made with a saw or a cutting disc in a handpiece. The mesial and distal cuts should angle slightly towards each other subgingivally, creating slight undercuts under the tooth.

The excess stone beneath the gingival margin is removed using a #12 round bur. Remove approximately 3-4 mm of material without undercutting the tooth or removing any of the line at the gingiva.

Using a straight Fisher bur, trim the sides of the subgingival preparation until they taper slightly inwards from the circumference of the gingival margin, undercutting it slightly. These preparations have to be at least parallel to each other and perpendicular to the occlusal plane, if they are not they will distort the band on seating. A slight undercut to the preparation ensures no interference with the model upon seating of the band. Prefabricated bands are formed to approximate the curved axial contours of the teeth. Shaping the preparations to match the subgingival contour of the teeth produces more accurate seating.

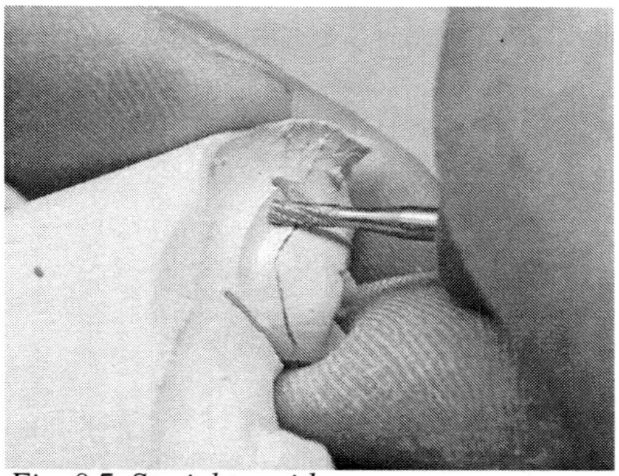

Fig. 8.7 Straighten sides of prep with fissure bur

The final trimming of the preparation is done with a scalpel or sharp knife. Remove any ledging around the margin and smooth the subgingival preparation.

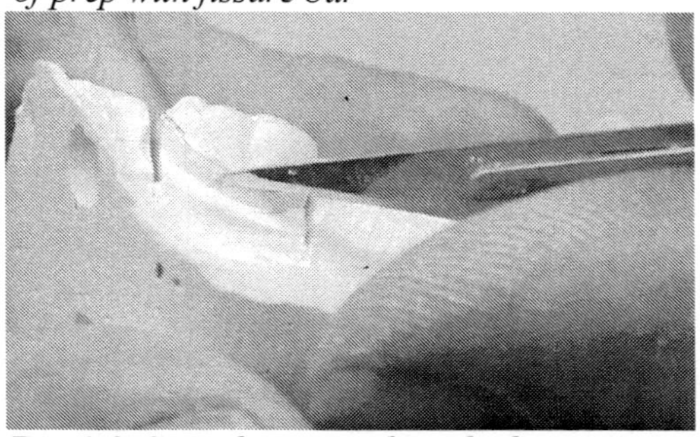

Fig. 8.8 Smooth prep with scalpel

When you have finished with the trimming of the margin, you should have a smooth transition between the supra and sub gingival areas. You must also still have intact all of the original pencil line you drew at the gingival margin.

A stainless steel orthodontic band may now be adapted to the preparation.

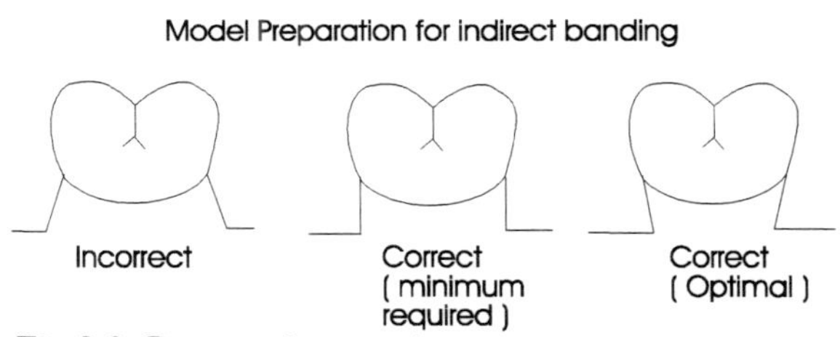

Fig 8.9 Preparation requirements

Fitting a prefabricated band

Prefabricated bands are very easy to seat on the model. It is a simple matter of finding the size of band that fits the particular tooth. Be sure to use a band for the correct tooth and quadrant before starting.

I find it better to start by choosing a band I think will be slightly large. This lets me see how close I am to the correct size without scraping the tooth. Forcing a small band down over a tooth will remove some of the clinical crown, making subsequent fittings less accurate. When you have found a band size which appears to be correct, gently push it down with an instrument. Often you will find that one side of the band will seat first — commonly the lingual — and then the other. The band should fit snugly all around the tooth.

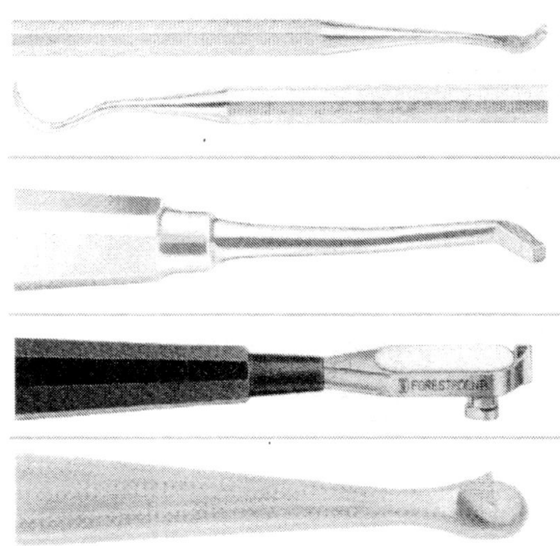

Courtesy of SNF-Forsestadent®

Fig. 8.10 Band seating tools

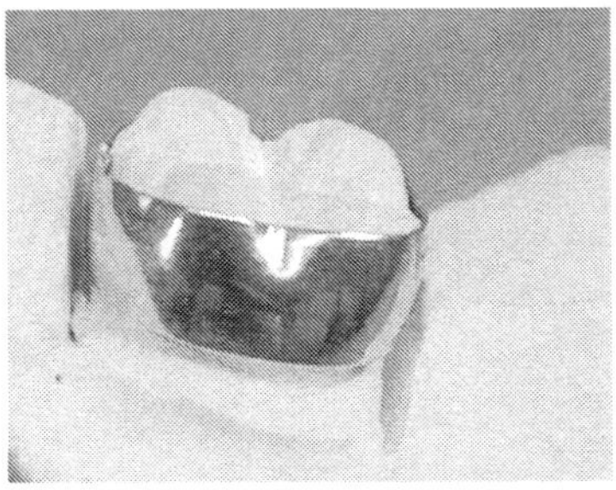

Fig. 8.11 Preformed band

The occlusal margin of the band should be at the marginal ridge or no more than 1 mm gingival to it. Any spaces between the band and the tooth at the occlusal of the band are removed by burnishing the band with an instrument until there is an even fit all around.

When a prefabricated band is fit to the model, it is a good idea to record the band size on both the model — on the tissue directly under the tooth — and on the prescription. If the band does not fit for any reason, or the patient requires another appliance, this will help you to fit the correct size band with minimum of guesswork.

Fabricating a custom band

A custom band is made with the ribbon-like, stainless steel band material. This material has a shiny side and a matte finish side. The matte finish is placed inside the band to provide better retention to the cement. The two most common sizes of band material used are .180x.005" for molar bands and .150x.004" for bicuspid bands.

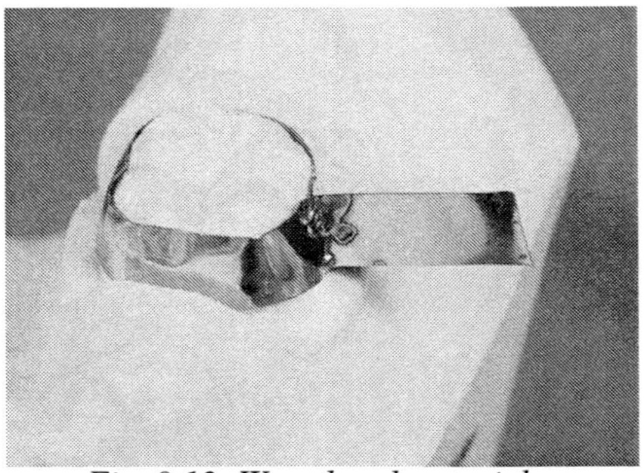

Fig. 8.12 Wrap band material about prep and spot weld

A custom formed band is made by wrapping a strip of band material around the tooth and then soldering the ends together. Cut a 5 cm strip of band material and form it into a U-shape the width of your finger. Place this around the tooth with the opening of the U to the buccal.

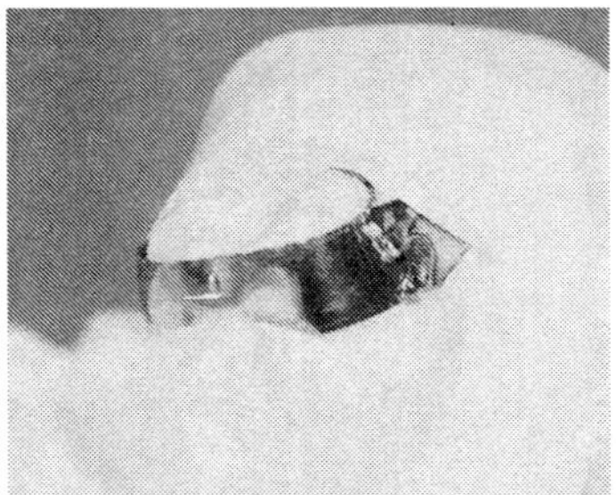

Fig. 8.13 Tighten band and cut excess material

Bend the band material to form a ring around the tooth with the joint in the centered on the buccal and the excess material projecting buccally. Spot weld the two sides of the band material together as close to the buccal surface of the tooth as possible. Using pliers, pull the excess tag of band material to take up any slack material around the tooth, and squeeze the tag close to the buccal of the tooth to tighten the band. Repeat this until the band fits the tooth as closely as possible. Spot weld again as close to the buccal surface as possible.

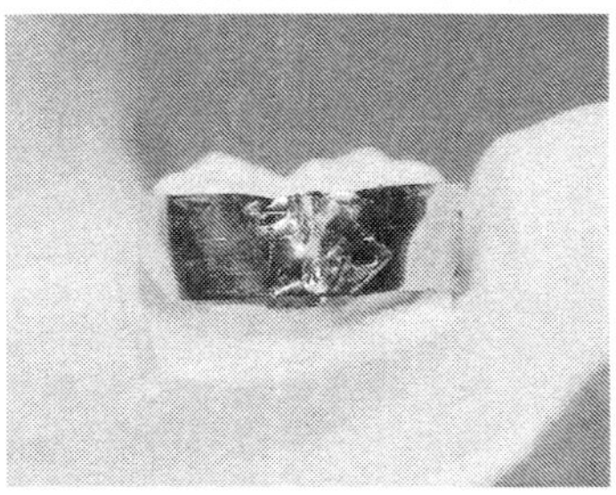

Fig. 8.14 Fold tag to buccal surface and solder

Cut the excess material of the tag, leaving 3-4 mm. Using an instrument, bend this small tag to the distal until it lays flat to the buccal surface of the band. This will help to tighten the band further. Spot weld the tag to the buccal surface of the band. The band is now ready for the joint to be soldered.

Bending the band loop

The loop portion of the band loop space maintainer (blsm) must meet three major requirements:

- It must be in contact with the proximal surface of the tooth on the other side of the edentulous area of the alveolar ridge (bracing tooth);
- It must not contact the tissue at any point and should have an even relief of approximately 1 mm at all points;
- The loop must be wide enough to permit the tooth for which the space is being held to erupt without interference.

To begin bending the loop, cut approximately 6 cm of 0.8 mm wire. The following directions are the steps in bending the loop for a blsm on the lower first molar.

The first bend is a gentle v bend in the center of the wire. This allows the wire to conform to the proximal surface of the bracing tooth. This V bend will lie parallel to the occlusal plane. This wire is generally placed just above the gingival margin of the tooth, as the teeth being contacted generally have short crowns and no undercuts. The contact joint must be occlusal to any height of contour for the tooth, otherwise the dentist will not be able to seat the blsm in the mouth.

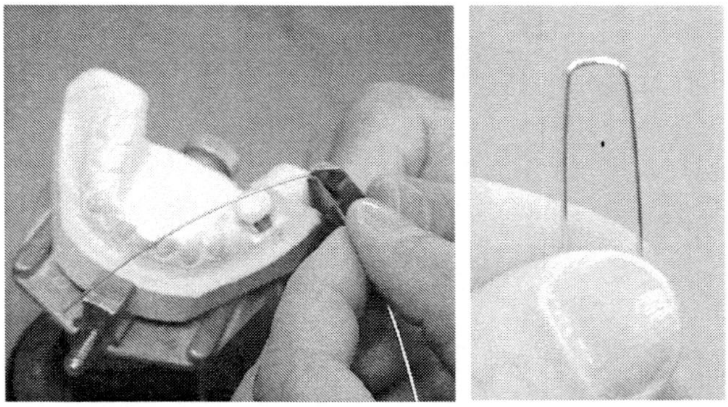

Fig. 8.15 First bends, small v and 90° bends

At a width of approximately 1 mm greater than the crest portion of the alveolar ridge, bend the ends of the wire down at 90° to the occlusal plane. This is done to make forming the loops easier.

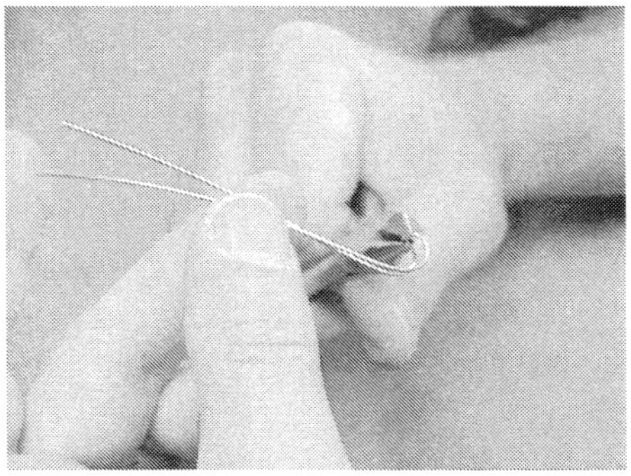

Fig. 8.16 Bend loops, 180°

Grasping the wire with the pliers immediately below the 90° bend. With your fingers at the far end of the wire, make a large gentle loop of 180°.

The 90° bends must now be increased (adjusted outwards) until the loops fit over the ridge without impinging on the tissue. The loops are adjusted so that they form a gentle curve from the proximal surface of the bracing tooth to the mesial of the band.

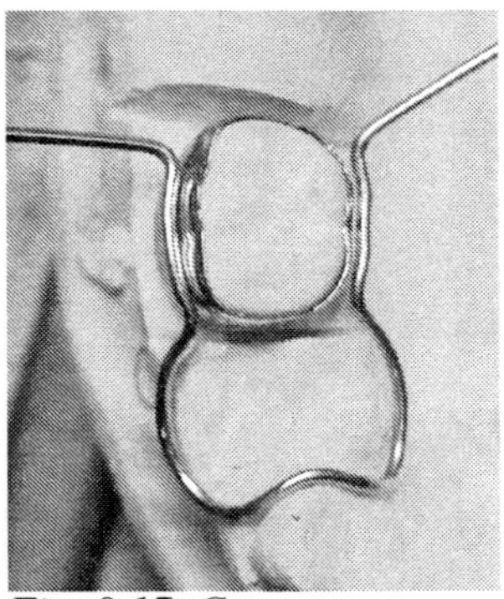

Fig. 8.17 Contour tags to band, buccal and lingual

The tags are bent to closely match the contour of the buccal and lingual sides of the band. They

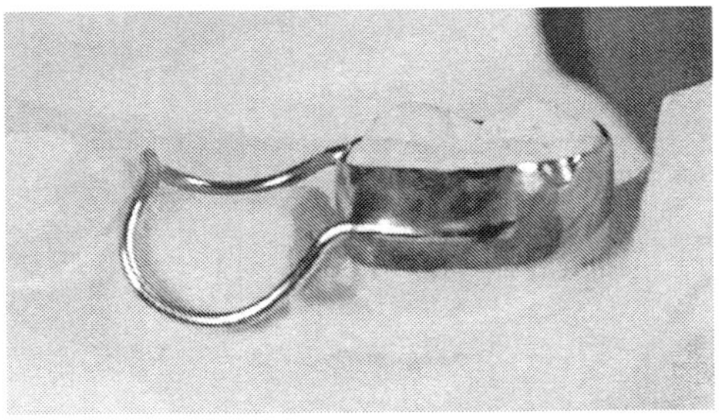

Fig. 8.18 Tag placement

should be parallel to the occlusal edge of the band. The tags on the buccal should be at the level of the center of the clinical height of the crown of the tooth. On the lingual, they can be slightly closer to the occlusal because this is a nonfunctional area and the lingual height of most teeth is less than the buccal height. The tags should extend ¾ of the mesial-distal length of the tooth.

Spot weld the loop to the band in at least two places on both the buccal and lingual to fix it to the band for soldering. Alternately, if a spot welder is not available the loop can be held in place with a mixture of plaster and pumice or waxed into position. If the wire is waxed into position, some type of thermal insulating material must be placed over the wax before soldering to prevent the wax from melting when heat is applied to the wire. Commercial thermal insulators are available, or a layer of wet ring liner will work.

If the band can be removed from the model for soldering, do so. This will result in a better solder joint. When bands are soldered on the model, the model acts as a heat sink, soaking up the heat from the torch. This makes it more difficult to warm the metal to accept the solder and burns the model.

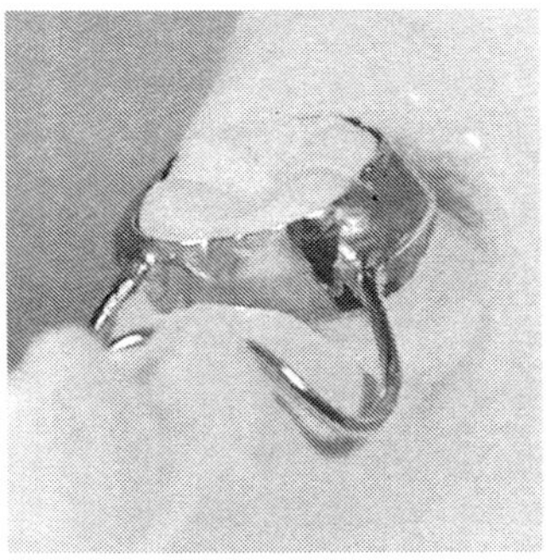

Fig. 8.19 Smooth solder joint, not bulky

Place sufficient solder over the joint to cover the wire. The solder should taper towards the gingival margin of the band. Too much bulk of solder in this area can result in tissue damage. Trim and polish the solder and the band.

For more detailed soldering and polishing instructions, see the section on *soldering* in Materials.

A rest can be placed on the bracing tooth by bending 0.7 mm wire over the distal marginal ridge into the distal fossa of the tooth. The rest is then soldered to the mesial of the loop where it contacts the bracing tooth.

Space maintainers and variations of the blsm

High contact blsm

There are several design variations that may be incorporated into the blsm when needed.

If the tooth being contacted by the loop has a height of contour significantly occlusal to the gingival margin, the shape of the loop must be modified to account for this. This is done by forming a small, sharp V-bend in the wire where it contacts the tooth. This V-bend is inverted and will sit approximately perpendicular to the occlusal plane, or vertically on the model. No portion of this V-bend should be placed in an undercut region. The point of the V will contact the tooth at or slightly above the height of contour. The V should be narrower than the bucco-lingual width of the tooth. Just above the gingiva, the V is bent outwards to form the beginning of the loop.

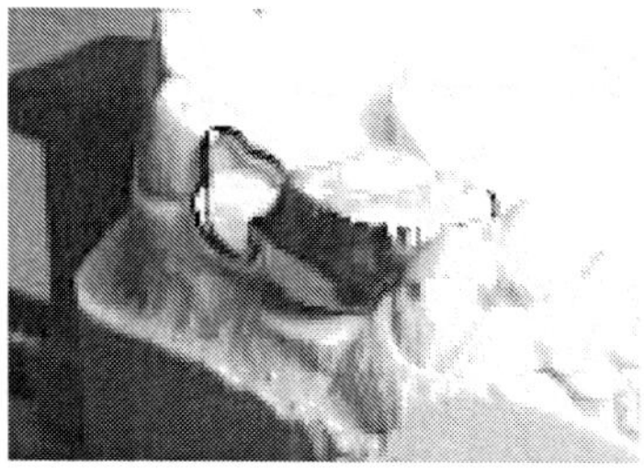

Fig. 8.20 High contact blsm

This form will allow the wire to contact the tooth above the height of contour without the wire being far enough from the tissue at any point to become an undue irritant.

Upper blsm

A blsm for the upper arch does not require the wide curved loop of the lower blsm. The palate of the upper causes the alveolar ridge to assume a wider form than the lower allowing the loop of a blsm to pass almost straight from one tooth to the other.

Intra alveolar space maintainer

A special situation exists when the deciduous second molar is lost before the eruption of the first permanent molar. The permanent molar can start to move mesially before it is even erupted. While it is under the tissue, we cannot place a band loop or a removable space maintainer on it. The tooth can therefore travel mesially and erupt in an incorrect position, blocking out the bicuspid.

A solution to this problem is known as an intra-alveolar space maintainer. It is resembles a blsm, with the band on the first deciduous molar and the loop running distally to the first permanent molar. The first permanent molar is still beneath the tissue, so in order to reach it we must employ an accessory that can go there also.

This is referred to as a blade. It is a projection of wire or doubled over band material or both which is placed into the tissue to con-

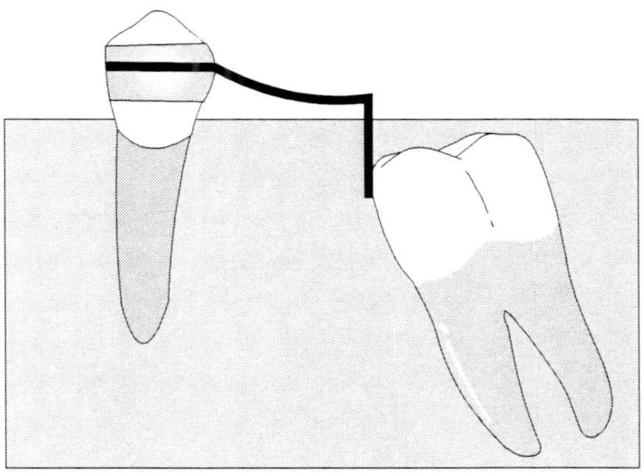

Fig. 8.21 Intra-alveolar space maintainer

tact the mesial of the first molar. The first molar will be guided in its eruption by this blade.

In order to construct this appliance the first information that is needed is the exact location of the unerupted tooth. The dentist obtains this by taking an x-ray and measuring the distance from the "d" to the mesial of the 6. This distance is transferred to the model and marked on the ridge. A groove is cut in the alveolar ridge at this location. The dentist can specify the depth of this cut to ensure that the blade reaches the unerupted tooth. If no depth is given, extend the blade 5 mm into the ridge. Bucco-lingually the blade should be placed in the center of the ridge.

Fixed Appliances

Lingual arches

The lingual arch can be used to accomplish a number of objectives, space maintenance, anchorage, or as a base for active components.

The lingual arch can be used as a space maintenance appliance when there are bilateral edentulous areas or multiple teeth missing from the arch, particularly in the mixed dentition stage. The bands on the first permanent molars act to hold these teeth from migrating mesially by anchoring against the linguals of the permanent incisors. It is generally better than multiple or long span blsm appliances if several teeth are missing. The lingual arch is also still effective if more deciduous teeth are lost while it is in the mouth because it is based on the permanent teeth in the mixed dentition. This is not necessarily true with the blsm.

The lingual arch may also be used as anchorage in some instances when there is an anterior pull on the molars — i.e.. Class II elastics — to prevent the molars from being mesialized.

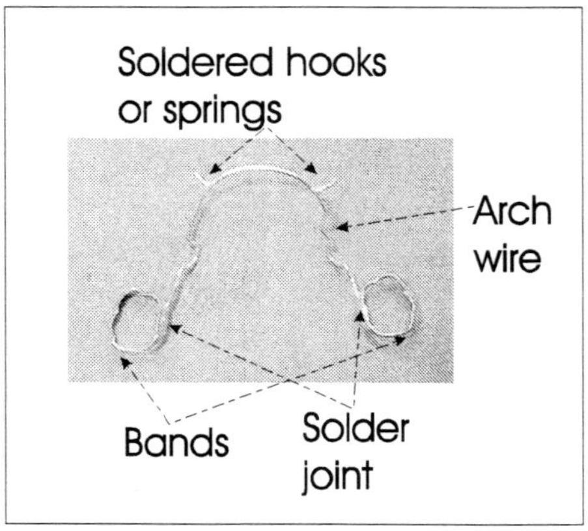

Fig. 8.22 Parts of the lingual arch

Springs can be soldered to the arch wire to exert forces from the lingual of the teeth. Most of these springs provide mesial-distal movement, however some can provide limited facial movement. Limited facial movement is generally preferable in a spring on a lingual arch, unless the appliance included has a labial arch to act as a control.

The basic soldered lingual arch has three parts:

- the arch wire
- the bands
- the solder joint.

Soldered lingual arch

The soldered lingual arch is placed in the mouth and left for the duration of treatment. As a soldered fixed appliance without attachments, it is difficult to adjust and virtually impossible to remove without damaging the appliance. It must, therefore, be extremely accurately constructed to ensure that no adjustments are necessary. The arch must fit the model exactly and passively. The soldered lingual arch is a staple appliance in many dentists treatment plans.

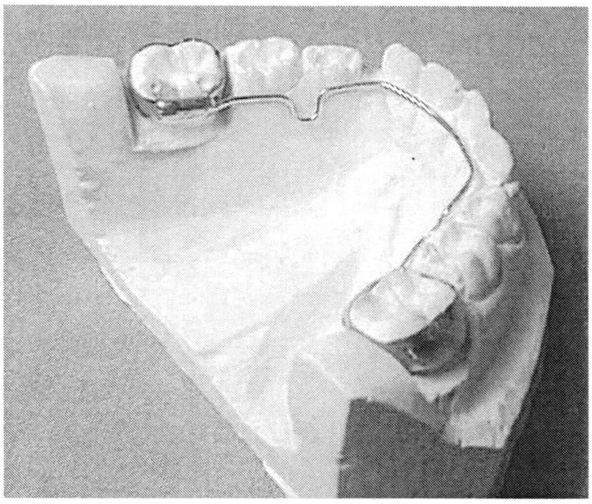

Fig. 8.23 Soldered lingual arch

Bending the arch wire

The lingual arch wire is bent with 0.9 mm wire.

In the anterior the wire should rest on the cingulums of the anterior teeth, and it should contact the lingual of the posteriors just above the gingiva.

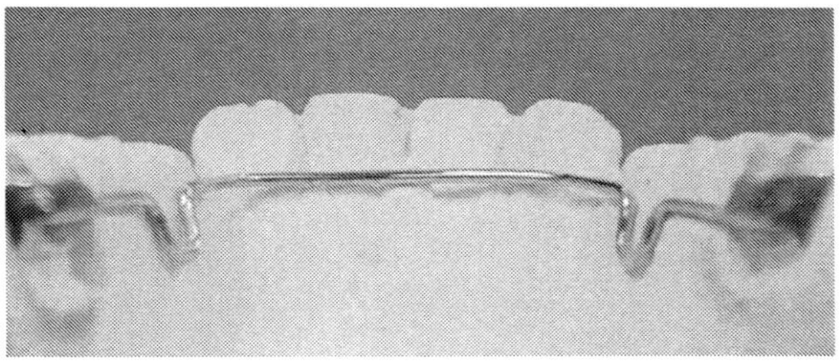

Fig. 8.24 Soldered lingual arch resting on cingulums

There is a Wilson loop placed between the first and second deciduous molars in mixed dentition, and between the first and second premolars in permanent dentition. This is to provide an adjustment point in the arch. Not all designs include the Wilson loops; some prefer the wire to follow along the linguals of the posteriors with no adjustment points.

As with any labial arch, the lingual arch may be bent from the center out, or from one end to the other. The shape of the anterior of the arch should be a smooth arc that compromises between conforming to the lingual surfaces of all teeth, and being symmetrical. When the lingual arch is used specifically as a space maintainer, the arch wire should conform closely to the linguals of all anterior teeth.

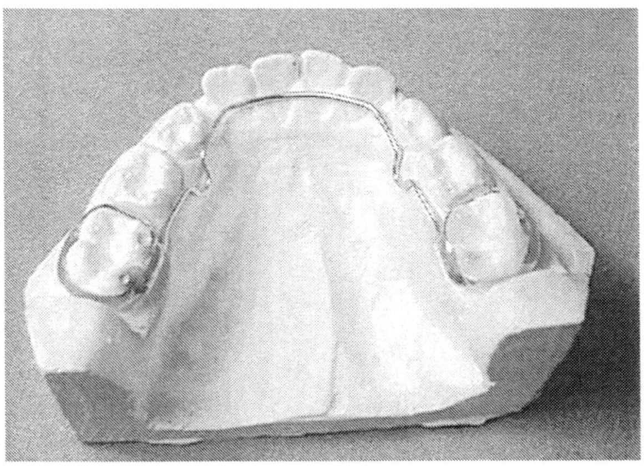

Fig. 8.25 Soldered lingual arch

When the deciduous molars have been lost, and the permanent incisors are standing by themselves, or with the deciduous cuspid, a spur or hook should be soldered to engage the distal of the last anterior. This will prevent the anteriors from drifting distally along the wire and opening anterior spaces.

The Wilson loops of the lingual arch are smaller than those of a labial arch, and they are angled to the lingual to prevent tissue impingement. These loops may be bent with parallel sides — as with the Hawley — or they can be closed more to the occlusal, creating a more pear shaped loop.

The appliance can be used to affect a slight labial tipping of the anteriors or distalization and uprighting of the molars by the opening of the Wilson loops. The pear shaped Wilson loops permit more activation for this purpose.

Fixed/Removable Lingual Arch

The fixed/removable (f/r) lingual arch has the ability to be removed from the mouth after the cementation of the bands without the necessity of removing the bands. This makes the post insertion adjustment of the appliance easier and more accurate.

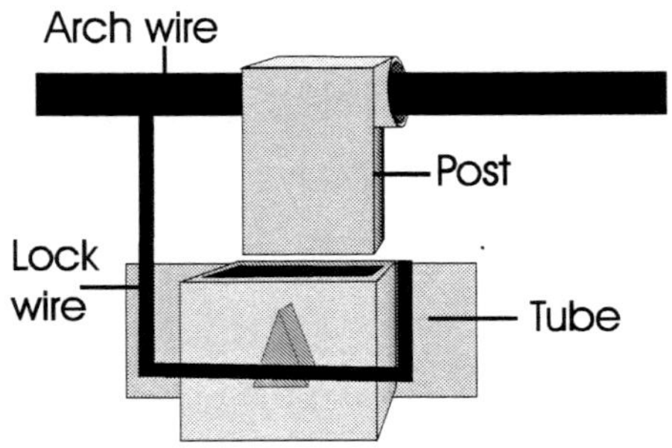

Fig. 8.26 Parts of post and tube attachment

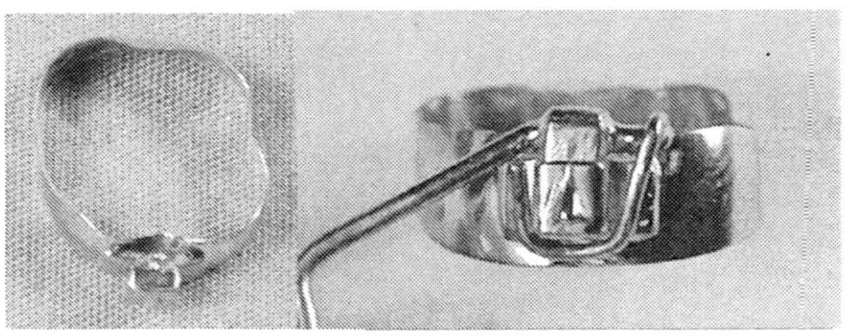

Fig. 8.27 Lingual tube soldered to band, attachment complete

The arch is fabricated using 0.9 mm (.036") wire. The removal is accomplished through the use of a post and tube assembly. This type of attachment is know as the “Ellis-type”. The post is soldered to the arch wire, and the tube soldered to the band. The arch wire continues distal to the tube on the band, and a dead soft lock wire is soldered from the posterior of the arch wire to pass anteriorly under the tube. This lock wire resists the unseating of the arch in the mouth.

Alternately there is a small raised triangle on the lingual surface of the tube. This triangle is always oriented with the base of the triangle to the gingival. The lock wire may be bent to engage either the undercut formed by the base of this triangle or the entire attachment.

Bending the fixed/removable lingual arch wire and soldering

The arch wire is formed to the same specifications as a soldered lingual arch.

The wire should rest on the cingulums of the anteriors, and contact the lingual of the posteriors just above the gingiva.

There is a Wilson Loop placed between the first and second deciduous molars in mixed dentition, and between the first and second premolars in permanent dentition.

The arch can be bent in one of two ways. The arch form may be bent to its shape so that the wire passes .5 mm lingual to the molar bands. The post and tubes are placed on the wires and positioned — angled toward the lingual surface of the tooth — so that the tubes contact the lingual surface of the bands. The tubes are then spot welded to the bands. The post is spot welded to the arch wire. The post is then removed from the tube and the lock wire spot welded to the distal of the arch. Solder the post and the tube to the arch wire and band respectively.

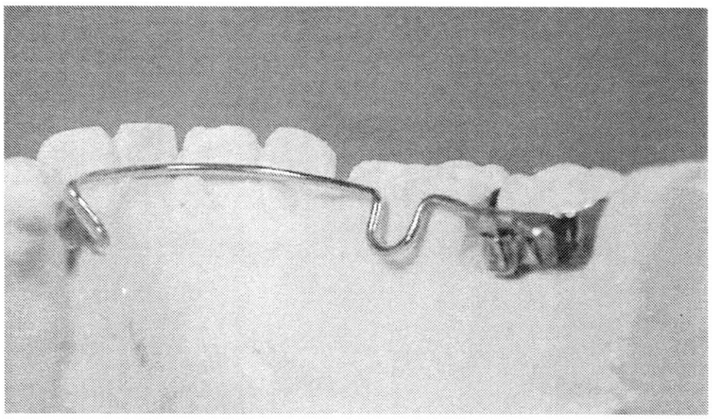

Fig. 8.28 F/r lingual arch

A second method is to position and solder the tubes onto the molar bands, and solder a post to a length of wire. The bands are seated on the model. The post is then placed into one of the tubes on the molar bands and the arch is bent. Starting at the end with the attachment, adapt the wire around the arch to the band on other side. The second post is then positioned on the wire to match the tube already on the band and soldered.

The lock wire is soldered at the same time as the attachments. The adaptation of the wire may be done after the soldering is completed.

The tubes and posts should be spot welded into place and then soldered with a minimum of excess solder. Any solder that is placed onto the post or into the tube will impede the seating of the appliance, probably requiring that the appliance be remade.

Active components and f/r attachments

Horizontal lingual sheath

The horizontal lingual sheath is a female attachment which is placed with the opening oriented parallel to the occlusal place, rather than perpendicular, such as the Ellis style attachment. This means that the appliance is inserted into the attachment from the anterior of posterior, depending on the design. This attachment has the advantage of having less

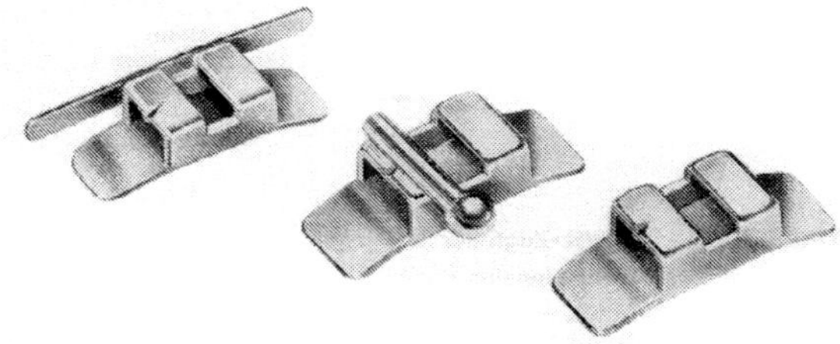

Fig. 8.29 Horizontal lingual sheathes. Courtesy of SNF-Forsestadent®

vertical height than the Ellis style attachment, therefore there is less chance of occlusal interference.

The lingual sheathes are available is sizes that accept 0.8 and 0.9 mm wire. The wire is doubled over so that it is two thicknesses wide oclusal-gingivally, and one thickness buccal-lingually.

This attachment design works well with appliances such as Trans-palatal arch, which exert forces transversely when activated. Such an appliance would work to unseat an Ellis style attachment.

Springs

Springs placed on the lingual arch are similar to those used on labial arches of removable appliances. The springs are soldered to the arch at one end and free to affect movement at the other. Several designs have an adjustment loop with the wire then coiled around the arch wire to improve stability of the spring.

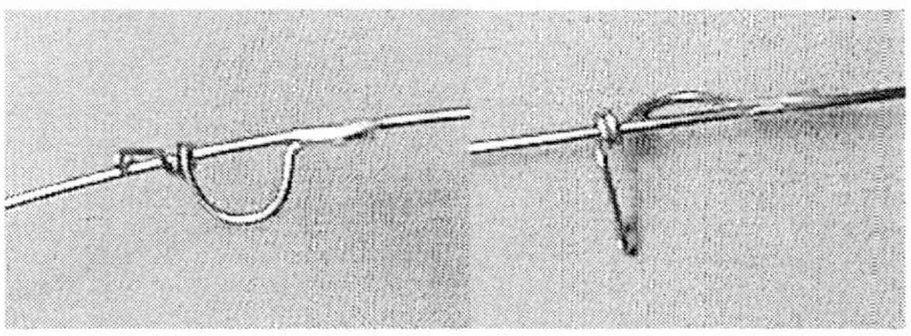

Fig. 8.30 Lingual loop finger spring

Springs can be placed on the lingual arch to produce mesial/distal tooth movements by having one fixed end on the arch, and the other end a coil around the arch wire that is free to move. A loop is formed between the two ends of the spring provides the adjustment point of the spring.

A spring to produce limited labial movement of the anteriors can be fabricated by soldering 0.5 mm wire to the arch lingual to the first bicuspid, bending an adjustment loop and then coiling the wire around the arch. The wire is then adapted to match the curve of the arch around to the other side, and then another coil and adjustment loop are bent. The tag on this side is also soldered to the arch. The spring is activated by compressing the adjustment loops between flat plier beaks.

Fixed retention appliances

A common retention appliance for the mandibular arch is the 3x3 lingual wire, or bonded lingual arch. This as a retainer which runs from the lingual of 3.3 to the lingual of 4.3 and is bonded to either all of the anterior teeth or just the two cuspids. This appliance acts to stabilize the anteriors, thereby stabilizing all of the mandibular teeth. As a bonded retainer there are no relapse problems associated with the patient not wearing their retainer. It is small, invisible and well accepted by patients. The bonded 3x3 can be used on the upper anteriors, but only in cases where there are no functional contacts between the lower anteriors and the linguals of the upper anterior.

Designs

There are a range of wires and designs used for these appliances, including different bonding methods.

The wires used can be a light braided wire (.016-.018") , a round wire (.5 mm) or a square wire (.016x.016"). The bonding attachment can be a mesh pad, or the wire itself can be covered with composite.

The simplest design is a piece of wire, usually braided, adapted to the lingual of the anteriors just incisal to the cingulum. This wire is then bonded to either the cuspids or all of the anteriors by covering it with composite. There is nothing added to the wire to enhance adhesion to the composite.

The mesh pad design of the 3x3 uses a round wire (.5 mm) which is soldered to the pads. The mesh pads are positioned over the lingual ridge of the cupid and the wire adapted along the linguals of the anteriors just incisal to the cingulums. The wire is then soldered to the pads. The mesh pads' style can also be purchased as preformed appliances in various sizes. The correct size is chosen and then adapted to the teeth.

The .5 mm round wire can be used to bend a lingual retainer that has a curly-q placed on the disto-lingual of each cuspid. Placing the bonding point to the distal of the cuspid helps to hold the cuspid against rotation. This design is normally bonded only to the cuspids.

Square wire (.016x.016") can be used to fabricate a 3x3 which includes a bonding point on each tooth in the anterior. In the center of the lingual of each tooth a small "v" is bent to lay flat to the tooth. Each of these will be covered with composite, splinting all of the anteriors together.

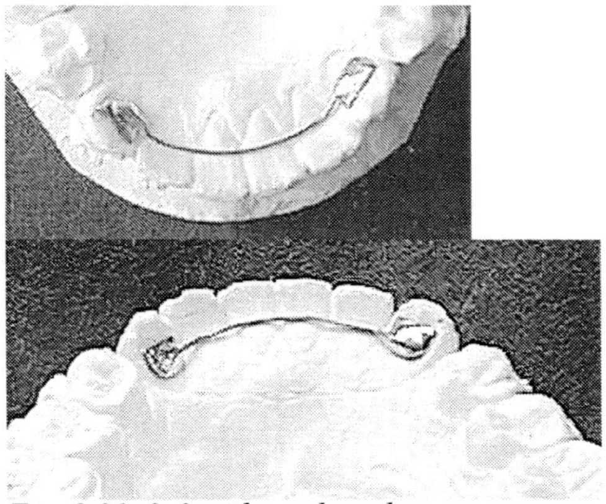

Fig. 8.31 3x3 with mesh pads

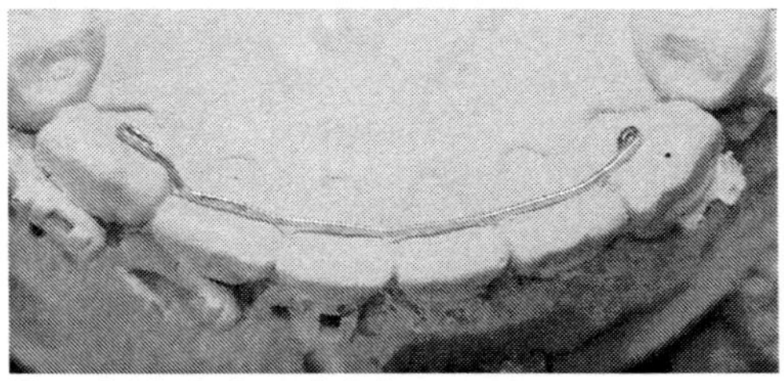

Fig. 8.32 3x3 with 0.5 mm wire

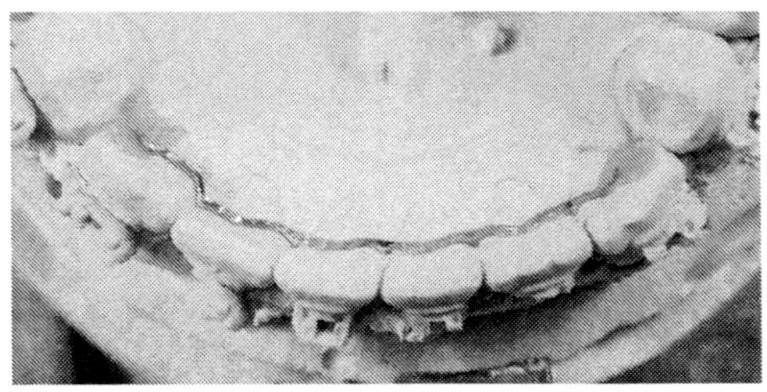

Fig. 8.33 3x3 with .016x.016 square wire, incisal view

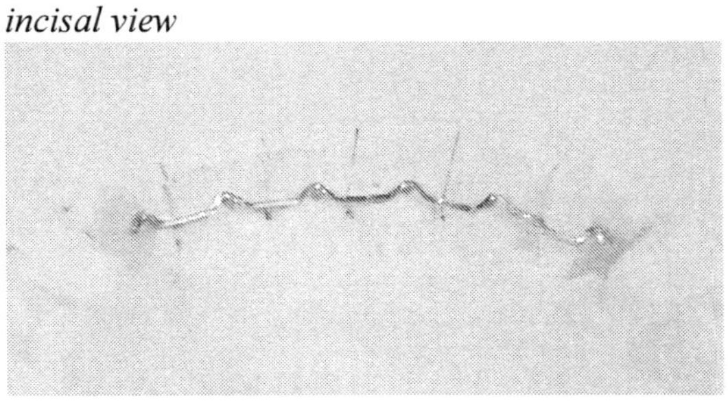

Fig. 8.34 3x3 with .016x.016 square wire, lingual view. Note v-bends on lingual of each tooth.

3x3 matrixes

Positioning the small wire that forms the 3x3 accurately can be a manual dexterity challenge for anyone. To assist in the insertion of the appliance, a matrix can be formed to transfer the wire's position from the model to the mouth. This matrix is made by adapting a heavy body polysiloxane impression material (lab putty consistency) over the wire and the teeth.

The matrix should cover the lingual surfaces and the wire from the lateral to lateral, leaving the lingual surface and wire exposed on the cuspids. The matrix must extend over the incisal and the buccal of the teeth to provide positive stops vertically. The wire, which is exposed on the lingual of the cuspids, allows the dentist to bond these teeth while the matrix is stabilizing the wire. The matrix can then be removed and the other teeth bonded, if desired.

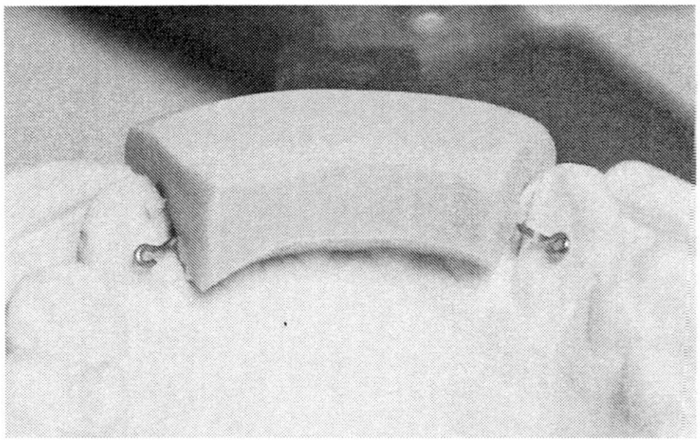

Fig. 8.35 3x3 fixed retainer with matrix

Fixed expansion appliances

Rapid palatal expanders (RPE)

Rapid palatal expanders (RPE's) perform a unique function for orthodontic appliances. Most expansion appliances are designed to slowly move the teeth. RPE's are designed to break a bone. The reason for this is to allow large amounts of lateral expansion to be created.

Not just any bone is broken, however RPE's exert their forces on the maxilla and cause the median suture — which joins the two halves of the maxilla — to fracture. In honour of this drastic ability, RPE's are affectionately called "skull-splitters"

While this may seem to be an extreme treatment, it works well, best in cases of children and adolescents. These young people have a suture that has not yet fully formed.

A suture is an immobile joint which is formed by the mechanical retention of small projections of bone interlocking, much like a zipper. All joints in the skull are sutures except for the TMJ. As we age, the sutures in our skulls continue to intermesh causing the joints to become stronger. In the young, the interlocking has not completely occurred and it is possible to break it fairly easily. Young people can also generate new bone more quickly once the expansion is complete, more quickly stabilizing the maxilla. This appliance is not restricted to younger patients. It has been successfully employed on many adult patients, however it does work better on younger people.

The RPE's work by placing a great deal of pressure on the maxilla in a short period of time. This is possible because the RPE's are fixed appliances. The pressure applied is much greater than any clasping system could resist.

The screw can be activated from 1 to 4 times a day at the dentist's discretion. In only a few days, the stresses induced by this expansion will break the suture. The quick application of the force means that the teeth do not have time to react by moving in the alveolar ridge. The fracture of the suture releases the pressure on the teeth ensuring that the tissue is not damaged beyond recovery.

Once the suture has broken, the two halves of the maxilla can be separated as necessary with little resistance, and then held at the desired separation until the palatal bone reforms. Retention in these cases is of paramount importance. Retention must be stable and worn continuously until new bone has filled the gap between the halves of the maxilla.

To work properly the design of the RPE must include a sturdy framework and strong expansion screw.

Banding an RPE

The RPE design is generally based on four bands. The appliance is soldered to bands on the 4's and 6's, although it may be placed on any other posterior teeth or just the 6's.

Prepare the teeth to be banded as usual (for detailed instructions see the "Basic banding techniques" at the beginning of this chapter).

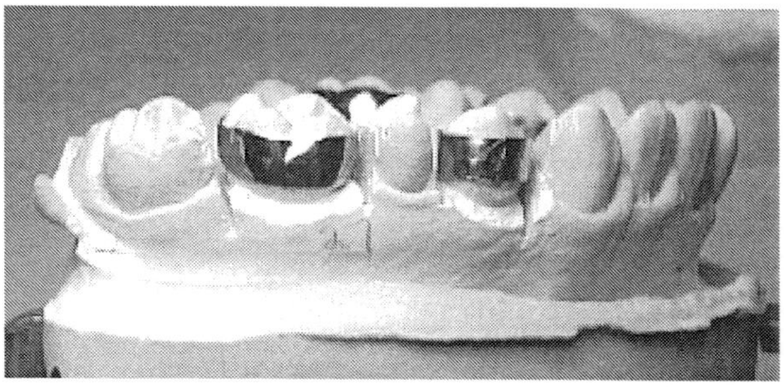

Fig. 8.36 Bands on 4's and 6's for RPE

With the RPE type appliances, it is preferable to use bands that are slightly larger than normal. When four bands are being placed into the mouth as a single unit, if they fit the teeth too tightly, the dentist will not be able to insert the appliance. A small amount of play is needed to facilitate insertion.

Types of RPE

The different types of RPE's are defined by their expansion screws. They are the Hyrax and Haas type RPE's.

One important point with regards to the expansion screw of an RPE is that the arrow of the screw must point to the posterior. The screw must open when the key is moved from anterior to posterior, otherwise the patient will not be able to activate the appliance themselves.

Hyrax

The Hyrax RPE derives its name from the Hyrax screw. The Hyrax is specifically designed for use in the RPE, although on some occasions it has been adapted for use in other designs. The Hyrax is a large heavily, built screw with four heavy wire arms attached to the body of the screw by either solder, welding or in some cases laser welding. The heavy wire arms must be bent using heavy pliers to avoid damage to your pliers.

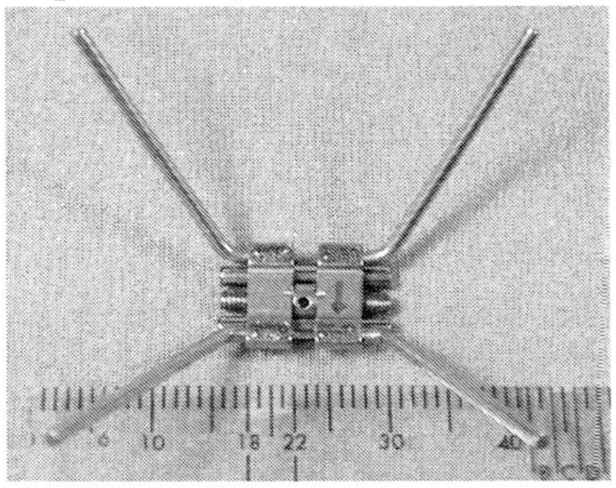

Fig. 8.37 Hyrax screw

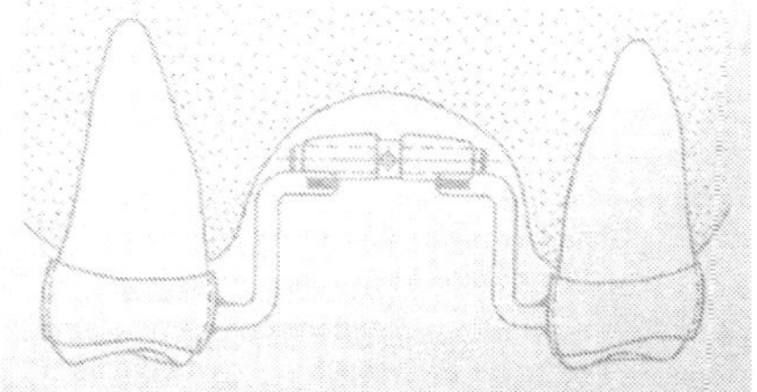

Fig. 8.38 Place screw high in palate. Courtesy of SNF-Forsestadent®

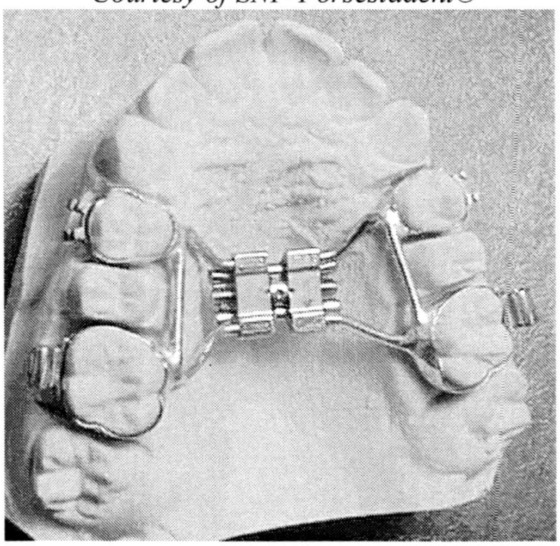

Fig. 8.39 Banded Hyrax appliance

The Hyrax is a relatively easy appliance to fabricate. The arms of the screw are bent to adapt to the bands and then it is soldered into place. The arms should be bent to allow the body of the screw to rest as high in the palate as possible for patient comfort. Placing the screw too close to the occlusal gives the patient little room for their tongue.

The posterior arms should contour to the distal of the 6's, with the anterior arms coming to the mesial of the 4's. The excess wire from one of the two arms can be cut off and then contoured to pass along the lingual of the teeth from 4-6, joining the bands together. This is usually easier than bending this wire continuously from one of the arms. The arms are then soldered solidly to the bands.

Haas

The Haas appliance is similar in design to the Hyrax, the difference being in the components used in each. While the Hyrax uses a special purpose screw which is soldered directly to the bands, the Haas employs a standard type screw which is placed in an acrylic body and joined to the bands with wire arms.

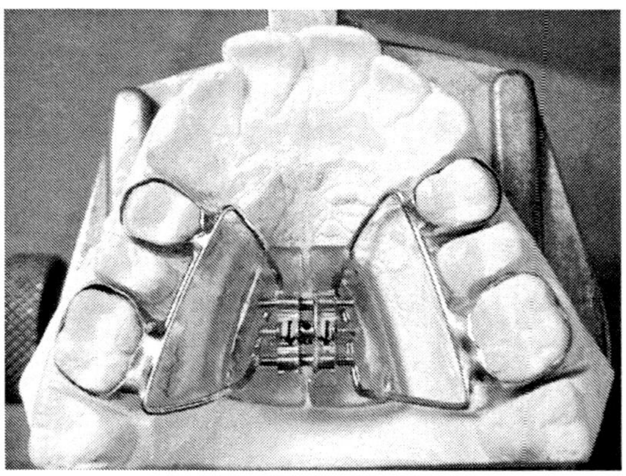

Fig. 8.40 Haas appliance

The Haas appliance again begins with four bands.

To these bands is soldered a wire arm of

1.0 mm wire. Using a 8 cm piece of wire, adapt the center section of the wire to contact the lingual of the bands on the 4 and 6. The wire may or may not contact the lingual of the 5. If the 5 is positioned buccally, do not contact it. The wire can extend distally to contact the lingual of the 7 if it is present.

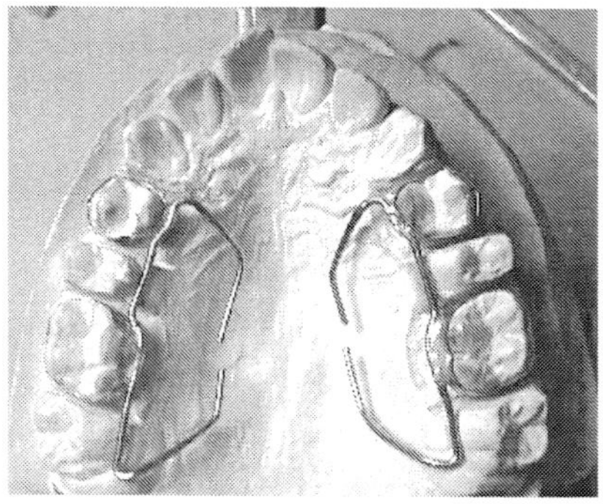

Fig. 8.41 Wires pass along lingual of posteriors

At the distal of the most posterior tooth, and the anterior of the 4, a bend is made which brings the wire down into the palate. These arms require at least 3 mm of relief from the palatal tissue. The distal arm should run slightly mesially and the mesial arm slightly distally. This will help to reduce the size of the acrylic body of the appliance.

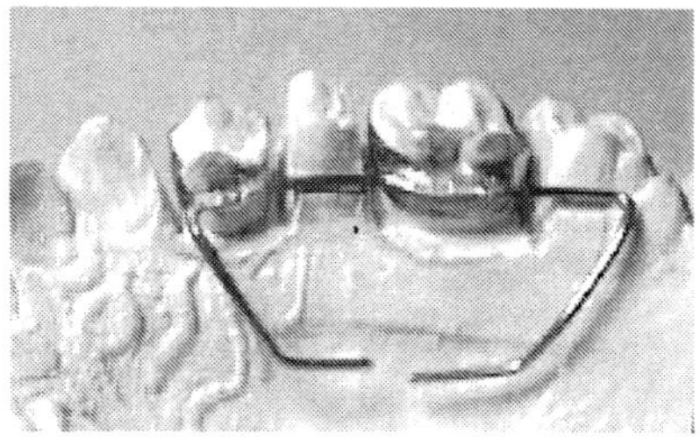

Fig. 8.42 Retentive tags

Approximately halfway between the gingival margin and the midline, both arms are bent 90° towards each other to form retentive tags. This distance will vary in accordance to the patient's palatal shape. The tags must be long enough to allow them to be encased in acrylic, yet the acrylic must come no closer than 3 mm to the gingiva margin. More relief from the gingival margin is preferable.

The arms are now spot welded and soldered to the bands. If possible, remove the bands from the model before soldering. With two bands per wire this can be difficult. Otherwise, solder on the model. This joint needs to withstand heavy forces, so add sufficient solder to ensure its strength.

Trim the joint, and return the bands to the model for the placement of the screw and application of the acrylic.

A large expansion screw is placed on the midline in the 5/6 region. The screw should be at least 3-4 mm from the tissue, but it should also be placed as high in the palate as possible without contacting the tissue on the lateral walls of the palate. On some patients, the palate is so narrow that the screw must be placed close to the occlusal plane in order for it to fit without contacting the tissue.

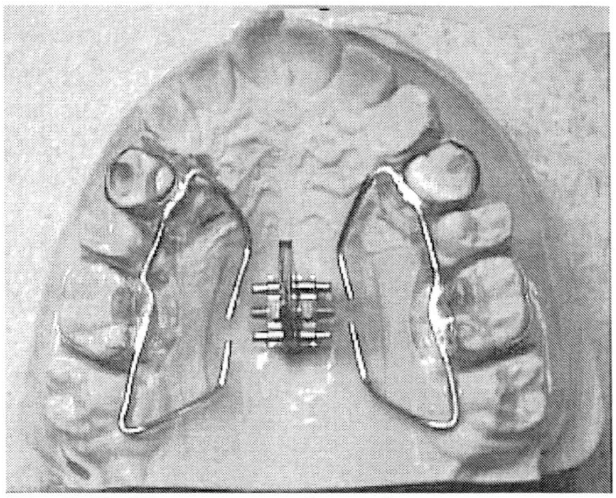

Fig. 8.43 Place screw under and between wires if possible

Ideally, the screw can be placed under the retentive tags of the wire arms (when viewed on the model), however, on cases with a narrow palate it is sometimes necessary to

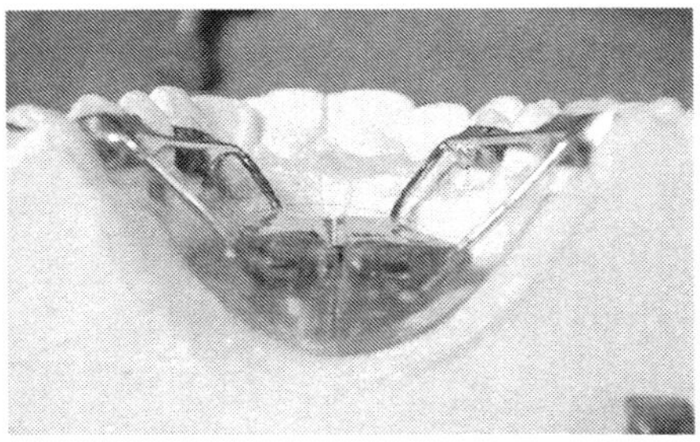

Fig. 8.44 Haas RPE acrylic must be relieved from tissue.

place the screw over these tags.

The acrylic body of the appliance has few design requirements. It must not be too close to the gingival margin — 3-5 mm relief — and have a minimum 2 mm relief from the palate. It must also completely encase the retentive tags of the wire arms and the expansion screw.

The palatal relief can be achieved by either trimming the tissue side of the acrylic after processing or by placing a layer of baseplate wax for relief on the palate before sprinkling.

The acrylic body is sprinkled, trimmed and polished as usual (for details see the section on acrylic processing in removable appliances). The acrylic is trimmed to be as small and unobtrusive as possible, while maintaining sufficient strength to withstand the forces placed on it.

A tip which can help you in placing and removing an RPE on the model is to open the expansion screw ¼ turn. This will generally make the appliance easier to work with.

Expansion key for RPE's

The last step in fabricating an RPE is to modify the expansion screw key of the appliance. Because the appliance is fixed in the mouth it cannot be removed when the patient needs to turn the screw. If the key is not modified two things can happen. First, the patient may not be able to open their mouth wide enough to insert the key. Second the wire key may slide through the screw and stab the patient's palatal tissue.

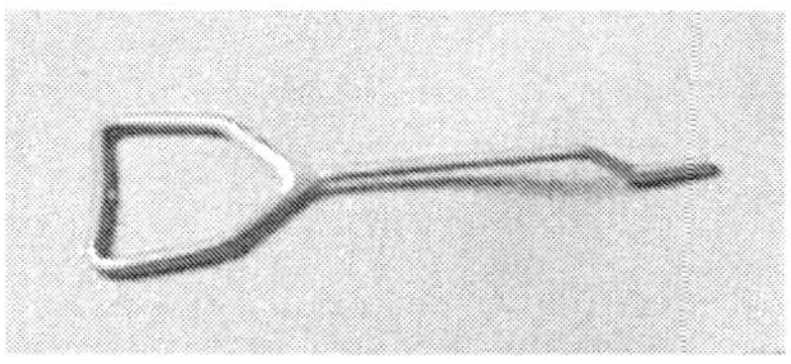

Fig. 8.45 Key modified for RPE

Therefore the key is modified by first shortening it to approximately 2/3 its original length, from approximately 35 mm to 25 mm. The last 5 mm of the key are then bent 45°, and 2 mm forward of this bend it is bent 45° in the opposite direction. This forms a bayonet bend in the end of the key and acts as an effective stop when the key is inserted into the screw.

The Bonded Hyrax

The Bonded Hyrax is a recent modification of the RPE. This design does not use bands as the retentive element, but instead has posterior bite pads which are bonded directly to the posterior teeth. These bite pads cover only the clinical crowns of the teeth, relieved 1-2 mm from the gingival margin. The doctor should prepare only the buccal and/or lingual surfaces of the teeth for bonding. If the occlusal surfaces are etched, the removal of the appliance and bonding material can be difficult and time consuming.

The hyrax screw is positioned as usual, high is the palate over the midline, with the arms approaching the lingual surfaces of the 4's and 6's. The attachment to the acrylic pads is by a wire (0.9 mm) which is adapted around the posterior teeth (buccal and lingual) and soldered to the arms of the screw. All soldering, trimming and polishing is done to the wires, and the wires are then embedded into the acrylic pads.

This design can produce occlusal pads which are excessively bulky, and can lead to tissue irritation by interfering with the patient's ablility to clean. An alternative design has a wire which is adapted from the mesial fossa of the first premolar (or first deciduous molar) to the distal fossa of the most posterior molar and closely contoured to the lingual surfaces of the teeth.This allows for a much less bulky acrylic pad, expecially on the buccal. The wire must provide enough relief from the lingual surface to ensure that it is completely embedded in the acrylic. By reducing the thickness of the acrylic pads the appliance is easier to keep clean as well as being more comfortable for the patient. The ends of the wire may be bent into contact with the occlu-

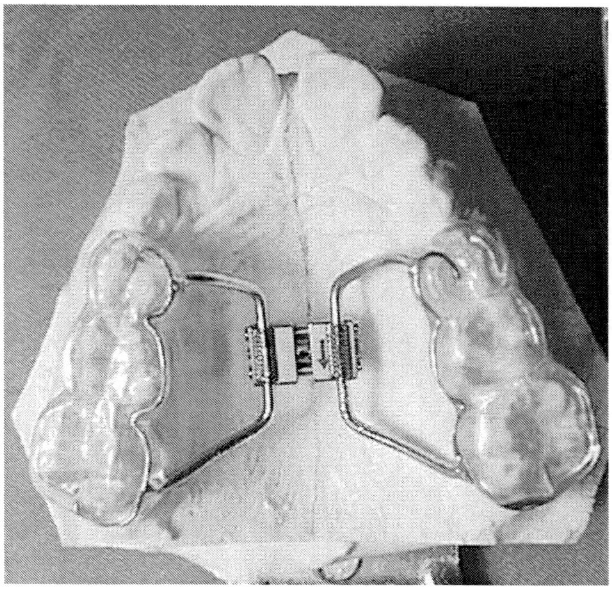

fig. 8.46 Bonded hyrax appliance

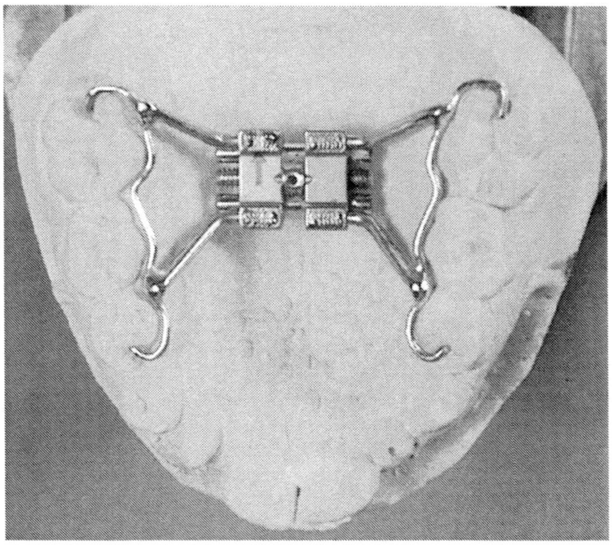

Fig. 8.47 wire for bonded hyrax. Note wires resting in fossaa supporting frame

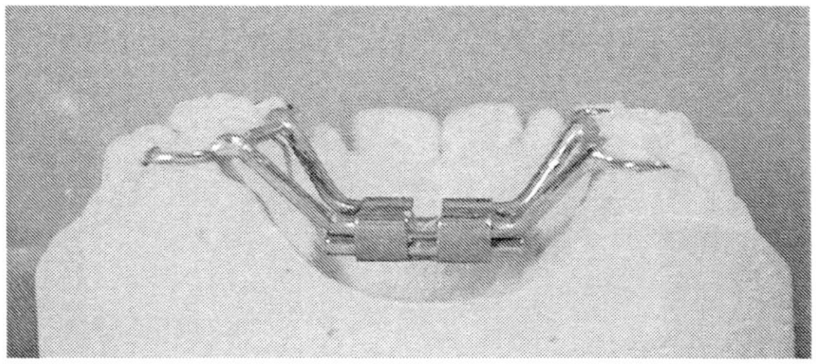

Fig. 8.48 bonded hyrax wires, posterior view. Note, wires are placed as high in the palate as possible.

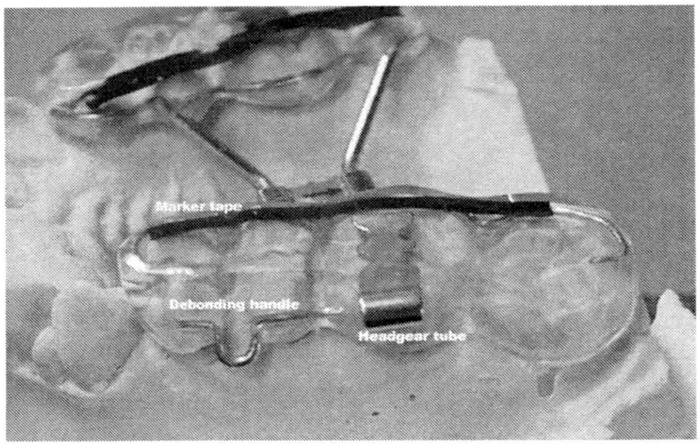

Fig. 8.49 bonded hyrax with headgear tube, debonding handle and marker over lingual cusps

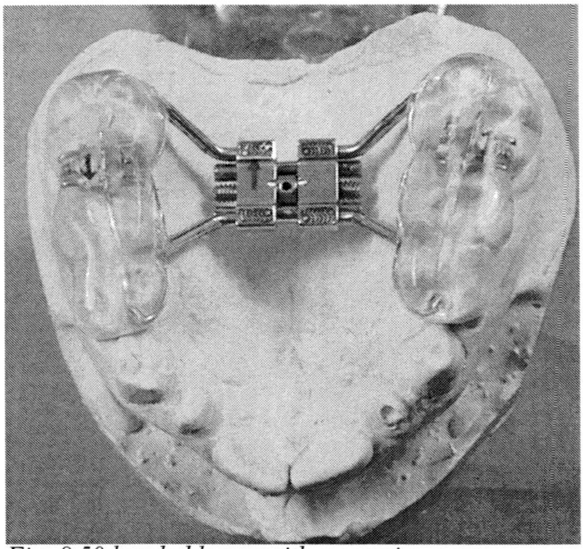

Fig. 8.50 bonded hyrax with expansion screw and band material placed into occlusal pads to aid debonding.

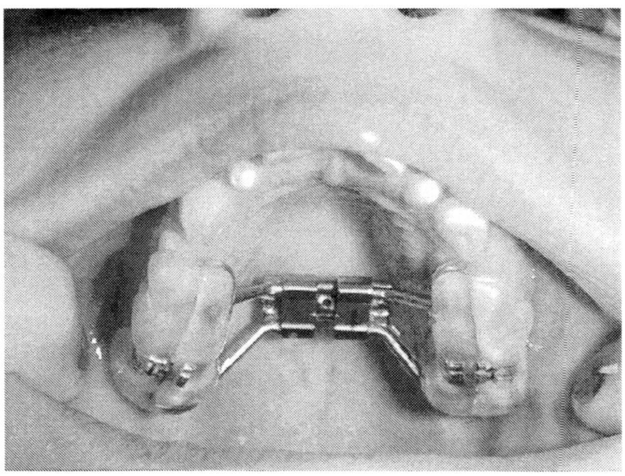

Fig. 8.50 Bonded hyrax cemented in mouth.

sal surfaces of the teeth in the fossas, acting as a positioning guide during acrylic application.

The wires are then waxed onto the model. Wax can be added to block out the buccal and lingual surfaces of the teeth for 1-2 mm occlusal to the gingival margin with a thickness of 1.5-2 mm. Baseplete wax can be attached to this bead of wax to extend vertically to the level of the opposing occlusion. This will assist in controlling and forming the acrylic as it is sprinkled onto the appliance.

Various components can be added to the acrylic pads; headgear tubes, Class III hooks, or wire handles for the doctor to hold during debonding. A marking strip can be added to the pads over the lingual cusps of the posteriors to aid the doctor in visualizing the amount of expansion that has occured.

Debonding this appliance can be a difficult procedure, involving cutting the occlusal surface of the pads with a bur and prying the halves apart. A modification suggested by Dr. Michael Alpern involves the inclusion of a small expansion screw and band material in the occlusal pad. The band material is placed along the central disectional goove of the posterior teeth, with the screw placed to act buccolingually in the anterio-posterior centre of the pad. The access area of the screw is covered with a temporary material before the appliance is inserted. When debonding, the this layer of acrylic over the band material is scored with a bur and the screw activated. The screw will split the acrylic pad and the appliance can be easily removed. This is one of those good ideas that the added expense and labour involved make unlikely to be used by many doctors or labs.

Expansion arches

Quad helix

The quad helix is a fixed upper expansion appliance fabricated entirely of wire. It can be either soldered or fixed/removable. It is attached to bands which are placed on the first molars. If it is to be fixed/removable, lingual sheathes are used.

The quad helix is bent with 0.9 mm wire. It derives its name from the four helixes, two formed in the anterior portion of the wire and two in the posterior.

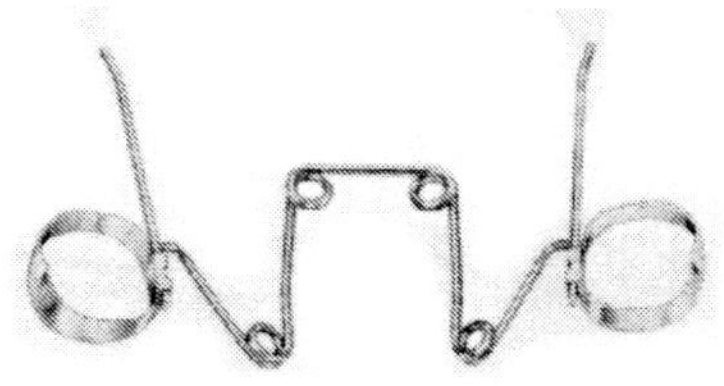

Fig. 8.51 Quad helix, courtesy of SNF- Forestadent

The two anterior helixes are positioned approximately 5 mm lingual to the cuspids, and are oriented parallel to the occlusal plane. The two posterior helixes are placed just distal to the banded molar to which the appliance will be attached. The posterior helixes should lay parallel to the palatal tissue.

The appliance is completed by an arm which runs along the lingual surfaces of the posterior teeth but does not need to be closely adapted to them. This arm is, however, adapted to the lingual surface of the cuspids.

As with many appliances, you can bend the quad helix by starting in either the center and bending out, or by bending from one end to the other, starting at the cuspid arms.

Trans-palatal arch

The trans-palatal arch is another all wire expansion appliance. It can be used to expand the arc slightly and rotate the molars. It can be a soldered of fixed/removable appliance. If it is to be f/r, then lingual sheathes are used.

The appliance is made with 0.9 mm wire. It passes laterally across the palate from first molar to first molar, with an omega spring centered over the midline. The wire is contoured to follow the palatal contours, 1-2 mm off of the tissue.

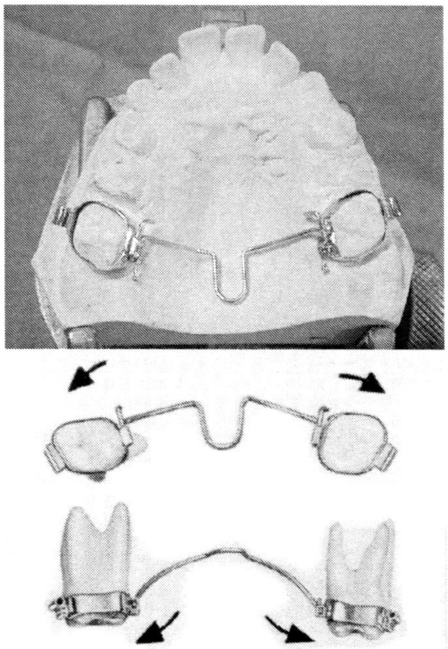

Fig. 8.52 Transpalatal arch, courtesy of SNF- Forestadent

Space regainers

Space regainers are used to regain space lost through mesial migration and distal tipping of teeth adjacent to an edentulous area. They are used to distallize a molar which has migrated mesially. Usually they are employed in the mixed dentition stage before the second bicuspid erupts. They can use springs, coil springs or expansion screws.

Band coil space regainer

The band coil space regainer is an active modification of the band loop space maintainer. The difference between the two is that the loop on the band coil passes through tubes on the molar band which allow it to slide freely. The loop also has open coil springs placed over it to the provide motive force.

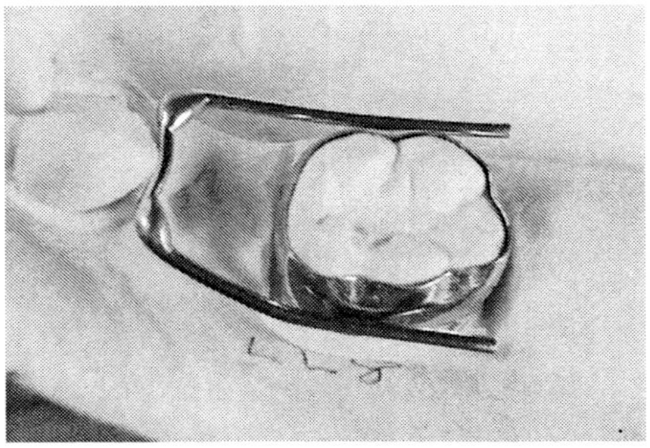

Fig. 8.53 Tags parallel and not too curved

The band is usually placed on the first molar with the loop contacting the distal of the first deciduous molar. If the permanent molar is not sufficiently erupted, the band can be placed on the deciduous molar with the loop working distally.

Start bending the loop in the same manner as the band loop space maintainer, using 0.8 mm wire. The loop should not be curved greatly. A straighter loop lets the coil spring work more easily.

The tag ends of the loop must be straight and parallel to each other and to the occlusal plane. Bend the tags to rest 0.5 mm from the buccal and lingual surfaces of the band.

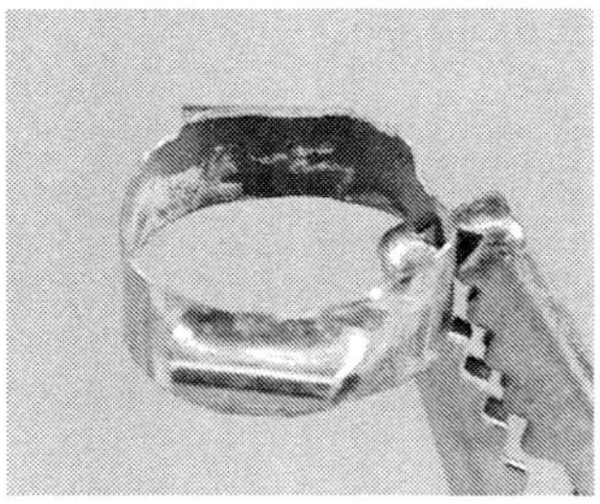

Fig. 8.54 Tubes soldered to band

Cut two 7 mm lengths of 0.9 mm tubing and slide them over the tags of the loop. Position the loop so that the tubes are in center on the clinical crown of the molar and spot weld them to the band. The tubes will project away from the mesial and distal surfaces of the band. This is normal if the tubes are parallel to each other.

Test that the loop slides freely in the tubes. The loop must be able to slide at least 2 mm into the tubes from the point where it would contact the bracing tooth. This is necessary to allow for the appliance to be inserted.

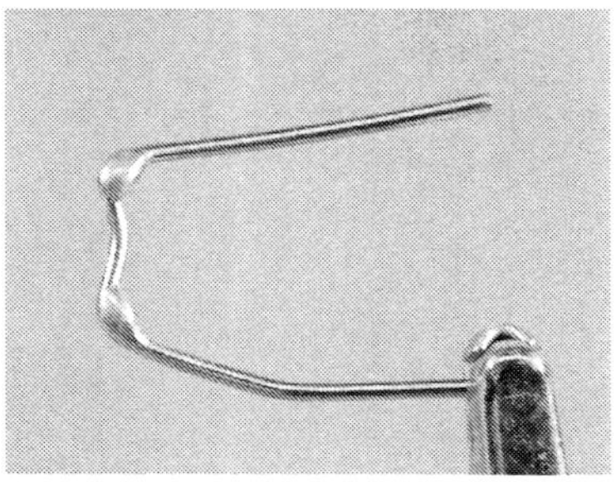

Fig. 8.55 Loop with solder stops

Once the tag orientation and the position of the tubes has been verified, solder the tubes to the band. The tubes may be trimmed so that they extend approximately from the mesial to the distal cusp of the molar.

Add small balls of solder to act as stops for springs onto the loop. These should be placed at buccal and lingual corners of the loop close to the bracing tooth.

Cut two lengths of 0.9 i.d. (inside diameter) open coil spring and place them over the buccal and lingual of the loop. The springs should be adjusted so that they have 3 mm of activation from their rest length to their position when compressed against the bracing tooth, or approximately ½ of the mesial-distal width of the tooth. The tags of the loop should be adjusted so that when the springs are fully extended they have at least 2 mm of wire inside the tubes. The length of the tags should also be such that when the springs are compressed, the tags project no more than 2 mm out of the distal of the tubes.

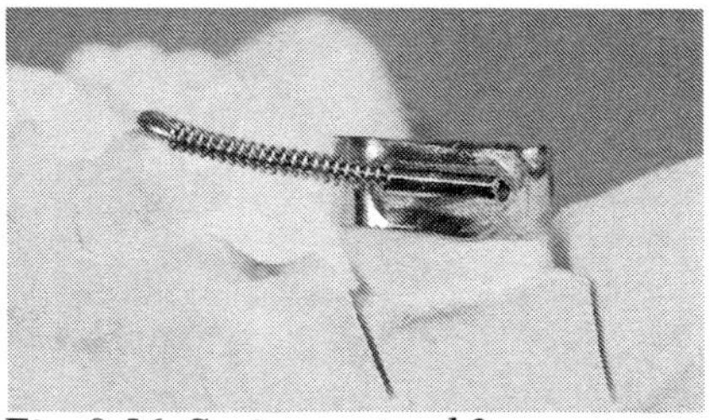

Fig. 8.56 Springs extend 3 mm at rest or ½ the mesial distal width of the tooth

Some technicians prefer to extend the loop through the tubes at rest and place a ball of solder to stop the loop from sliding through the tubes and separating from the band. This is a good idea, provided the tags do not extend so far when the spring is compressed that they project into the tissue.

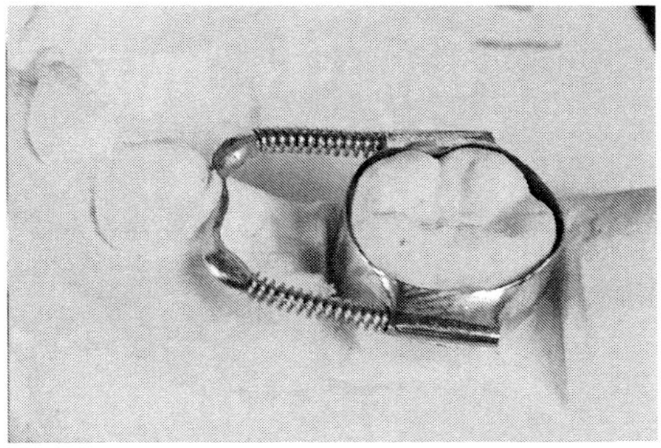

Fig. 8.57 Finished band coil space regainer

Jack screw space regainer

The jack screw space regainer uses two small nuts — one for adjustment and the other a locking nut — on a threaded shaft to apply force to the teeth. Both of the teeth involved in the appliance are banded, the permanent first molar and the first deciduous molar.

A 0.9 mm tube is soldered to the buccal surface of the band on the permanent molar. It is aligned in the center of the clinical crown and with the buccal surface of the deciduous molar.

The thread shaft is not threaded over its entire length. The nuts are moved against the section which is not threaded and then the threaded portion is placed into the tube on the molar. The unthreaded portion is spot welded to the deciduous molar band. The nuts are moved to sit against the tube and then the threaded post is soldered to the deciduous molar. The appliance is activated by threading the nuts along the shaft and allowing them to separate the teeth.

Unilateral spring space regainer

This is a simple appliance which can be used to mesialized a bicuspid or deciduous molar. It consists of a band on the permanent molar, a 0.9 mm wire guide, which runs to the lingual of the tooth being moved, and a lingual loop spring soldered to the guide wire. The spring is activated by pressing on the loop with a pair of flat beak pliers.

Fixed appliances to distallize impacted molars

The first permanent molar can erupt in a position which causes it to be impacted under the second deciduous molar. This can cause resorption of the distal root of the deciduous molar further impacting the permanent tooth. Several appliances can be employed to push the permanent molar distally, allowing it to erupt and the deciduous molar to retain its root until the bicuspid begins to erupt under it.

These designs begin with a band on the deciduous molar and an attachment point on the permanent molar. The attachment point is needed to give the appliances something to work against. There is nothing on the occlusal surface of the molar that can be used to anchor a spring or elastic. The attachment point may be a bonded button on a mesh pad or a ledge formed by the dentist from composite.

The most common designs use either springs or elastics to move the tooth. If springs are used there may be one or two. A single spring, resembling a z-spring or double helix, can be soldered to the band and bent to engage the attachment point. Two springs, each with a single helix positioned beside the attachment point, may also be used.

Elastics are employed with an appliance which is called a "Halterman" or "skyhook" appliance. This has a wire soldered usually to the buccal of the band which curves past the permanent molar and ends in a hook several millimeters to the distal of the tooth. The hook should be aligned with the central disectional groove of the molar. A bonded button is placed on the occlusal surface of the tooth, and chain elastic is stretched from the button to the hook pulling the tooth distally.

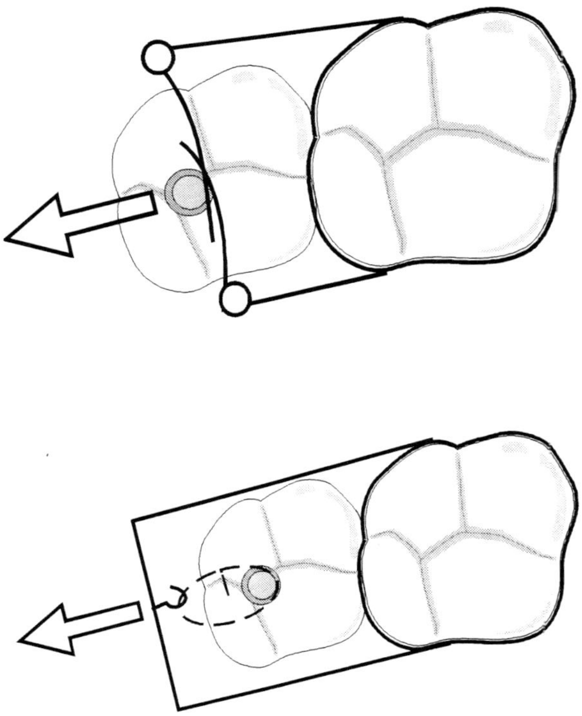

Fig. 8.58 Designs to distalize impacted molar

Miscellaneous fixed appliances

Nance button

The nance appliance is a maxillary fixed or f/r appliance. It is used as a bilateral space maintainer or to provide anchorage for the molars against a mesializing force. It consists of: molar bands, a wire passing anterior to the cuspids and then crossing the arch to the other side, and an acrylic button.

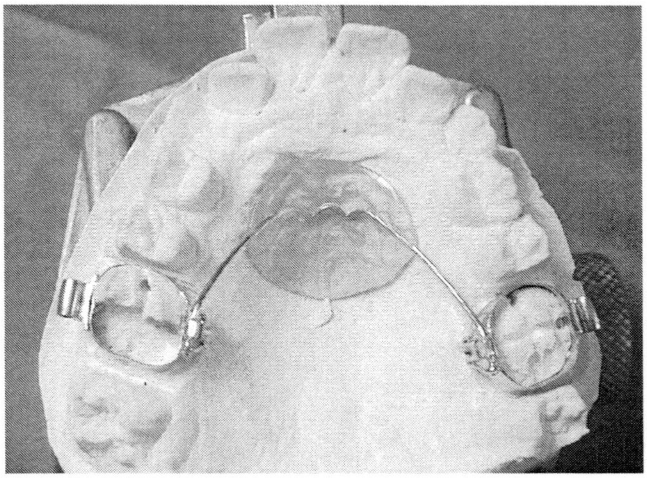

Fig. 8.59 Nance button

The nance is similar to the lower lingual arch. While in some cases a lingual arch can be used on the upper, in most the function of the lower anteriors would interfere with a wire on the linguals of the upper anterior. The nance performs the same space maintenance functions as the lower lingual arch by bracing the molars against the palatal tissue in the rugae area. This keeps the appliance from interfering with the occlusion.

The acrylic button must be sufficiently large to spread the force over the tissue; a button the size of a quarter, 20 mm, is good.

The wire runs from the bands along the lingual surfaces of the posterior teeth and then bends medially into the palate. It is best if this bend of the wire can rest on the lingual surface of the cuspid, but this is not always possible.

The wire crosses the palate over the rugae area. Over the midline, the wire should have a bend included in it to provide a retentive region for the acrylic. A W or sharp V bend over the midline accomplishes this. The wire should be 1 mm off of the tissue at all points.

The acrylic button is sprinkled and processed. The button is trimmed to a smooth shape approximating a circle as the tissue contour permits. The periphery of the button should be bevelled slightly to blend with the tissue, but not thinned to a sharp edge.

If the nance is to be made as a f/r appliance, the vertical Ellis type attachment should be used.

Fixed habit breaker

The fixed habit breaker works the same as the removable habit breaker discussed earlier. It interferes with the patient's habit and protects the linguals of the anterior teeth from unwanted forces. The fixed habit breaker has the advantage of being fixed in the mouth, therefore almost ensuring the patient's cooperation. Almost ensuring because a determined child will manage to remove the appliance.

The appliance is based on molar bands and a 0.9 mm wire — similar to a lingual arch — which run along the linguals of the posterior teeth and across the palatal tissue several millimeters lingual to the anterior teeth. Just distal to the cuspids, the wire crosses the palate, contoured to the tissue.

The portion of the appliance that interferes with the habit is called the fence. The fence for a thumb sucking appliance can be made to sit just off of the tissue in the rugae region, thereby making it impossible for the patient to create a seal and preventing suction.

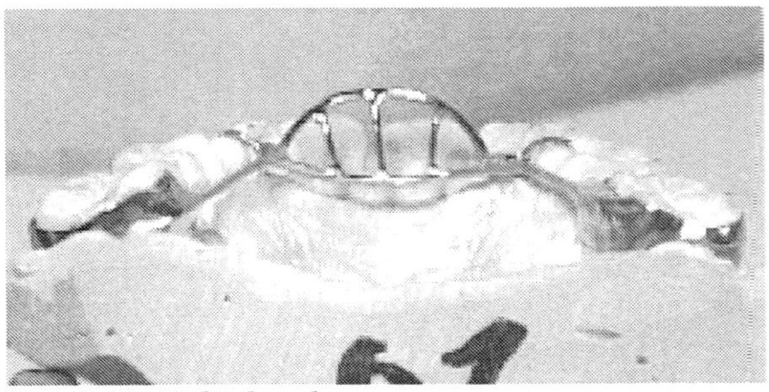

Fig. 8.60 Habit breaker fence, lingual view

A fence for a tongue thrust habit should cover the lingual of the upper anteriors and sit just lingual to the cingulums of the lower anteriors in centric. In this position it protects the lingual of these teeth from the tongue and encourages the tongue to move posteriorly to a more normal posture.

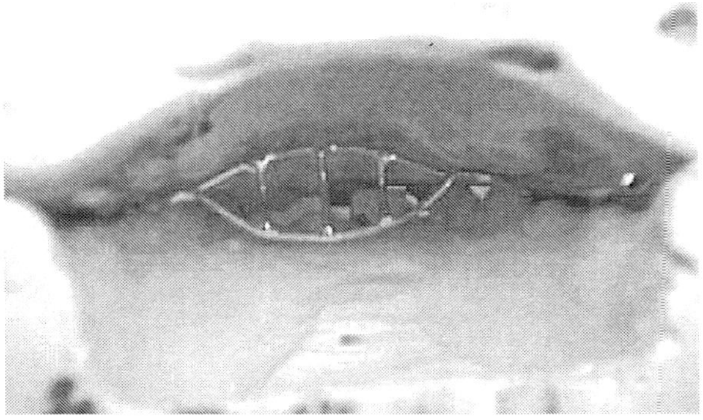

Fig. 8.61 Habit fence in occlusion, sitting just off lower cingulums

Most fences have a top member that defines the longest extent of the fence and vertical bars running from the lingual arch to the top member. In some case, the vertical bars will be ball clasps that continue past the top member, however few people still use the sharpened spurs that were once standard on these appliances. Three vertical bars evenly spaced across the fence are usually sufficient. The bars should be slightly concave or bowed out to the anterior to provide more room for the tongue.

The easiest way to assemble a habit breaking fence is to use a spot welder to tack all the pieces into place before soldering. If this is not possible each wire must be soldered one at a time, being sure not to melt the joint on the last wire — causing it to more — when soldering the next.

It is good practice to add an occlusal rest to this appliance. The rest is made with 0.7 mm wire and placed in the mesial fossa of the first bicuspid. This rest helps to support the fence and keep it off of the tissue.

Lip bumper

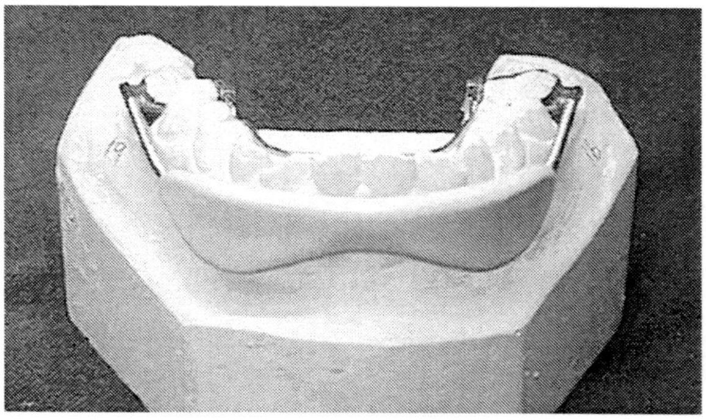

Fig. 8.62 Lip bumper, labial view

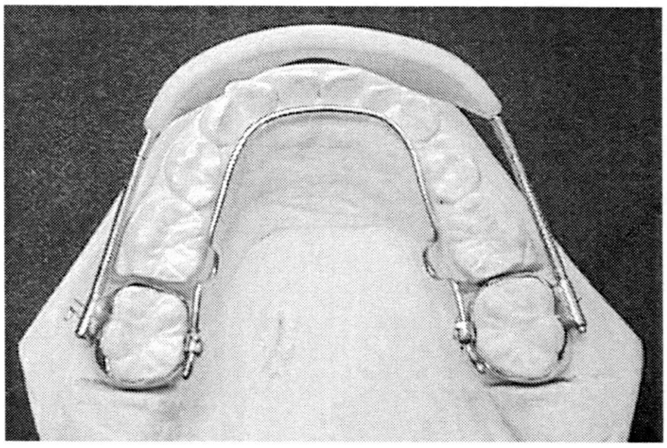

Fig. 8.63 Lip bumper, occlusal view

The lip bumper is used to keep the lips off of the labial surface of the anterior. On the lower, this is usually to allow the anterior teeth to move labially, but also to a degree it can result in distalization of the molars. On the upper, it can be worn as an adjunct to the facebow at times when the patient does not want to wear the headgear. It is based on molar bands, and consists of a prefabricated guard formed about an 0.9 mm wire called the Denholtz muscle anchorage appliance. The guard includes an open coil spring on either side which provides the force used to remove the lip from the teeth.

The 0.9 mm wire is placed into a 1.0 - 1.1 mm tube soldered to the buccal of the molar band. The lip bumper is bent to allow the wires to move freely in these tubes. The coil springs are adjusted to hold the lip bumper approximately 3 mm off of the labial surface of the teeth.

Straight wire brackets

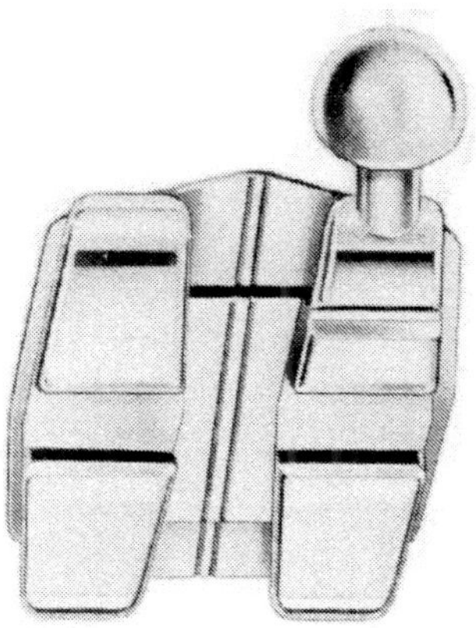

Courtesy of SNF-Forsestadent®

Fig. 8.64 Straight wire bracket

Straight wire brackets are the orthodontic appliance most familiar to people. Then are commonly called braces. They are bonded directly to the labial surfaces of the teeth. Straight wire brackets derive their name from the fact that when the wire connecting the brackets to each other is straight, the teeth have been moved into their correct positions.

The original edgewise brackets developed by Angle around the turn of the century, had a slot cut into the bracket that was perpendicular to the wing of the bracket both horizontally and vertically. All the adjustments that were needed to align the teeth had to be bent into the wires. This was an extremely difficult task, requiring great skill and much practice.

The straight wire brackets used today have slots which are milled at a precise angle to reflect the correct position of each tooth. That is why the wire now straightens as the teeth are corrected. The challenge lies in correctly positioning each bracket on the tooth so that the bracket can bring that tooth into its proper alignment.

Bracketing systems are highly complex with a huge variety of treatment options and accessories. We cannot possibly cover them properly in the context of this book. Therefore we will only briefly discuss brackets here.

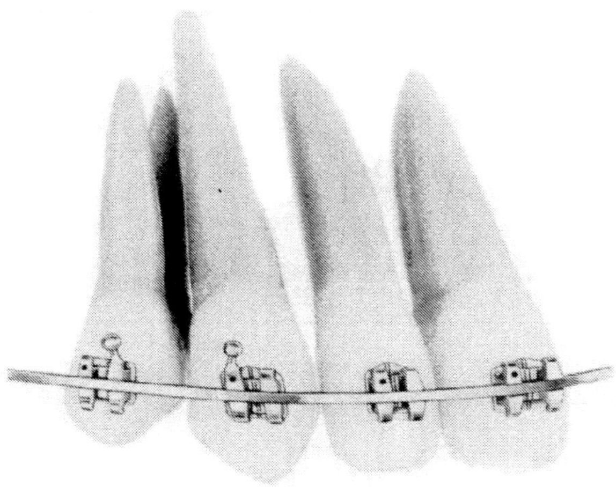

Courtesy of SNF-Forsestadent®

Fig. 8.65 Straight wire brackets on aligned teeth

The brackets

Brackets have two general configurations, one for the anteriors and bicuspids, and another for the molars.

On the anteriors and bicuspids, the bracket has a generally rectangular base, which is placed with its long axis perpendicular to the long axis of the tooth, and two t-shaped tie-down wings, placed mesially and distally, parallel to the long axis of the tooth. A precision milled slot (0.22 x 0.25 or .018x.022) is cut through the wings to accommodate the arch wires used in treatment. Arch wires are secured to the brackets with wire or elastic ligatures. These ligatures pass over the wire mesial and distal to the bracket wings and then run under the t-wings occlusally and gingivally. This holds the wire firmly to the bracket. The slots are manufactured with preset angulation both mesio-distally and occluo-gingivally.

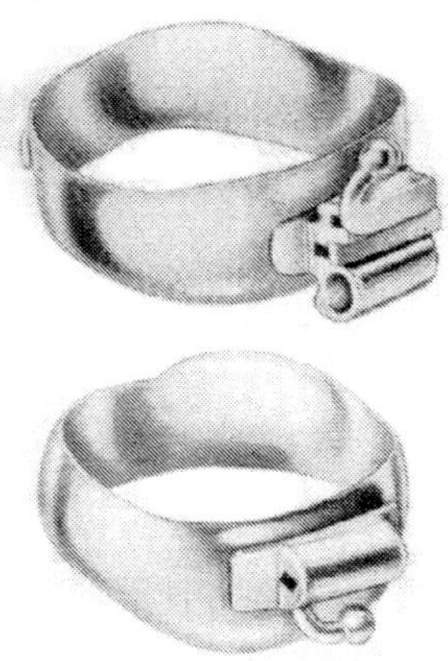

Courtesy of SNF-Forsestadent®

Fig. 8.66 Upper and lower molar bands with buccal tubes

Molar brackets have tubes rather than slots, and are called molar tubes. The wires are slid through the tubes from the mesial, and then seated in the rest of the brackets on the arch.

Some molar brackets have "convertible" tubes. This means that the buccal wall of the tube is a separate piece that is spot welded into place and can be removed by the dentist. The brackets can then have the wire inserted buccally and tied in with a ligature much like an anterior bracket.

Many molar tubes, particularly maxillary molar tubes, include a large .045" tube on the outside (buccal) of the bracket. This is called a headgear tube and is used to insert extraoral attachments such as facebows.

"Whether you think you can or you think you can't, you are right."
Henry Ford

9 Nightguards

"Always do right. This will gratify some people, and astonish the rest"
Samuel Langhorne Clemens (Mark Twain) 1835-1910

"Real integrity is doing the right thing, knowing that nobody's going to know whether you did it or not."
Oprah Winfrey (1954 -), in Good Housekeeping

Splints and night guards are commonly used in two types of treatment. One is the case of patient's who grind their teeth, particularly at night, which is called bruxism. The other is as a tool for treating pain related to temporo-mandibular dysfunction — a disruption of the healthy function of the TMJ. This temporo-mandibular condition is also known as myofacial pain dysfunction syndrome.

A number of theories have been advanced as to why people grind their teeth, or have pain related to, but not confined to, the TMJ. However, for the purposes of fabricating a splint to be used in the treatment of either of these conditions we are not going to cover the factors leading to these conditions in any depth at this time.

Suffice to say that the most commonly held theory states that these are the effects of imbalances in the occlusion. These imbalances disrupt the smooth working of the muscles of mastication, which can then displace the meniscus in the joint. These two factors can work together or separately to induce discomfort in the patient.

The idea of the nightguard or splint is to provide an artificial occlusal surface on which the patient can function, removing any occlusal imbalances from the system. This gives the patient relief and provides the muscles a time to return to their normal functional patterns.

In order for this to be successful the occlusal surface of the splint needs to accurately reflect the opposing dentition.

Each tooth on the opposing arch must have at least one contact point on the acrylic occlusal surface.

On eccentric movement — any movement of the mandible from the centric position — the posterior teeth must be discluded by guidance from the anterior teeth. In other words, when the patient moves their jaw, the anterior teeth must contact the acrylic occlusal surface and the posterior teeth must not. The best teeth to guide this disclusion are the cuspids, this is their function in natural dentition. This is known as a cupid protected occlusion.

The occlusal surface should be smooth, offering no indentations that the opposing teeth can settle into and adopt as a habitual bite. The surface does not need to be flat, only smooth. Some people characterize this as a skating rink occlusion, the teeth being free to slide over the occlusal surface with no interference.

All teeth on the arch wearing the splint must be included in the splint. Even if only half of the most posterior tooth can be covered, it must be. This is to avoid any supraeruption of the teeth when they lose contact with their opposition because the vertical has been opened by the acrylic occlusal surface.

The acrylic occlusal surface must be thick enough to resist breakage. The absolute minimum thickness is 1 mm, 1½ mm is better for strength.

Splints can be placed on the mandible or maxilla. A common trend is to place night wear splints on the maxilla and splints which are to be worn through the day on the mandible. The mandibular splint can be less obtrusive and more comfortable for the patient. The dentist and patient will decide which arch the splint should be on.

Mounting and bites

To fabricate a splint you should have an upper and lower model or impression, and a bite taken at the desired vertical opening. These will let you mount the models accurately and provide you with the opportunity to make an accurate splint. Fabricating a splint without an opposing model is no easier for the laboratory and will force the dentist to spend an excessive amount of time adjusting the bite chairside.

The articulator used to mount a splint must have a positive vertical stop which is adjustable. This can be a thumbscrew in the posterior, although an anterior pin is more accurate. By definition a nightguard is made to a bite which has the patients vertical opened so that the occlusal surfaces do not touch, This is why the vertical stop of the articulator is so important.

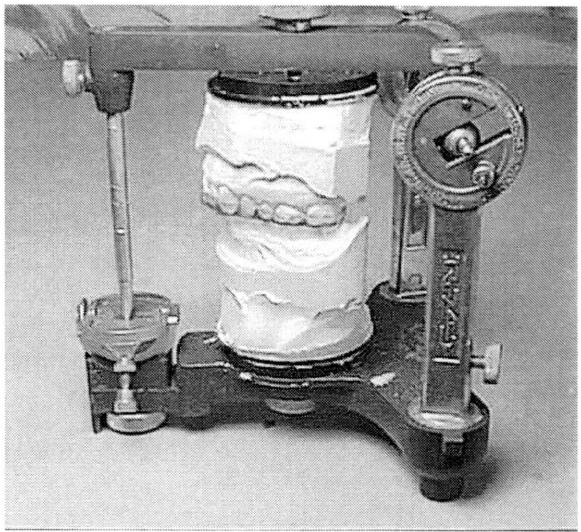

Fig. 9.1 Nightguard mounted on Hanua articulator

If the bite (occlusal registration) can be taken with the patient at an open vertical, the mounting will be more accurate. The act of opening the vertical from centric to approximately 2 mm on an articulator introduces errors into the splint. The articulators arc of movement on opening can never match that of the patient's TMJ.

When seating the models in any bite, it is imperative that the bite be cut down to ensure proper seating of the models. Cut the bite along the bucco-occlusal line angle of the lower and the incisal edge of the upper until only the cusp tips and incisal edges of the teeth engage the bite, whether it is wax or silicone. If the bite is an elastic material, trim back any material that has cured in undercut regions of the teeth. These will not be able to enter the same undercuts on the models and will act to open the vertical. Models will not seat completely in an uncut bite. To see this mount a set of models using an uncut bite and then cut the bite down and check the mounting against it. You will see that the teeth did not settle completely into their position in the uncut bite.

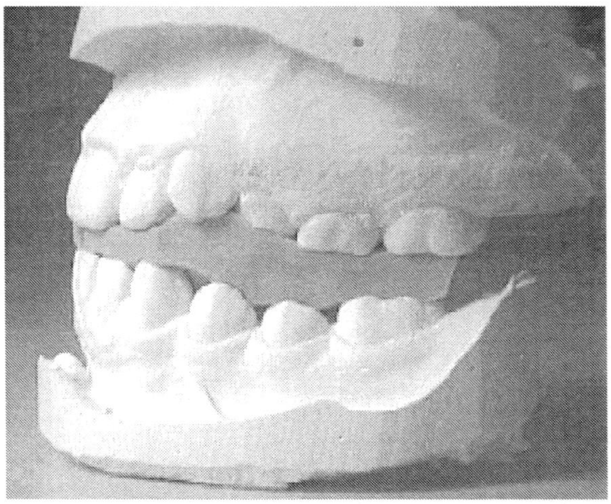

Fig. 9.2 Occlusal registration cut to allow models to seat properly

If the bite must be opened on the articulator, open it only enough to provide sufficient acrylic thickness to be created in the posterior, under the lowest hanging cusp of the upper.

Fabricating a nightguard

Processing methods

Nightguards can be heat cured, processed with the dough method, or sprinkled.

To heat cure a night guard it is processed in the same manner as a denture would be. This method is generally used by denture laboratories when they process a night guard. It requires that duplicate models be made, the case be flasked and deflasked, and complicates fitting the appliance back to the master model. This method can be very accurate, however overall it is time and labour intensive without providing any additional benefits. The old assumption that the heat cure acrylic is more stable no longer holds true with the improvements to self curing materials. If a laboratory is already processing quantities of prosthesis using heat cure methods, then nightguards can be slipstreamed into the process with little additional effort. The average small orthodontic laboratory, however, is usually best served using one of the other methods.

The sprinkling and dough application methods work almost identically. We will therefore discuss the sprinkle method and use the same basic technique for the dough application.

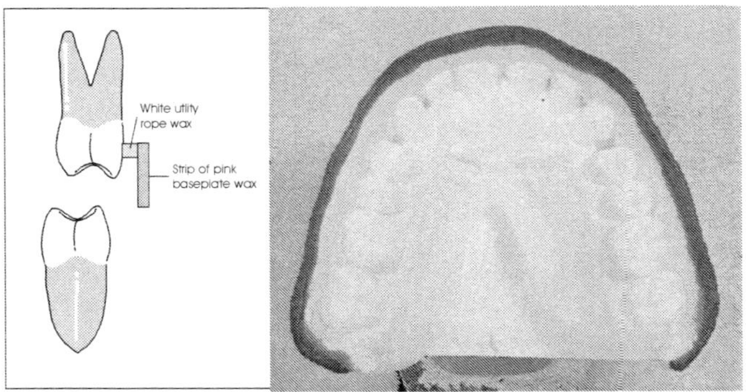

Fig. 9.3 Wax block out for acrylic on buccal surfaces

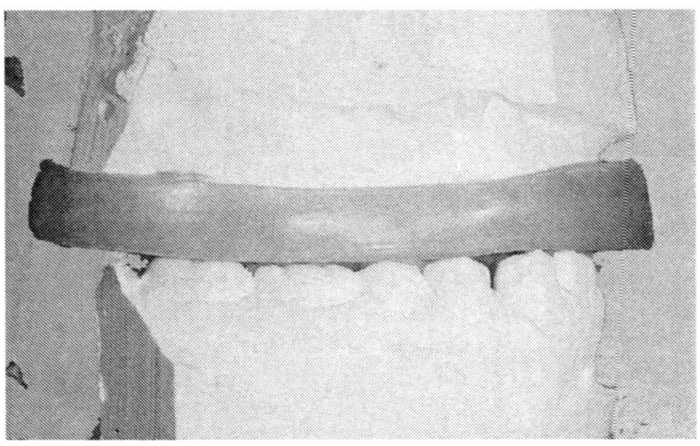

Fig. 9.4 Wax extends to occlusion of the opposing arch.

I advocate using wax to define and control the acrylic application for a nightguard. Some people prefer to apply the acrylic without so constraining it and then trim off the excess.

White rope wax is placed on the buccal surface of the teeth, 2 mm cervical to the incisal edges and cusp tips. Pink baseplate wax is then positioned vertically on the buccal of the rope wax and extended occlusally to the level of the occlusal surface of the opposing teeth. This wax acts to control and shape the acrylic as it is being sprinkled and as a gauge to the thickness of the occlusal pads. When the acrylic is sprinkled level with the top of the baseplate wax, it is close to the final thickness needed. The articulator can be closed to the bite, and the opposing occlusal surfaces should just contact the occlusal pad.

The nightguard is soaked, separated and sprinkled as any other acrylic appliance. The order in which to sprinkle is; the lingual tissue areas first, then the buccal area defined by the wax up, and finally the occlusal surface.

After processing the appliance is trimmed to shape; a horseshoe palate with the occlusal pads extending 1½ mm over the buccal surface and 1½ mm thick. The occlusion is trimmed down until only the impressions left by the tips of the opposing cusps are visible. The occlusal surface is then refined using articulating paper and a #12 round bur. Using the articulating paper, lightly tap the opposing model against the occlusal surface. Use the round bur to grind in any points of occlusion on the occlusal surface until the opposing teeth all contact the surface simultaneously and with even pressure. Use a straight sided carbide bur to smooth the occlusal surface, being careful not to remove the marks indicating the centric stops. Pumice and polish the appliance taking care not to polish away any of the centric stops.

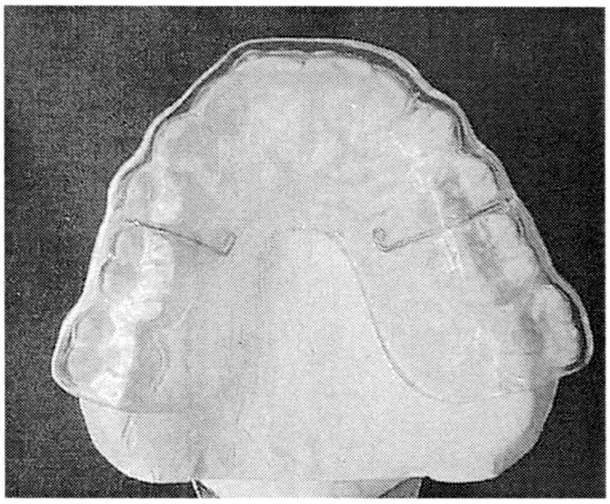

Fig. 9.5 Finished nightguard, occlusal view

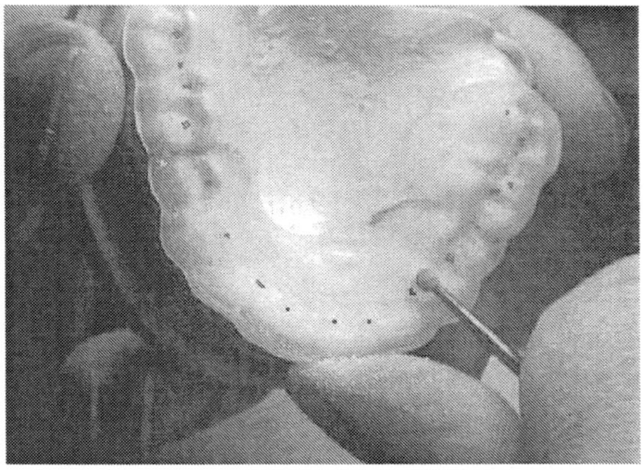

Fig. 9.6 Grind in occlusal surface. One contact point per opposing tooth. even and simultaneous contact.

The night guard is an adequately retentive appliance for most patients without any clasping. The friction created by the close fit is effective at holding the appliance in the mouth. If additional retention is needed, almost any clasp design can be incorporated. The most common clasp in the nightguard is a ball clasp placed between the 1st and 2nd bicuspids, or between the 2nd bicuspid and 1st molar.

Gelb splint

The Gelb splint is a small TMJ appliance for the mandibular arch. The design of the Gelb includes a wrought lingual bar, this helps to reduce the bulk of the appliance making it a more comfortable for the patient.

The original Gelb design called for mandibular advancement. This advancement is not always included in the appliance, it is a matter of the prescribing dentists preference.

The Gelb was designed to be a daytime appliance for patient's requiring full-time wear for pain management. It must be accompanied by a night wear full arch maxillary splint to avoid supraeruption of the mandibular incisors.

The Gelb consists of the lingual bar, a posterior bite pad in each quadrant,

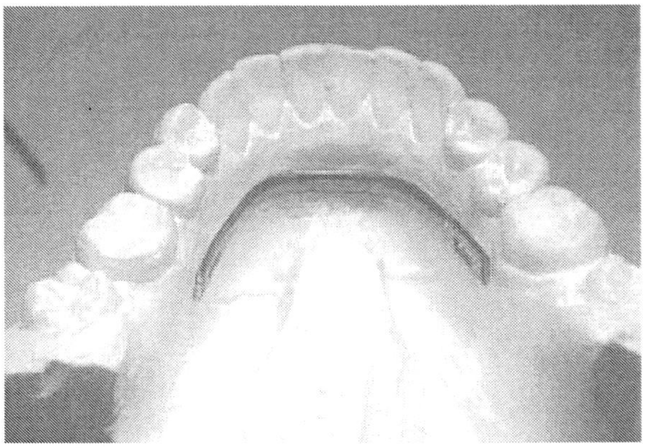

Fig. 9.7 Wrought lingual bar

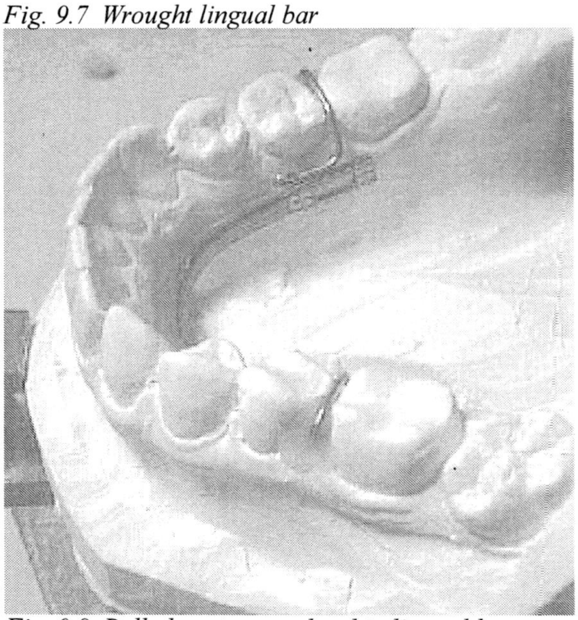

Fig. 9.8 Ball clasp tags occlusal to lingual bar

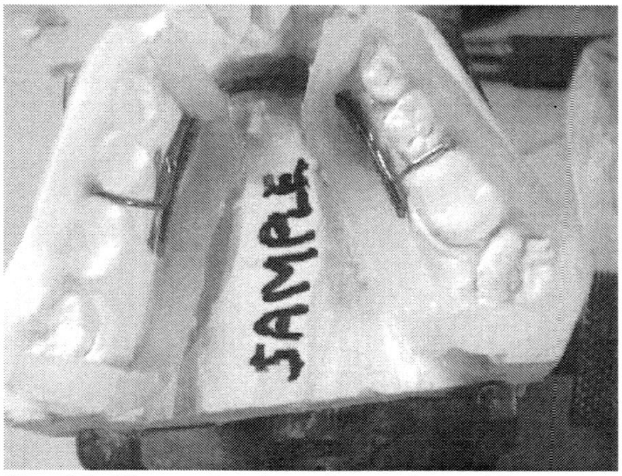

Fig. 9.9 Wax out borders of posterior saddles

"Have you had a kindness shown?
Pass it on."
Henry Burton, 1840-1930

"We make a living by what we get,
we make a life by what we give."
Sir Winston Churchill (1874 - 1965)

and ball clasps for retention.

The lingual bar is a 1.5x3.0 mm oval wire, they may be purchased in lengths or as performed lingual bars. It is bent to lay 1 mm off of the lingual tissue. The ball clasps are bent with their tags laying occlusal or lingual to the lingual bar.

The posterior bite pads are called saddles, and run from the first bicuspids to the most posterior teeth, contacting all posterior teeth in the opposing arch. The acrylic saddles can be defined with rope wax before sprinkling to reduce excess acrylic. If the mandible is advanced in the construction bite, the occlusal surface of the saddles should have indexing for the opposing cusp tips to hold the patient in the protruded position.

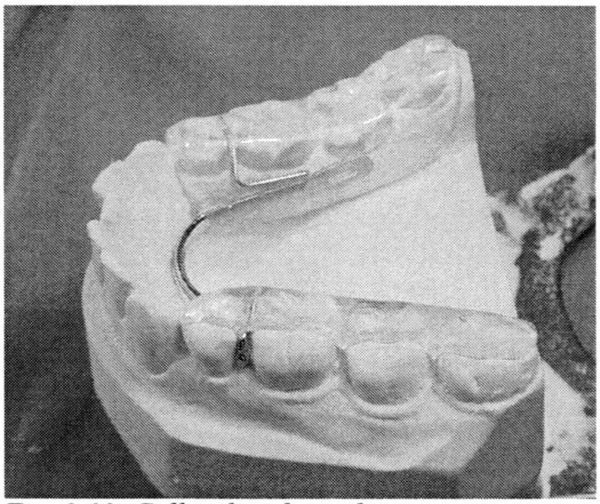

Fig. 9.10 Gelb splint, lateral view

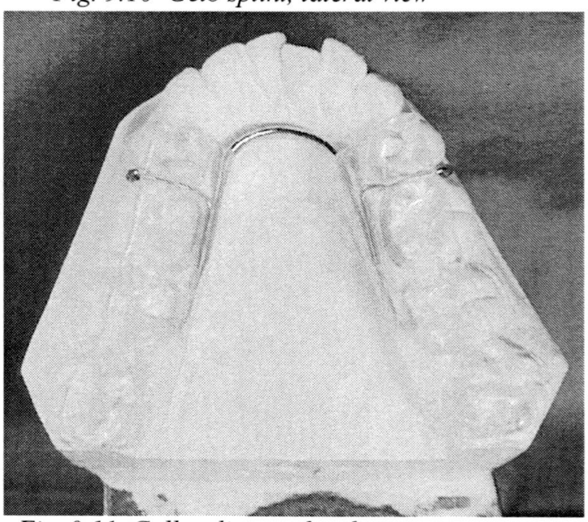

Fig. 9.11 Gelb splint, occlusal view

Colour and patterns in acrylic

10

People can have the Model T in any colour--so long as it's black.
Henry Ford (1863 - 1947)

When was the last time that you were asked to make a fluorescent purple crown? With sparkles? Or to include a dinosaur in a complete denture? One of the things that contributes to the fun of doing orthodontics has been the call by doctors and patients for designs and colours in their appliances.

There are several ways that this can be done. Some are simple, requiring almost no change in technique. Some require an artists skill and eye.

The most basic change that can be made is to the colour of the appliance (Fig. 1). Most labs use a transparent orthodontic acrylic, applied by the sprinkle or "salt and pepper" technique. Most ortho acrylics come in clear, with some also available in pink. The colour of the acrylic is usually in the monomer. To change the colour you can obtain either coloured monomers or monomer dyes from several companies (Forestadent's from Swiss NF Metals, or from Great Lakes Orthodontics (Fig. 2)). Colours available include blue, green, red yellow, orange, purple, black, neon colours and fluorescent colours.

We always purchase our monomer as clear, then add the monomer dyes to achieve the desired colours. With most colours a few drops of dye goes a long way. The more dye added, the deeper the colour of the acrylic (Fig. 3).

The first thing to try is making your clear acrylic look clearer. this is done by adding just a few drops of blue dye to the clear monomer. As our grandmothers knew when they added blueing to their wash, a slight blue tint makes white (or clear) look whiter. This gives your acrylic a crystal clear appearance.

To make an appliance all one colour, simply use the correct colour of monomer when sprinkling it. In order to make an appliance with two or more colours, each colour should be added in turn (Fig. 4). The order in which they are added is dependant on the darkness (saturation) of the colour and its position. Generally the darker colours should be added first and the lighter colours after. In a design with three colour stripes, the two outside colours would be sprinkled first, their inside edges cut square with a sharp knife if needed, and the third colour filled in between them.

Some labs will create intricate designs in the acrylic with the different colours, sunrises or baseballs (Fig. 5). This can be done by scoring and cutting the wet acrylic during sprinkling and added each additional colour. Or by laying down a base colour and curing it, then trimming in the design into this base and adding successive layers of different colours. Personally, I find these methods to be too time consuming and labour intensive. They also require quite an artistic eye, something to which I lay little claim.

Computers have given us access to an almost infinite range of designs to include in or appliances. Most computer graphics program comes with thousands of pieces of clipart that can printed out and included into our appliances (Fig. 7). Alternately, there are many commercially available stickers and decals that can be used. Some from ortho supply houses, others from local toy and educational stores. Popular characters such as Bugs Bunny and Mickey Mouse can be found this way. Using decals or clipart gives consistency to the art. These decals are included into the appliance by first laying down a layer of acrylic, positioning the decal, and then covering it with subsequent layers.

The colours of the appliances can be modified by using an opaque polymer (Fig. 7). This works well with dark or fluorescent colours. When using the opaque polymers you must remember that any portion of the appliance that must be visible through the appliance, such as the arrows on expansion screws or decals, need to be covered with clear acrylic after they are embedded into the coloured (Fig. 6).

Another type of opaque acrylic popular with the kids is the "glow-in-the-

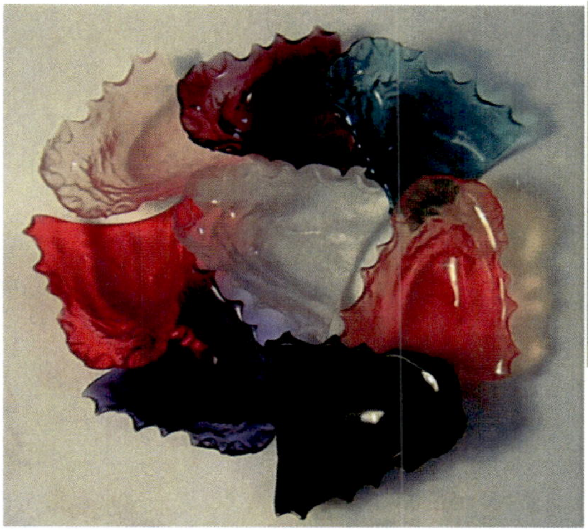

Fig 1. Some of the colours for acrylic

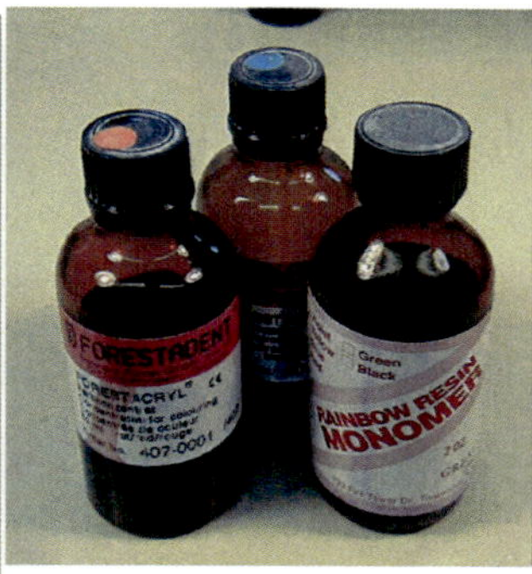

Fig 2. Monomer dyes

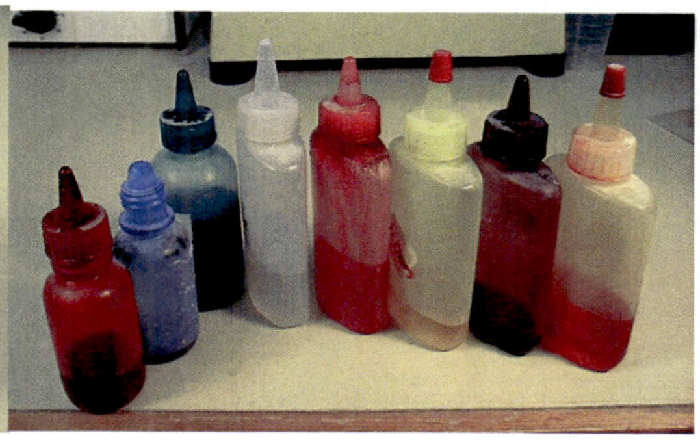

Fig 3. Clear monomer dyed to colors

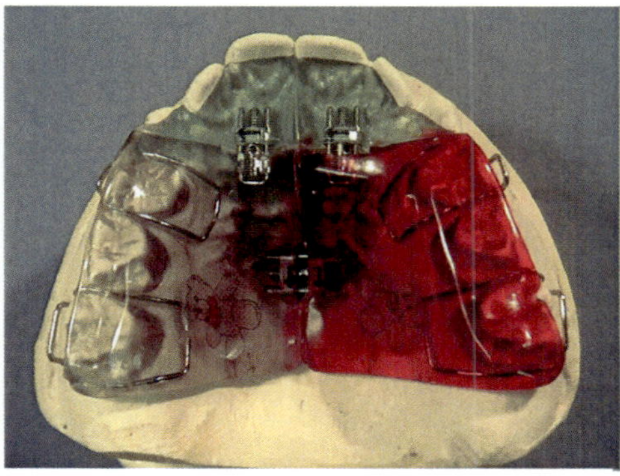

Fig 4 3-colour appliance with teddy bears

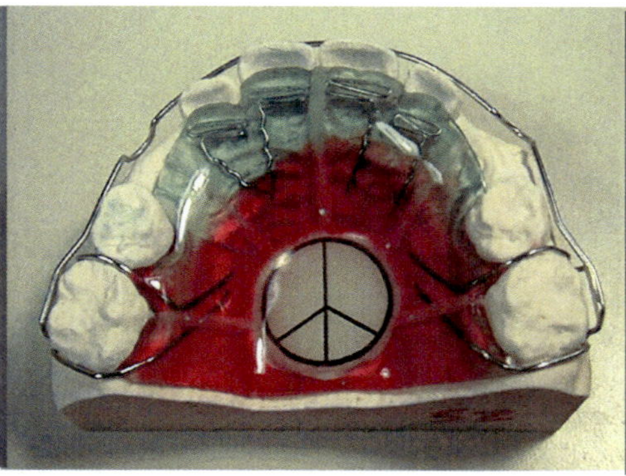

Fig 5. Glow-in-the-dark Ying-yang with rays

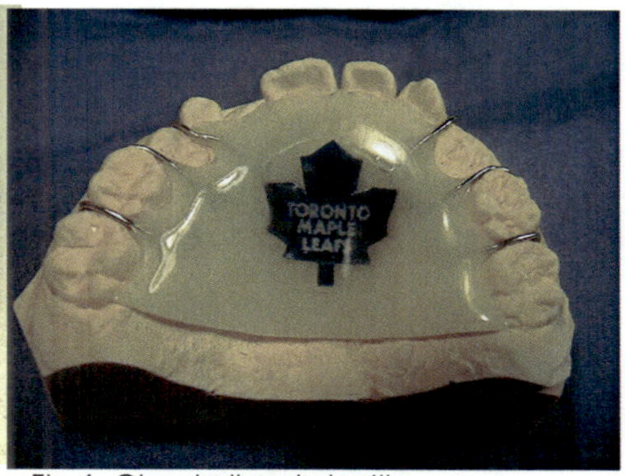

Fig 6. Glow-in-the-dark with Toronto Maple Leaf logo

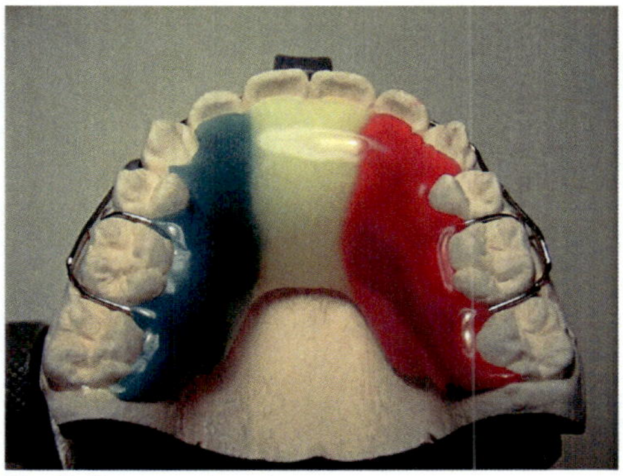

Fig 7. Three colour opaque

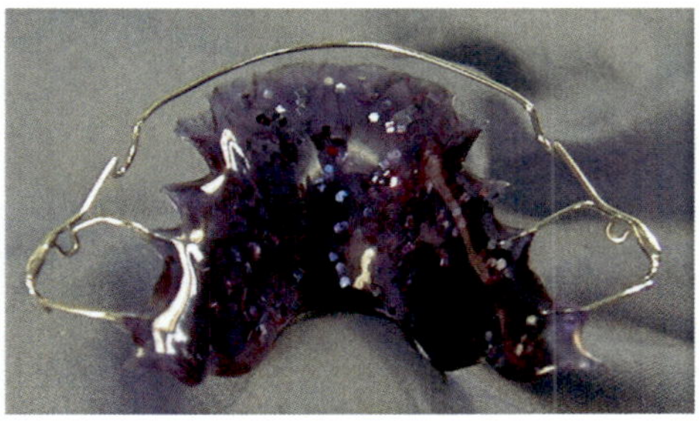

Fig 8. Purple with sliver sparkles

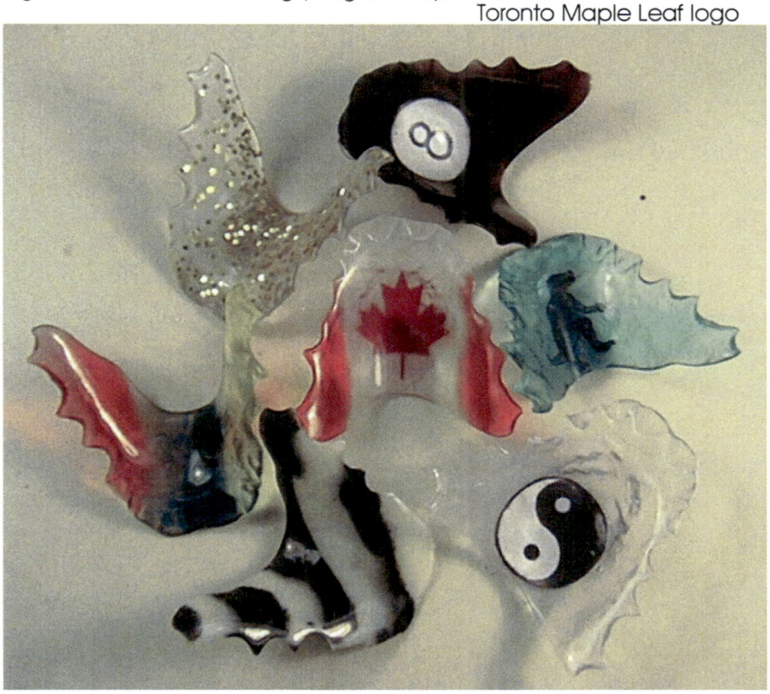

Fig 9. Enjoy making your own designs

dark" type. Why? I'm not entirely sure, but it is cool. Every time we make one, someone takes it into a dark room just to see that it really does glow. Some manufacturers suggest using this acrylic as a dough(mixing the monomer and polymer in a mixing bowl and applying the resulting dough to the model), rather than by sprinkling. This avoids a marbling effect caused by thin layers of clear polymer separating from the more opaque glowing particles. With practice you can sprinkle this acrylic without marbling, it's very fine particles just make it more of a challenge. Remember to always shake the container well before sprinkling. The "glow-in-the-dark" acrylic can also be coloured, however, the darker the colour the less the glow. The natural colour is a slight greenish tint.

Other materials such as sparkles and bits of coloured acrylic can be added to the appliance during sprinkling to characterize it (Fig. 8).

The limit of what can be created is bounded only by your imagination and inventiveness (Fig. 9). Have fun!

When choosing between two evils,
I always like to take the one I've
never tried before.
Mae West, Actress, 1892-1980

11 Appliance glossary

"What's another word for Thesaurus?"
Steven Wright

This section contains prescriptions for common designs of appliances. The appliance names may vary from place to place, however these designs are fairly universal.

- Hawley retainer
- Schwarz expansion appliance
- Habit breaker and automatic Hawley arch
- Transverse appliance
- Saggital appliance
- Gelb splint (Mora)
- Spring Retainer
- Modified Spring Retainer
- Bionator
- Band Loop Space Maintainer
- Lingual Arch
- Bonded 3x3 retainers
- Nance appliance
- Rapid palatal expander
- Crozat
- Jackson
- Twin Block
- Frankel III
- Headgear and facebow

Hawley retainer

Wires
Adams Clasps - 0.7 mm
3x3 Hawley Arch - 0.8 mm
Horseshoe palate

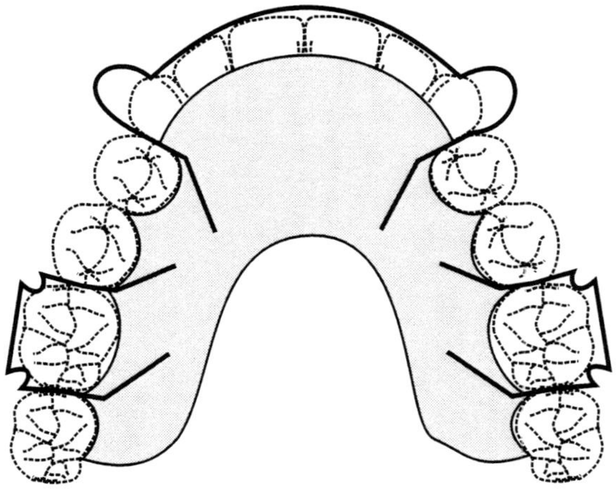

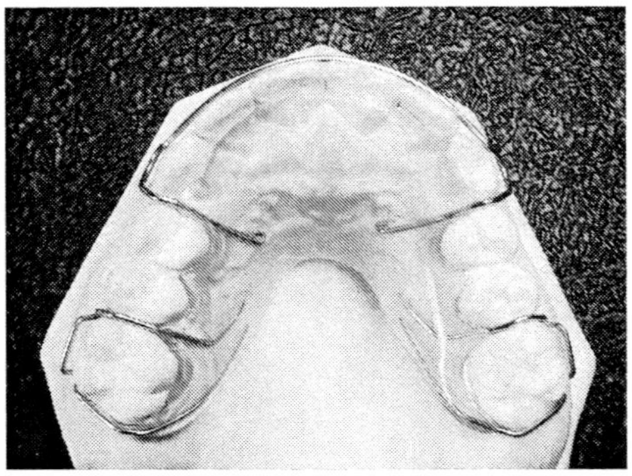

Expansion appliance with double helix springs (Schwartz)

Wires
Adams Clasps - 0.7 mm
Hawley Arch - 0.8 mm
Z-spring - 0.5-0.6 mm

Posterior Bite Pads 4 to 7
1 ½ to 2 mm thick

Midpalatal expansion screw

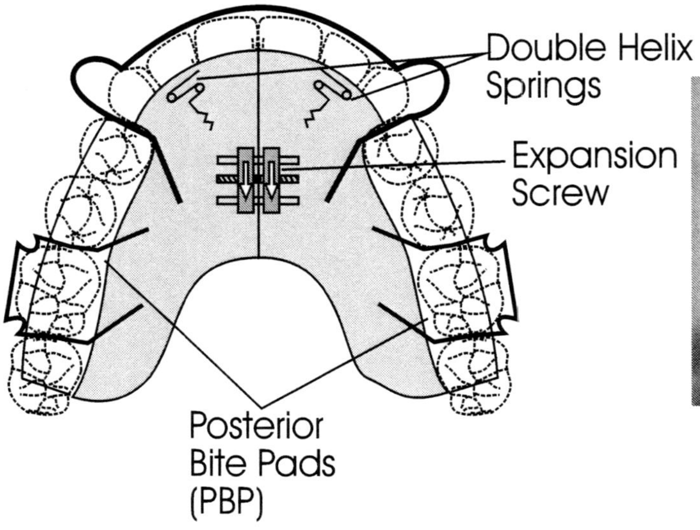

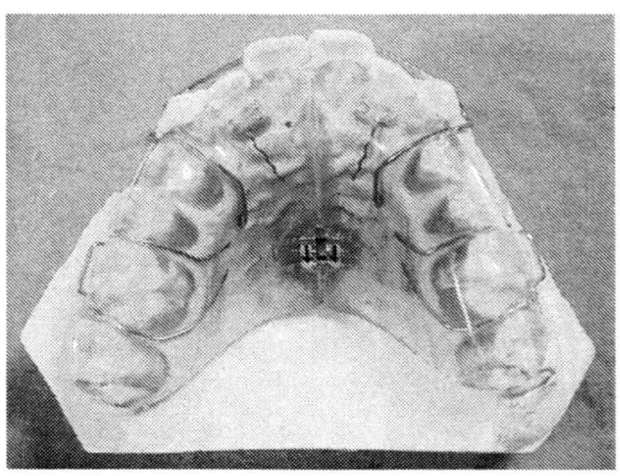

Habit breaker with automatic Hawley arch

Wires:
Auto Hawley
  Arch - 0.9 mm
  Spring - .012 to .016"
  Tube - .020 to .024"
Habit Breaker
  - 0.8 or 0.9 mm
Adams Clasp
  - 0.7 mm

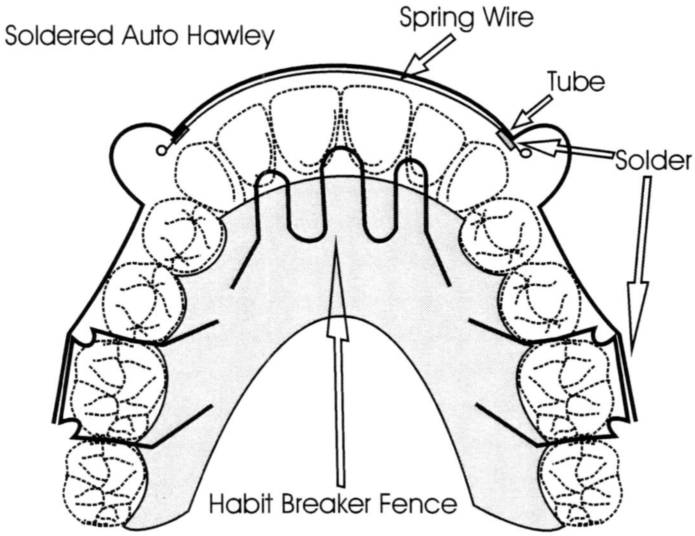

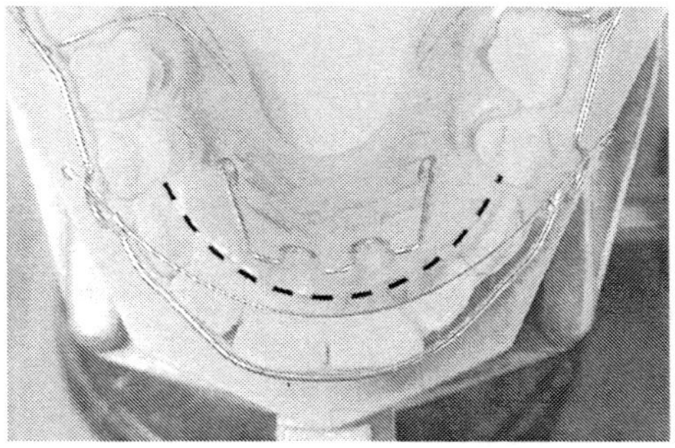

Transverse appliance

Adams or ball clasp on 4's
  - 0.6 or 0.7 mm for adams clasp
  -0.7 or 0.8 for ball clasp
Adams clasp on 6's
  - 0.7 mm
Midpalatine screw

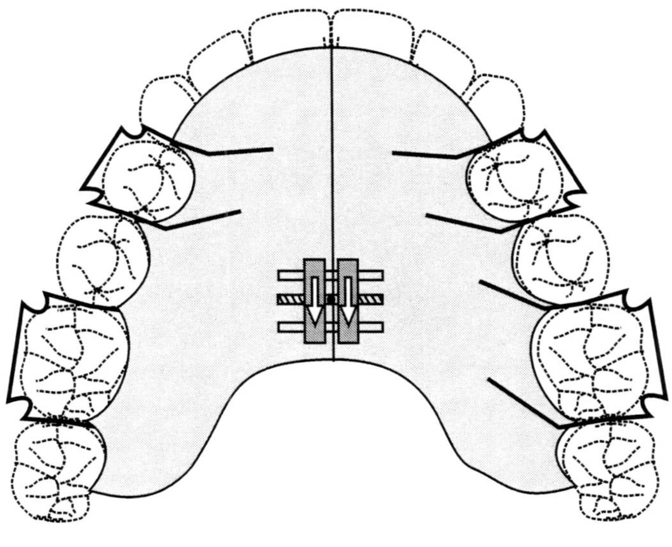

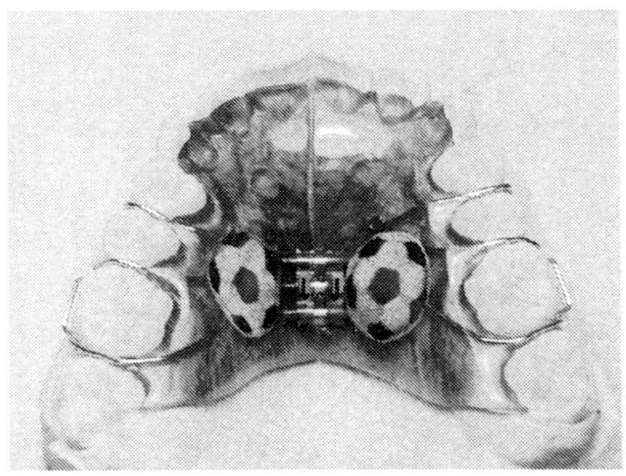

Saggital appliance

Wires
Adams 1.4,2.4 - 0.6 or 0.7
Adams 1.6,2.6 - 0.7

2 expansion screws - parallel to long axis of the Alveolar ridge. Cuts for screws must be non-binding
Posterior bite pads

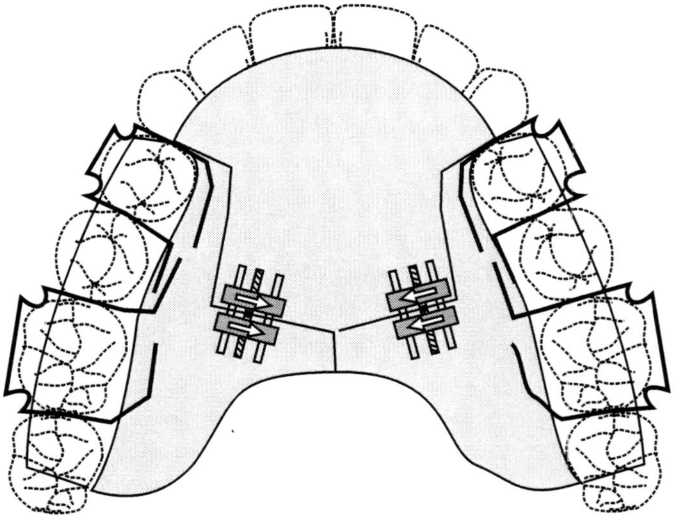

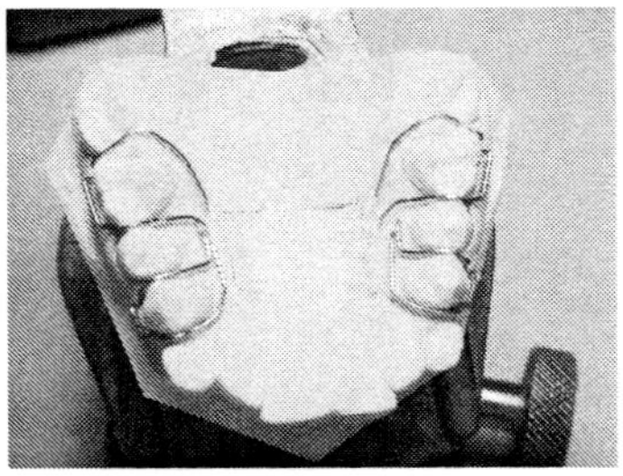

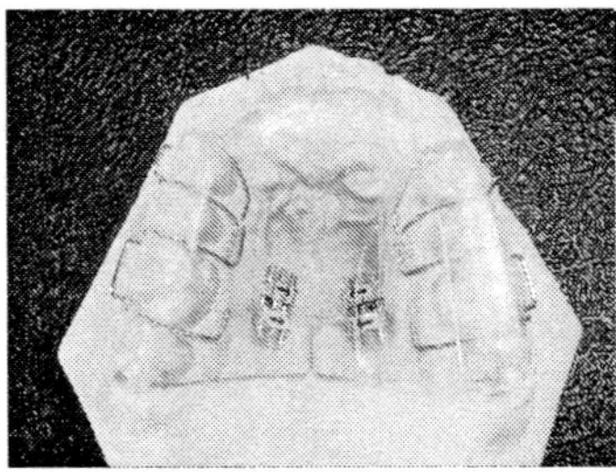

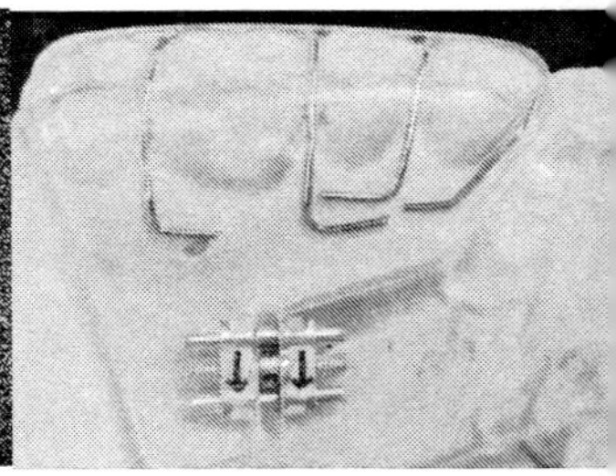

Gelb splint (Mora)

Wires
Lingual Arch - 1.50 x 3.00 mm
Ball Clasps - 0.7 to 0.9 mm

Construction bite can be taken in a mandibular advanced position

Posterior bite pads from 4's to 7's, ending at bucco-occlusal line angle.

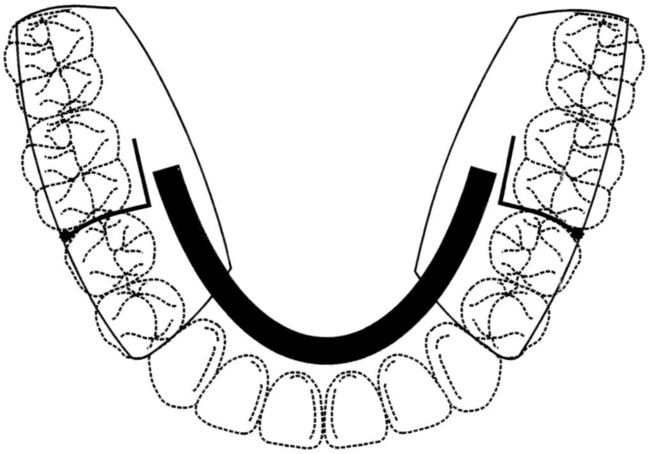

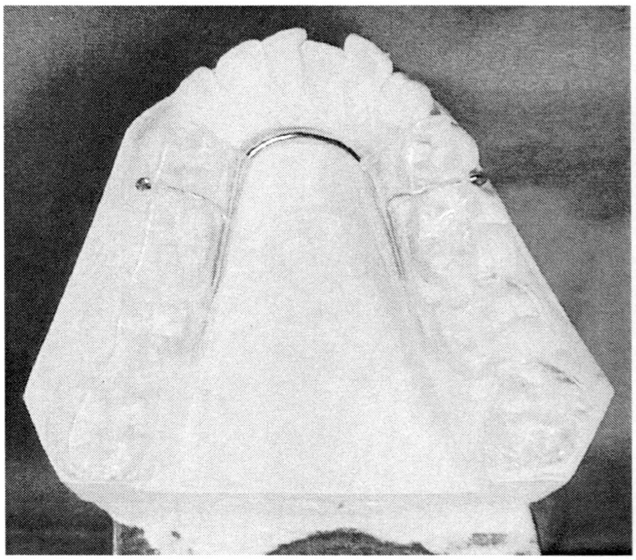

Spring Retainer

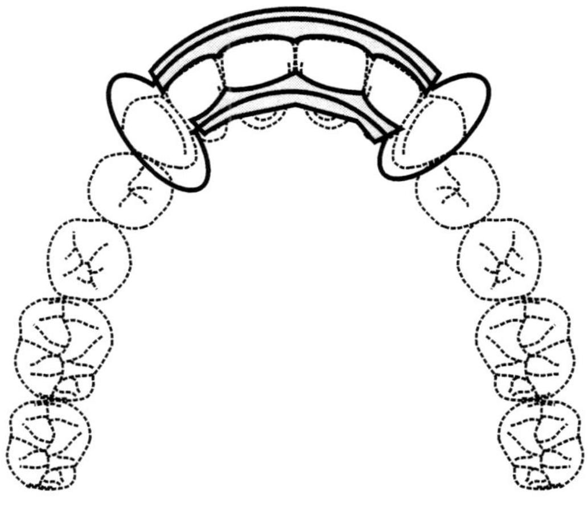

Wire: 0.5-0.8 mm
Indications:
Works well on minor anterior rotations and buccolingual displacements
Contra-indications:
Will not move teeth mesio-distally.

Appliance is visually unobstrusive and the patient may be comfortable with it's small size. However, its size also introduces the possibility of accidental aspiration. As the teeth straighten, appliance loses its retention and loosens in the mouth.

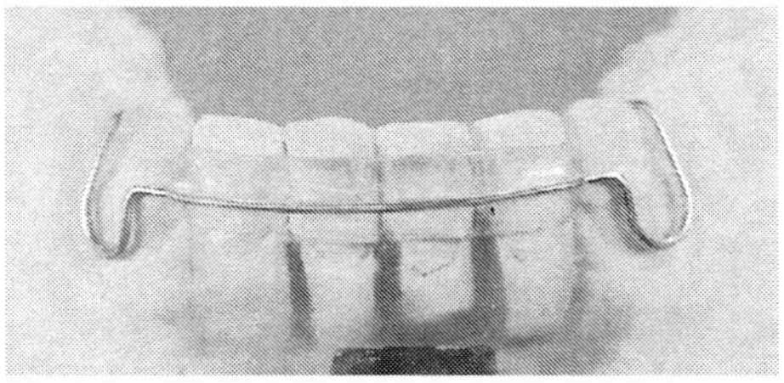

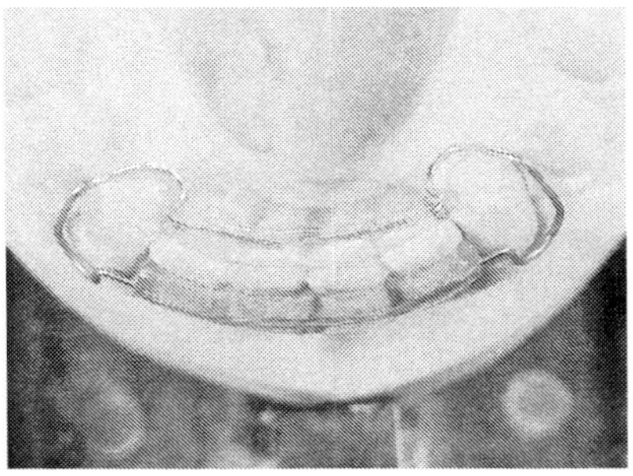

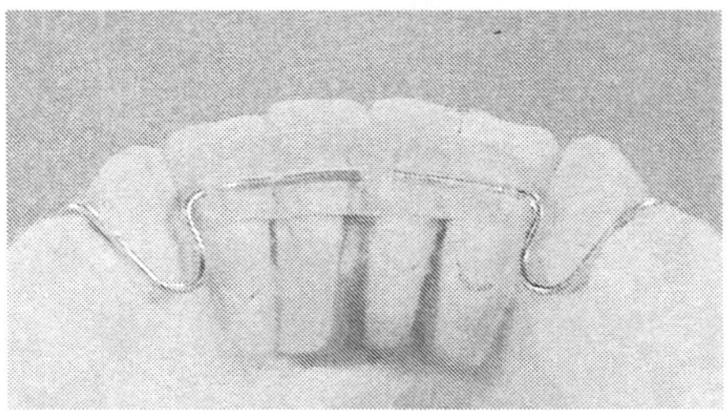

Modified Spring Retainer

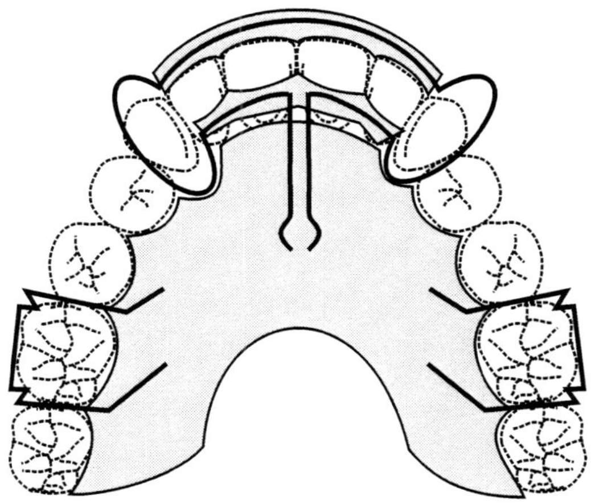

Wire:
Arch - 0.5 to 0.8 mm
Adams - 0.7 mm
Indications and Contra-indications:
Same as Spring Retainer, but not as effective on lingual displacements because of limited flexibility to lingual.
Because of the acrylic plate and clasps this appliance has better retention and no danger of aspiration.

Bionator

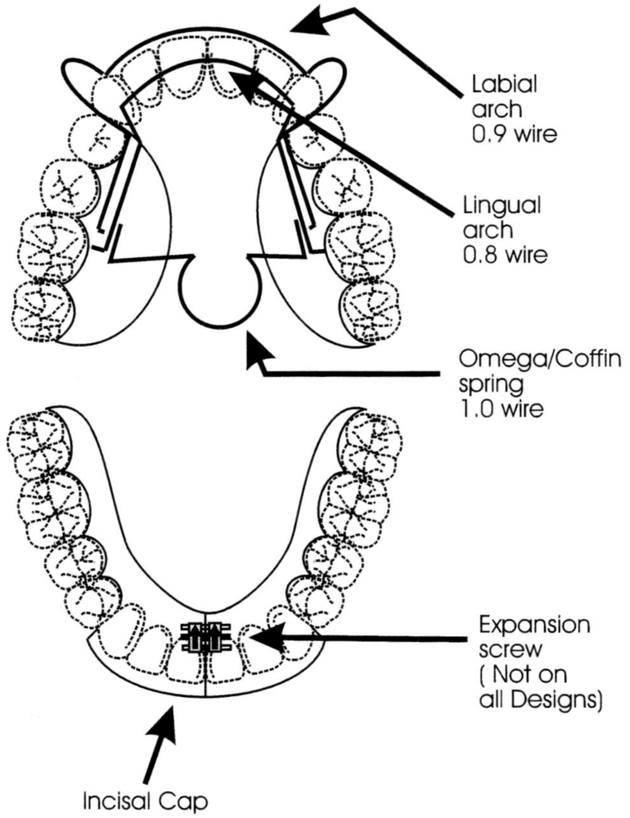

It can be used in a Class II occlusion to advance the mandible, a deep bite occlusion to open the vertical, an open bite to close the vertical, and also has a design that attempts to restrain the mandibular growth in a Class III.

Fabrication of Bionator requires maxillary and mandibular impressions, as well as a bite.
The bite must have a minimum of 2 mm opening between the upper and lower incisors.

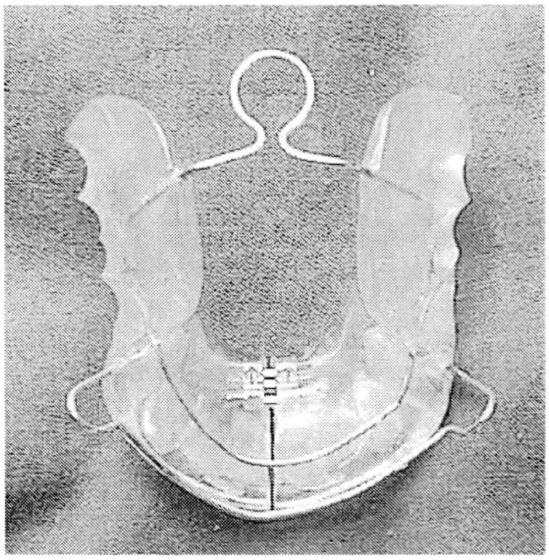

Band loop space maintainer

Band - .180"x.005" material for custom bands
Wire - 0.8 mm, 0.32"

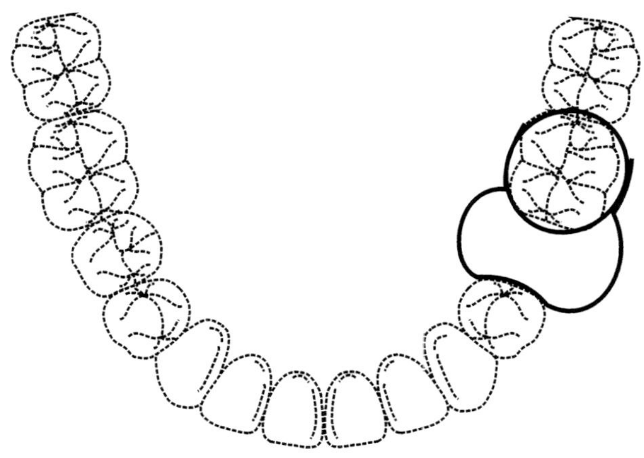

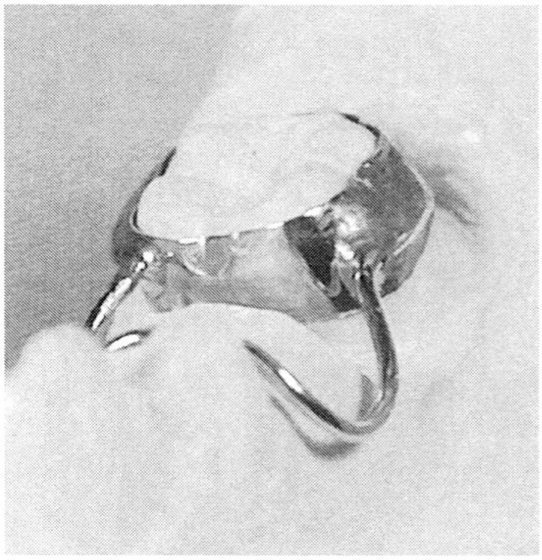

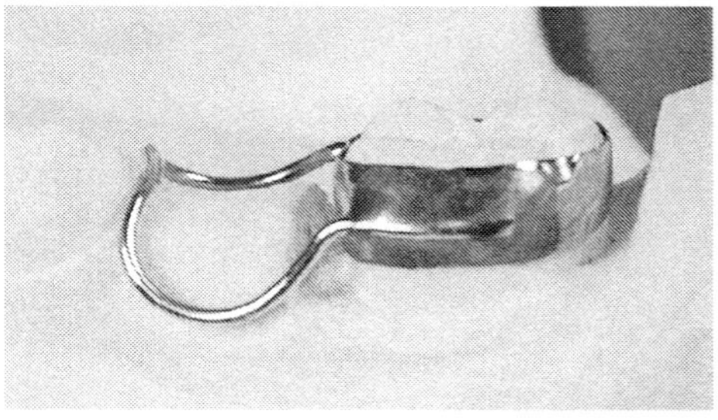

Soldered Lingual Arch (Bilateral Space Maintainer)

Arch wire - 0.9 mm
arch rests on cingulums
of anteriors.

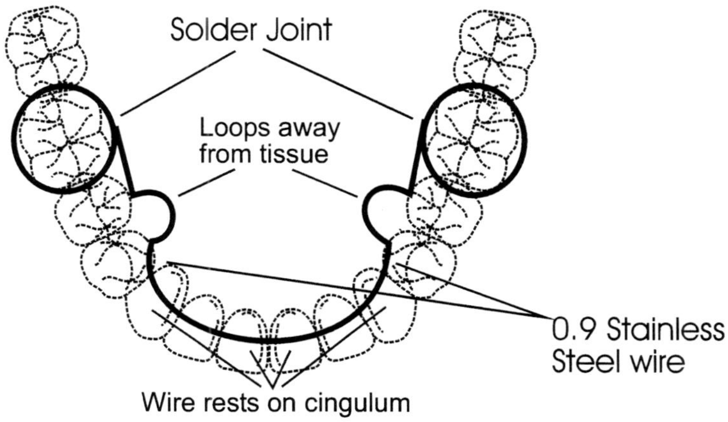

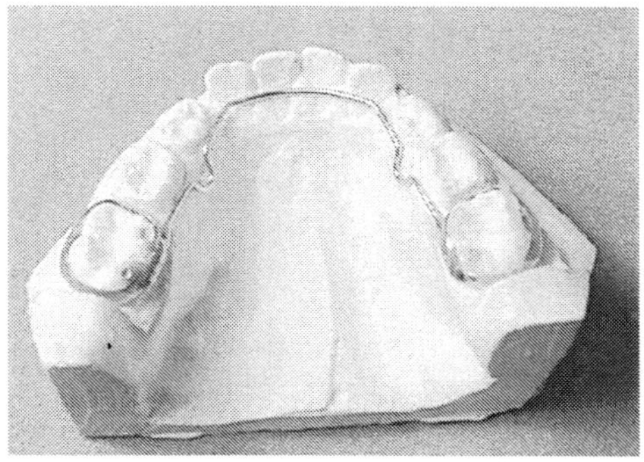

3x3 Lingual arch

Wires
-on mesh pad attachment; 0.5-0.6 mm
-braided wire; 0.016" (0.4 mm)
-round wire; 0.5 -0.6 mm
-square wire; 0.016"x0.016" wire

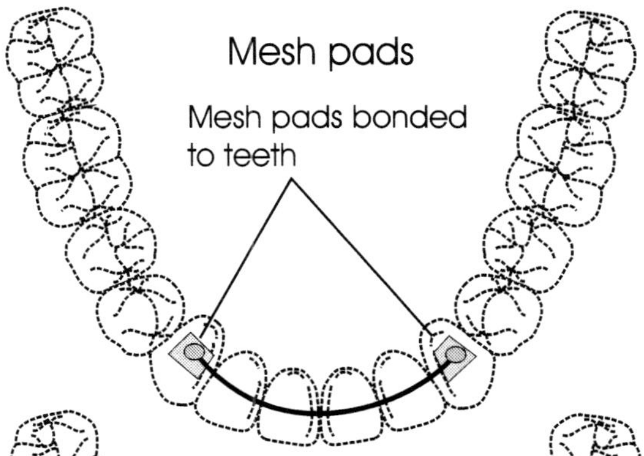

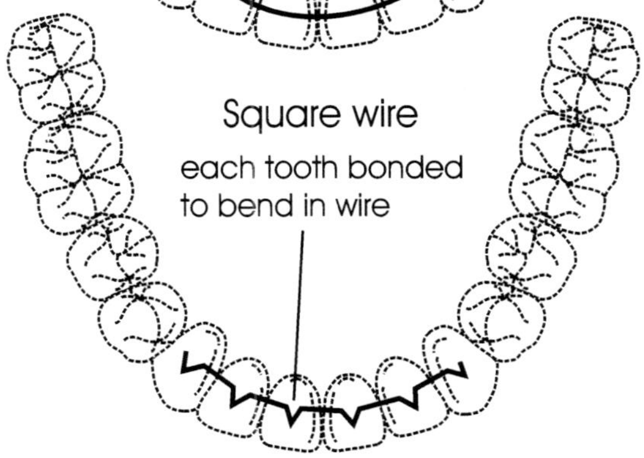

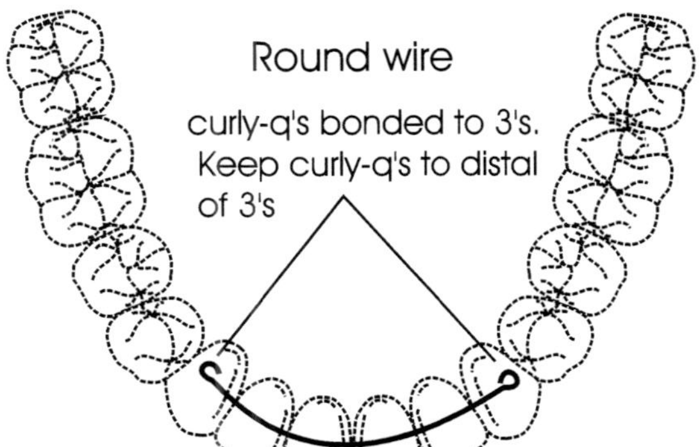

Nance appliance

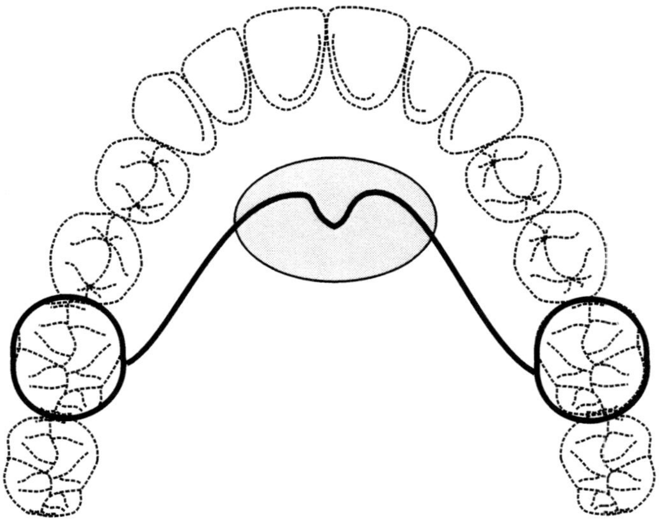

Stainless Steel bands on 1.6
and 2.6 - .180x.005"
lingual wire - 0.9 wire

Provides space maintenance
for molars. Can also be used
for anchorage to retract anteriors

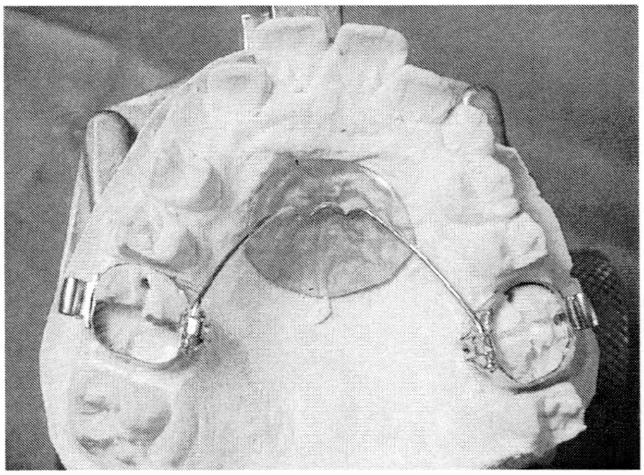

Rapid palatal expander

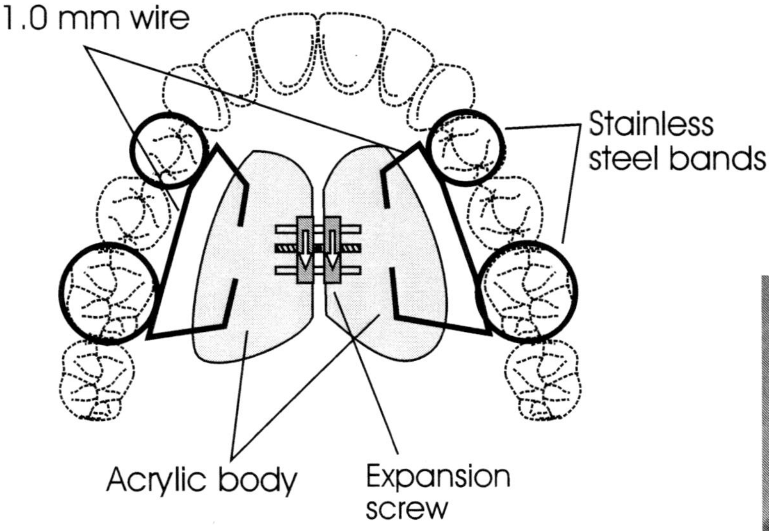

Molar bands - .180x.005
Premolar bands - .150x.004
Wire - 1.0 or 0.9 mm

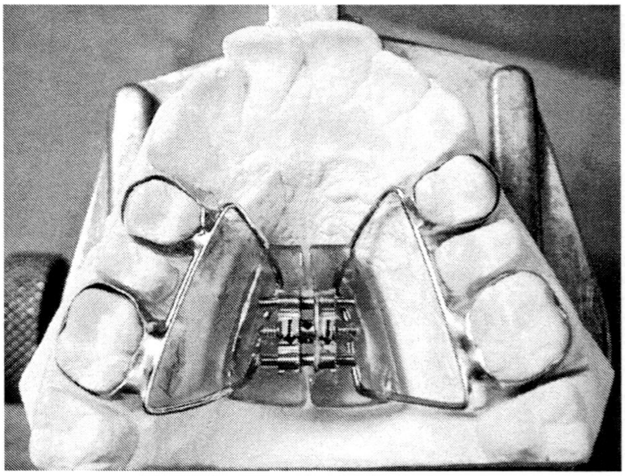

Crozat

Wires
Clasps - 0.7 mm
Lingual arms - 0.7 mm
Body wire - 1.27 mm (.050")
Lingual springs - .7 mm

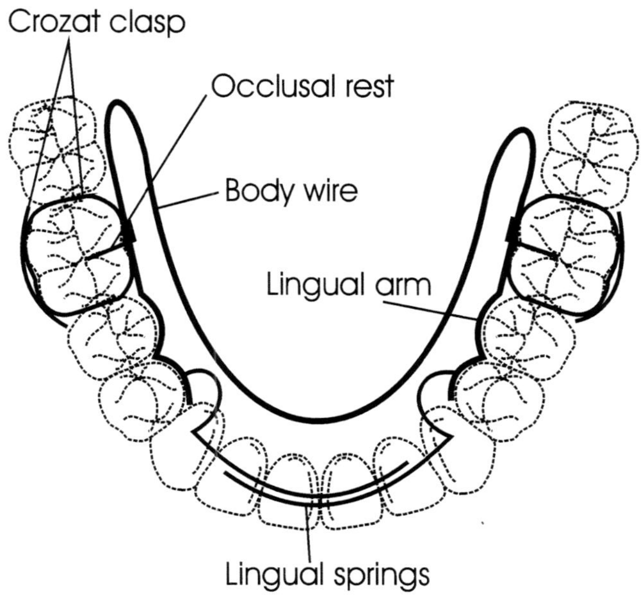

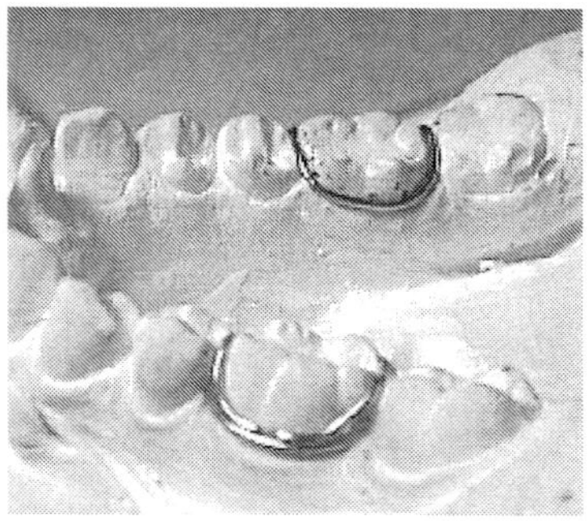

Crozat clasp buccal and lingual view

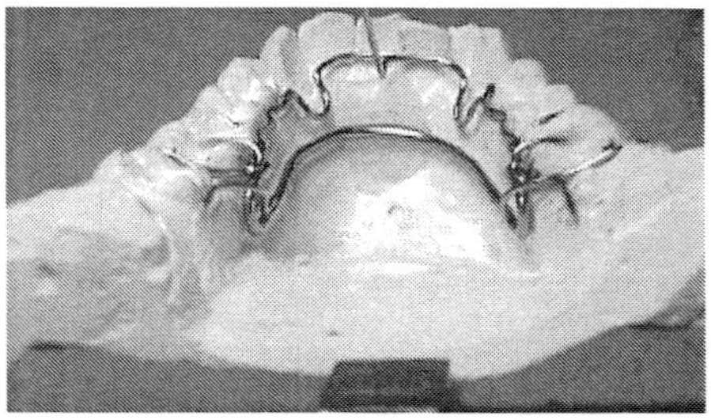

Crozat wires, lingual view

Jackson

Wires
Adams clasp - .7 mm
Body wire - 1.0 mm
Lingual springs - 0.5 mm

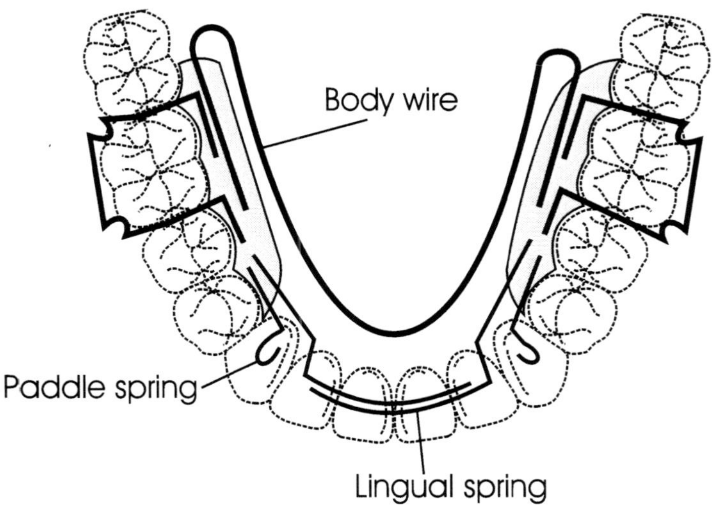

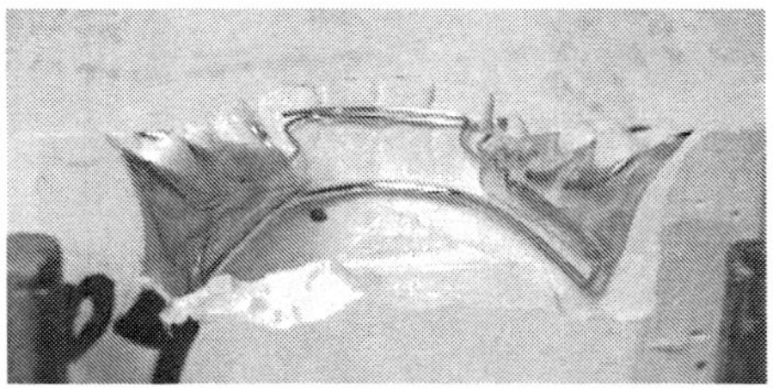

Jackson, lingual view

Twin Block

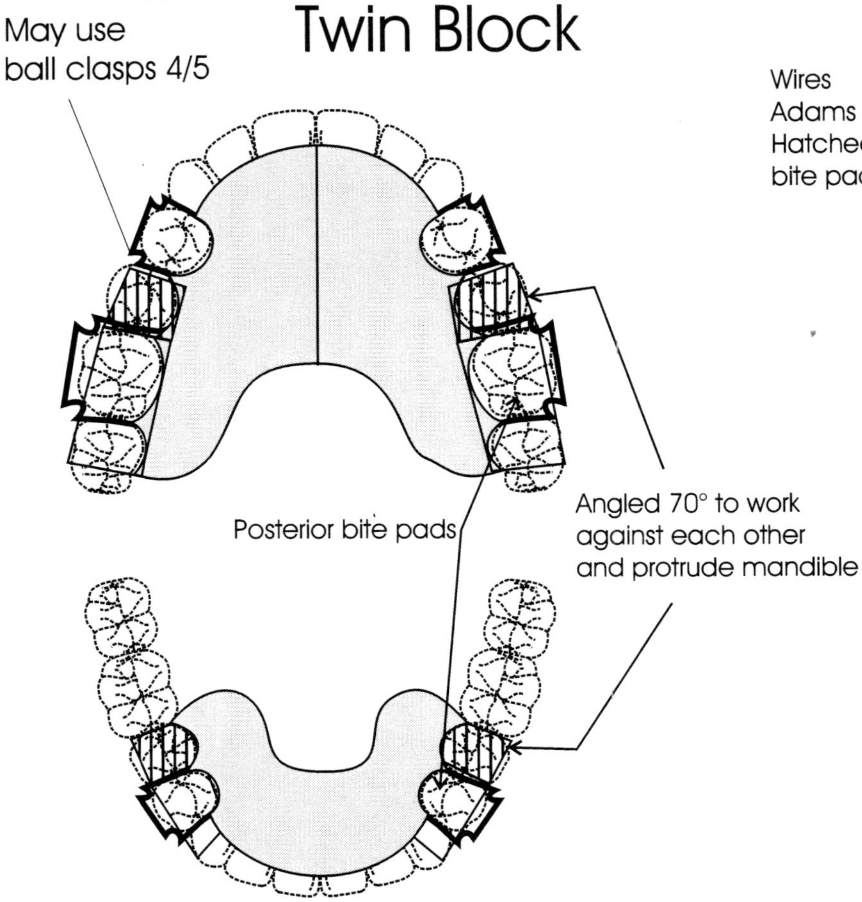

Wires
Adams - 0.7 mm
Hatched areas of
bite pads articulate at 70° angle

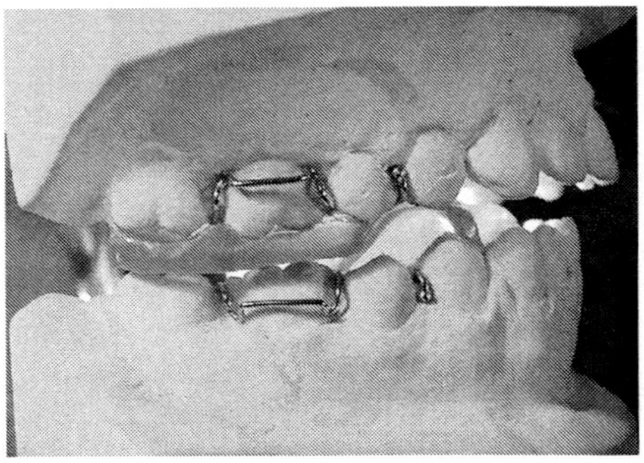

Frankel III (for Class III)

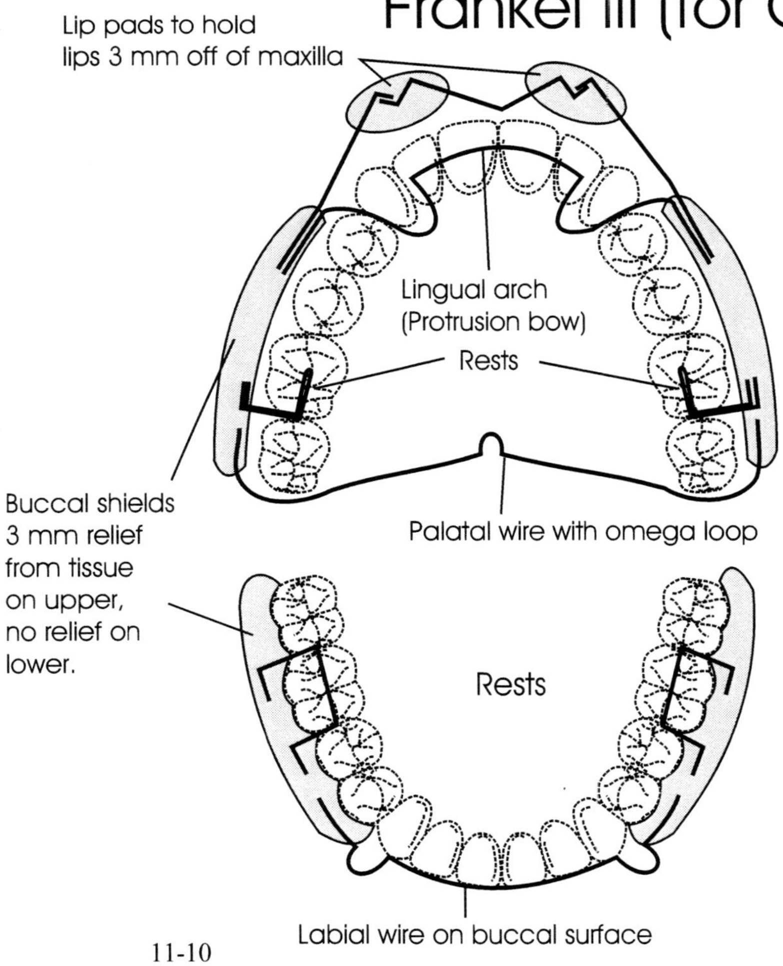

Wires
Palatal wire - 1.0 mm
Rests - 0.8 mm
Lingual arch - 0.7 mm
Wire for lips pads - 1.0 mm

Relief
Buccal shields 3 mm off maxillary posterior, contacting mandibular posterior. Lip pads 3 mm off maxillary anterior.
Mandibular labial wire placed in groove cut 1 mm into buccal surface of mandibular anteriors

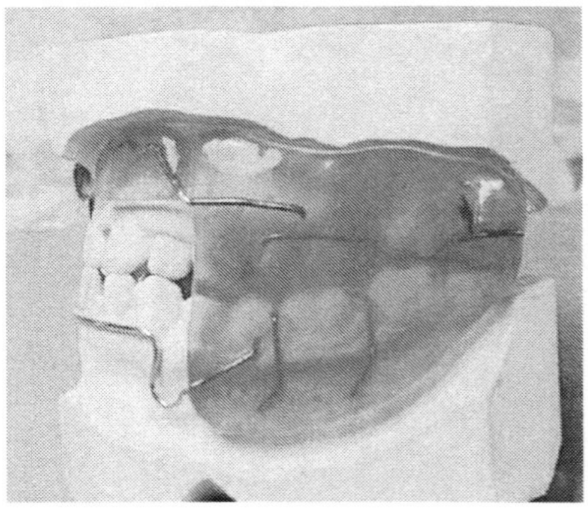

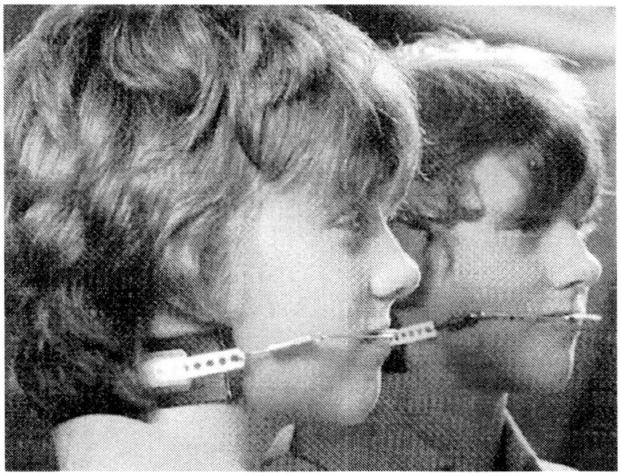

Cervical headgear

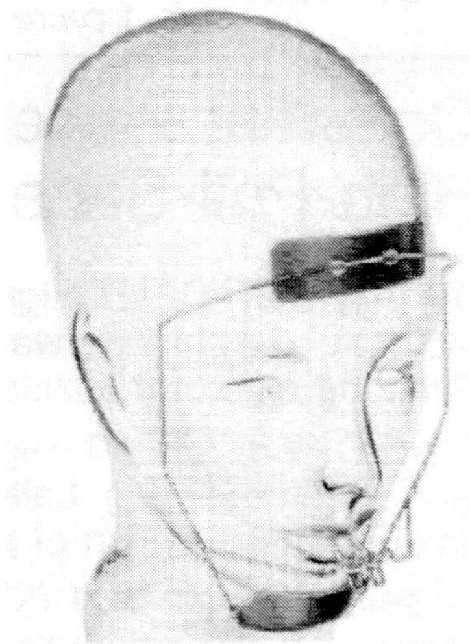

Reverse pull headgear

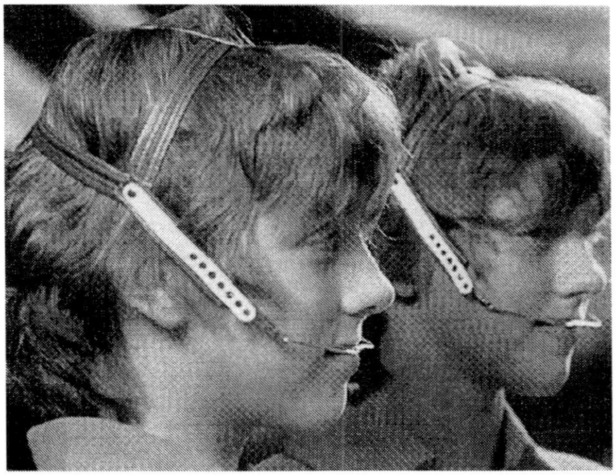

High pull headgear

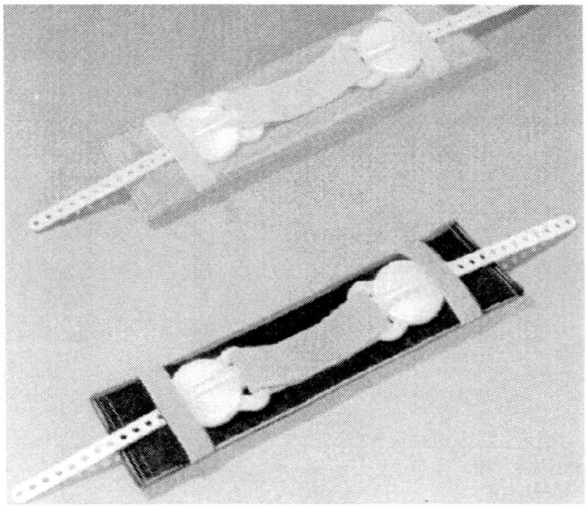

Cervical headgear with safety release

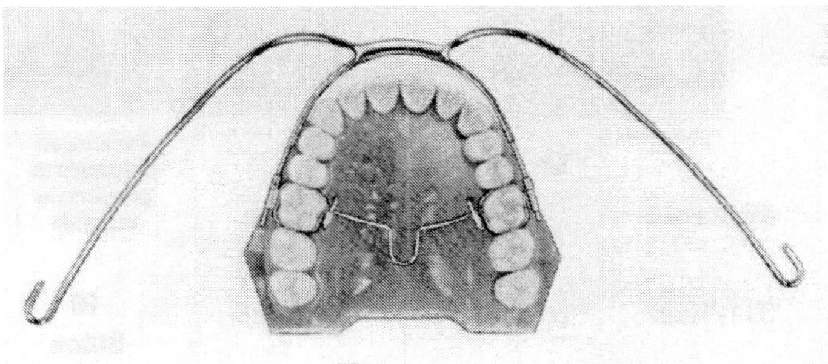

Transpalatal arch with facebow

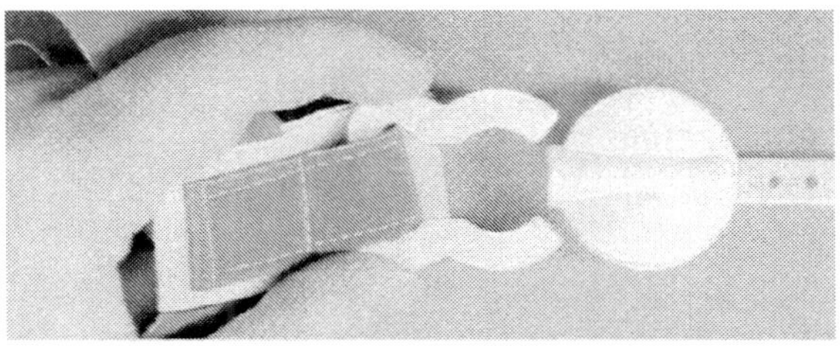

Safety release disengaged

Headgear and facebows for extraoral forces.
The facebow is inserted into .045" headgear tubes placed on molars or in appliances.
The facebow is attached to the headgear by a hook which engages a spring mechanism.
Safety headgear contain a breakaway mechanism to protect the patient from injury
in case the facebow is pulled from the mouth.

Photographs courtesy of SNF-Forestadent

References

ANDERSON, John N., (1976), Applied Dental Materials, Blackwell Scientific Publications, Great Britain.

BOIKESS, Robert S. and EDELSON, Edward, (1981), Chemical Principals, Harper & Row Publishers, New York.

FOSTER, T.D., (1980), A Textbook of Orthodontics, Blackwell Scientific Publications, Great Britain.

GRABER, T.M. and NEUMANN, Bedrick, (1977), Removable Orthodontic Appliances, W.B. Saunders Company, Philadelphia.

LAWSON, Harvey W., AA, CDT and BLAZUCKI, Joan L., R.G, BS, (1990), Bench-Top Orthodontics, Quintessence Publishing Co., Ltd., Chicago, Illinois.

PHILLIPS, Ralph W., (1994), Elements of Dental Materials, W.B. Saunders Company, Philadelphia.

SALZMANN, J.A., D.D.S., F.A., P.H.A., (1974), Orthodontics in Daily Practice, J.B. Lippincott Company, Philadelphia . Toronto.

SIM, Joseph M., (1972), Minor tooth movement in children, The C.V. Mosby Company, Saint Louis.

WHITE, T.C., GARDINER, J.H. and LEIGHTON, B.C., (1967), Orthodontics for Dental Students, Warren H. Green, Inc., St. Louise, Missouri, U.S.A.

WITT, Dr. Emil; GEHRKE, M.D.T.; SHAYE and Dr. Robert SHAYE, B.A., D.D.S.; (1988), Removable Appliance Fabrication, Quintessence Publishing Co., Inc., Chicago, Illinois.

WITZIG, John W.and SPAHL, Terrance J., (1987), The Clinical Management of Basic Maxillofacial Orthopedic Appliances, PSG Publishing Company, Inc., Littleton, Massachusetts.

Index

Afterword

While I was busy writing this book, I came across this quote by Aldous Leonard Huxley (1894-1963), the author of "Brave New World". It was a book that I had to read in high school English class, and was one of the better of the books that we had to study. After the past several months of working on this text, this quote touches me, containing a simple and elegant and generous truth that I will always remember whenever I open a book by any author.

I hope that this book will provide everyone who reads it with some help in their own search for knowledge.

"A bad book is as much of a labor to write as a good one; it comes as sincerely from the author's soul."
Aldous Leonard Huxley

WD Publishing
517 Powell Rd,
Whitby, Ontario, Canada
L1N 2H5
1-800-668-4652 or (905) 725-4652
Fax (905) 725-9348
www.mcodental.com

Suggested Retail
$75.95 Cdn or $60.00 US

ISBN 0-9681430-1-6